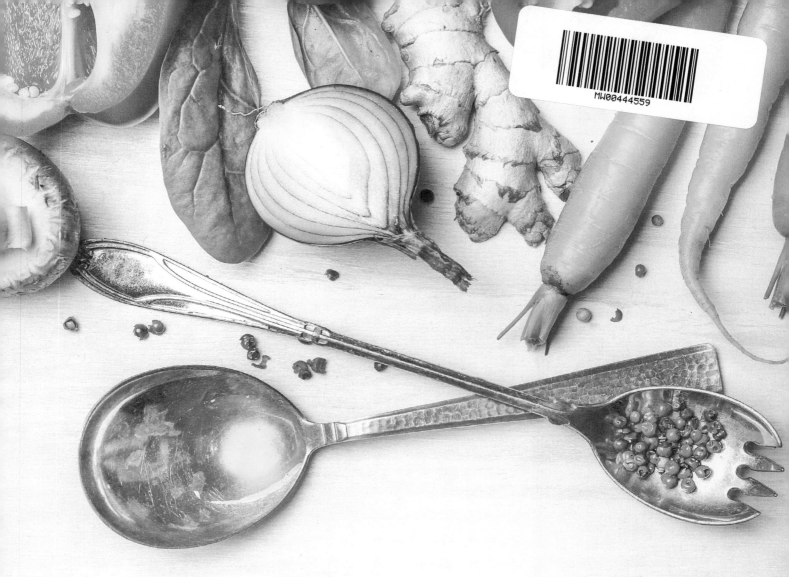

FOOD, NUTRITION, & CULINARY ARTS

MARY ANN EATON • JANET ROUSLIN

Kendall Hunt
publishing company

Cover image © Shutterstock.com

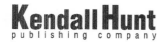

www.kendallhunt.com
Send all inquiries to:
4050 Westmark Drive
Dubuque, IA 52004-1840

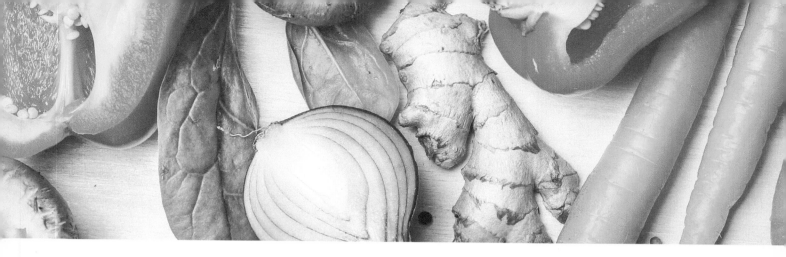

Brief Contents

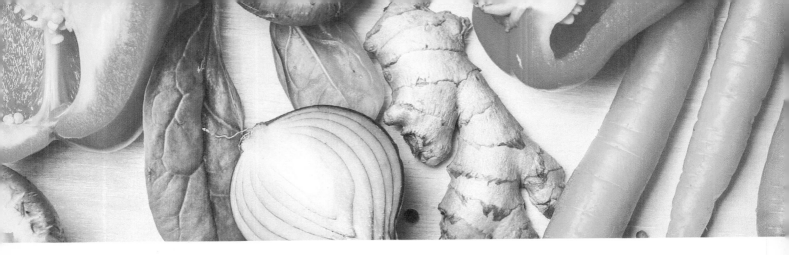

Contents

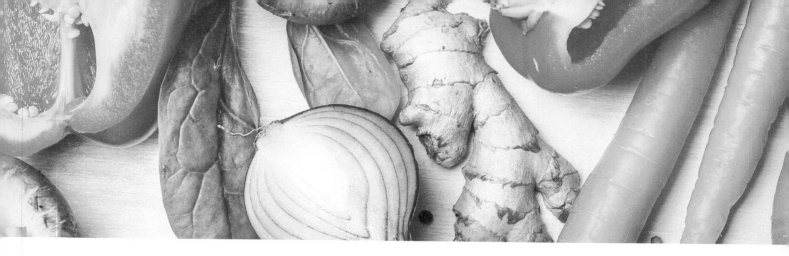

Acknowledgements

We would like to thank the following contributing authors and reviewers for their support in making this textbook revision a reality: Allison Acquisto, M.A., R.D., L.D.N., Patricia Blenkiron, Ed.D., R.D., C.D.E., Laura Brieser-Smith, M.P.H., R.D., C.H.F.S., Kara J. Cucinotta, M.S., R.D., L.D.N., Barbara Kamp, M.S., R.D., L.D., Emily A. LaRose, M.S., R.D., C.N.S.C., C.S.P., Branden Lewis, M.B.A., Mary Etta Moorachian, Ph.D., R.D., L.D., C.C.P., C.F.C.S., Barbara Robinson, M.P.H., R.D., L.D.N., C.N.S.C., Todd Seyfarth, M.S., R.D, and Marleen Swanson, M.S., R.D., M.B.A., and Suzanne Vieira, M.S., R.D. We appreciate the valuable professional expertise they provided in compiling a text that contains the latest information on the science of nutrition and its integral relationship to culinary arts.

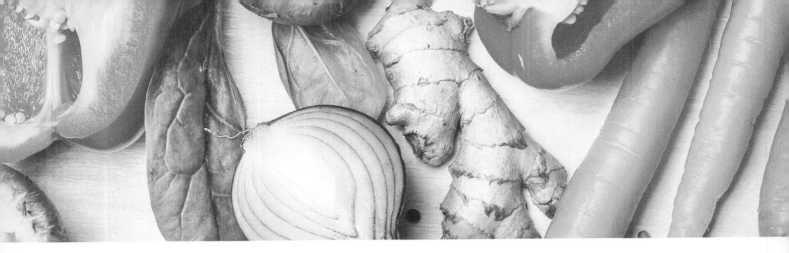

About the Authors

Mary Anne Eaton, PhD., RDN, CFS

Mary Anne Eaton is an Adjunct Professor at Manchester Community College where she teaches various nutrition courses. She has a Doctorate in Nutrition and Food Science from the University of Rhode Island. Her interest is in the field of aquaculture where she has done research using flaxseed in salmon feed to retain EPA and DHA levels in salmon flesh. She also supports an interest in lipid chemistry with a focus on specialty oils in the culinary industry. Mary Anne is a Registered Dietitian and a Certified Food Scientist. Her experiences include a variety of clinical work in healthcare settings.

Mary Anne is an active member in several professional organizations including the Academy of Nutrition and Dietetics (AND), the Dietetics Educators Practice Group of AND, and the New Hampshire Dietetics Association. She participates yearly at conferences to increase her knowledge in the areas of nutrigenomics and healthful oils.

Janet Rouslin, MA, RDN, LDN

Janet Rouslin is a retired Associate Professor of Culinary Nutrition at Johnson & Wales University where she taught Culinary Nutrition Students for over 20 years. A Registered Dietitian, she holds a Bachelor of Science Degree in Food and Nutrition from the University of Maine at Orono, and a Master of Arts in Teaching specializing in Culinary Arts. She has extensive background in clinical dietetics in hospitals, and long-term care facilities.

Janet is an active member of numerous professional organizations including The Academy of Nutrition and Dietetics (AND), The Rhode Island Dietetic Association, The Culinary Professionals Practice Group of the AND, The Dietetic Educators Practice Group of the AND, and The American Society for Parenteral and Enteral Nutrition. Janet has presented workshops throughout the U.S. and abroad, on the Mediterranean diet and the culinary uses and health benefits of olive oil. Janet was instrumental in developing the first didactic program for Nutrition and Dietetics accredited by the AND, combining Culinary Arts and Nutrition at Johnson & Wales University.

Exploring Nutrition

1

KEY TERMS

Academy of Nutrition and
  Dietetics (AND)
Anthropometry
Biochemical analysis
Biological
Calorie
Clinical methods
Diet
Dietary methods
Dietary standards
Energy-yielding
Empty calorie

Essential nutrient
Gram
Inorganic
Licensure
Malnutrition
Non-energy yielding
Non-nutrient
Nutrient dense
Nutrition
Nutrient
Nutrigenomics
Nutritional assessment

Nutritional status
Organic
Overnutrition
Phytochemical
Psychological
Registered Dietitian/
  Nutritionist (RDN)
Dietetic Technician
  Registered (DTR)
Sociological
Undernutrition

Introduction

The study of **nutrition** is a fast-growing and ever-changing science. The importance of the relationship between food and nutrition is now recognized both in the nutrition field and in the area of culinary arts. An analogy of the body's need for food can be made to a car's need for fuel and oil. Fuel and oil are needed to keep an engine well maintained, while fuel in the form of food is required to keep the body running at peak levels. The quality and quantity of fuel, whether for a car or for a body, is the key to optimum performance. The natural blending of culinary arts and nutrition brings the value of nutritious foods to new heights for health and sensory well-being. This first chapter discusses the three W's of nutrition: What? Why? and Who?

What Is Nutrition?

Nutrition is a complex science that studies the substances in food and their corresponding interactions in the body. When an individual consumes nourishment of any type (solids or fluids), the body transforms these components by either physically or chemically changing them. These processes enable our bodies to utilize the food's components in the best way possible. These interactions include ingestion, digestion, absorption, transportation, metabolism, storage, and excretion. Food substances can have a positive or negative impact on health depending on the types and quantities selected. When studying food intake, it is necessary to evaluate an individual's diet. **Diet** is a summation of all the foods and fluids consumed. A broader scope of nutrition also includes a cultural, social, and environmental association with food.

Terminology of Nutrition

The substances or compounds that make up food are called **nutrients**. The six essential nutrients are carbohydrates, lipids (fats), proteins, vitamins, minerals, and water. These **essential nutrients** provide the body with energy, and help in its growth and maintenance. Essential nutrients must be supplied by the diet. Some nutrients are **energy-yielding** and provide needed energy for the body to remain active, while others are **non-energy yielding** and assist in the energy production process but do not supply energy in and of themselves. Carbohydrates, lipids, and proteins are classified as energy-yielding, whereas vitamins, minerals, and water are non-energy yielding. Essential nutrients also serve to provide the body with the necessary substances for growth and maintenance. They form new structures such as bones, organs, and cells and allow the body to repair and replace cells and structures that have been damaged. The chemical nature of the essential nutrients necessitates further categorization. Nutrients can be either **organic** or **inorganic**. Organic nutrients contain the element carbon while inorganic nutrients do not. The four organic nutrients are carbohydrates, lipids, proteins, and vitamins, while minerals and water are inorganic.

Two terms are generally used in the measurement of food energy: **calorie** and **gram**. Calorie is a measurement of heat energy and gram is the unit used to measure weight (in this case the weight of food quantities). The measurement of calories per gram of a food is the amount of energy provided by a given quantity of food. Energy-yielding nutrients each provide a particular amount of energy. Carbohydrates and proteins provide 4 calories per gram, while lipids supply more than twice this amount of energy at 9 calories per gram. Alcohol contributes calories, 7 per gram, but is not classified as a nutrient as it interferes with the growth, maintenance, and repair of body tissue.[1] Table 1.1 shows the average caloric value for each nutrient.

TABLE 1.1 The Six Classes of Nutrients		
Nutrient	Energy Value (Cal/Gm)	Inorganic/Organic
Carbohydrates	4	Organic
Proteins	4	Organic
Lipids (fats)	9	Organic
Vitamins	0	Organic
Minerals	0	Inorganic
Water	0	Inorganic

The following example shows how to determine the caloric value of energy-yielding nutrients. Follow steps 1 to 3 to determine the caloric value of an apple, a teaspoon of butter, and a slice of bread.

1. An apple contains 15 grams of carbohydrate. How many calories does this represent?
    1 gram of carbohydrate = 4 calories
    Answer: 15 grams of carbohydrate × 4 calories/gram = 60 calories

2. One teaspoon of butter contains 5 grams of lipid. How many calories does this represent?
    1 gram of lipid = 9 calories
    Answer: 5 grams of lipid × 9 calories/gram = 45 calories

3. A slice of bread contains 15 grams of carbohydrate, 1 gram of lipid, and 3 grams of protein. How many calories does this represent?
    1 gram of carbohydrate = 4 calories
       15 grams of carbohydrate × 4 calories/gram = **60** calories
    1 gram of lipid = 9 calories
       1 gram of lipid × 9 calories = **9** calories
    1 gram of protein = 4 calories
       3 grams of protein × 4 calories calories/gram = **12** calories
    Answer: 60 calories + **9** calories + **12** calories = **81** calories

Anything that is not a nutrient is incorporated into the broad category of **non-nutrient**. A non-nutrient is any compound found in food other than the six essential nutrients, including those compounds found in herbs and spices. The variety of herbs and spices also make a significant contribution to the diet by adding beneficial phytochemicals to the body. A **phytochemical** is a non-nutrient compound in plant-derived foods that displays biological activity in the body. This biological activity is usually beneficial, although the positive contributions of compounds such as St. John's Wort, Ginkgo biloba, and Ginseng are controversial. Ingredients used by chefs to enhance flavor often contain phytochemicals as well. Hot peppers contain capsaicin, the same non-nutrient used medicinally as an anti-inflammatory agent. The pungent flavor found in garlic (allium sativum) is a potent phytochemical that is known to lower cholesterol.[2] Polyphenols are also non-nutrients that contribute to health and well-being. Studies on high polyphenol content in dark chocolate have indicated a decrease in blood pressure and an improvement in insulin sensitivity in healthy people.[3] It has recently become apparent that food must be evaluated as a whole rather than assessed as a collection of isolated nutrients. When foods and their corresponding substances are blended in flavorful combinations they allow us to enjoy eating and to derive healthy benefits as well.

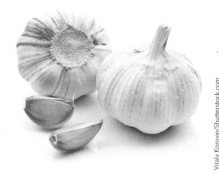

Garlic enhances the flavor of many dishes and contains phytochemicals such as allium derivatives.

Vitaly Korovin/Shutterstock.com

Nutritional Status

Nutritional status is defined as a person's health, as influenced by both the intake and utilization of nutrients. The consumption of either an inadequate amount of nutrients or an excessive quantity may contribute to health concerns. Consuming an insufficient amount of iron-rich foods may bring about iron deficiency anemia. A diet high in sodium may cause hypertension, or high blood pressure. Both of the aforementioned are examples of problems connected with nutritional status involving the intake of certain nutrients.

Inadequate utilization of a nutrient can also be a problem. Although the intake may be adequate, an individual's health status may be negatively impacted if the body is unable to efficiently process a particular nutrient. For example, a carrier known as the intrinsic factor must be present for the absorption of vitamin B_{12}. An individual who consumes a sufficient amount of vitamin B_{12} may still develop a health condition known as pernicious anemia, if absorption is inadequate.

Health conditions, such as iron deficiency anemia, hypertension, and pernicious anemia are all considered forms of **malnutrition**. The word malnutrition's prefix, mal, means bad. Malnutrition is poor nutrition resulting from a dietary intake either above or below the amount required to meet the body's needs. Malnutrition caused by an intake or condition that results in suboptimal levels of a nutrient is referred to as **undernutrition** (as seen in the anemias mentioned), while malnutrition resulting from an excess intake of a nutrient is referred to as **overnutrition** (as evidenced in the health condition known as hypertension). Knowledge of foods that contain needed beneficial nutrients, and those containing excess, potentially harmful nutrients, is invaluable. Chefs can greatly improve the quality of meals by adjusting a recipe to either incorporate or remove food sources based on need.

Why Is Nutrition So Important?

So why is it so important to consume a healthy, well-balanced diet? How much of an impact does food choice have on one's health status? Nutrition research in the first half of the twentieth century focused on identification and prevention of nutrient-deficient diseases. In the second half of the century, research shifted to the role of diet in maintaining health and reducing the risk of chronic diseases, such as heart disease and cancer. A healthy, well-balanced diet can profoundly affect how a person feels. Do you feel better when you consciously consume foods that are full of energy, vitamins, and minerals, or when you are rushing around and have very little time to think about what you are eating? The body reacts daily to the nutrients with which it is provided. High energy and a feeling of well-being result from a good nutrient intake while a poor nutrient intake causes a low energy level and a lesser feeling of well-being. A lifetime of poor food choices can impact both emotional and physical well-being. Health implications of poor dietary choices and their effects on the aging process will be discussed later. The health of older individuals is directly related to chronic disease development and quality of life issues.[4]

Community Nutrition

Individuals are usually considered to be responsible for their food intake, health and how they live their lives. Realistically, this assumption is not always accurate. Persons with physical and psychological illnesses, the elderly and low-income earners frequently need assistance in creating appropriately nutritious meals. Community nutrition programs focus on the nutritional needs of these select population groups. Community-based programs exist at the federal level, the state level and also at the city or town level.

The Food Stamp Program was renamed the Supplemental Nutrition Assistance Program (SNAP) on October 1, 2008. This new name was designed to reflect the goal of the program, which was to better accommodate the nutritional needs of clients. The SNAP program helps low-income people purchase food that they need for good health. An electronic card is provided to buy food at participating grocery stores. The benefits allocated are issued based on Gross and Net Income levels. Additional Federal programs include: School Breakfast and Lunch Programs, The Food Distribution Program, the Women, Infants and Children Program (WIC) and the Farmers' Market Nutrition Program (FMNP).[5] In New Jersey, the Department of Agriculture works with the Women, Infants and Children Program (WIC) and the Farmers' Market Nutrition Program (FMNP) to provide locally grown, fresh fruits, vegetables and herbs to nutritionally at-risk pregnant, breast-feeding, or post-partum women, children 2–5 years old, as well as eligible seniors over 60 years old.[6] Additional States have similar programs to those found in New Jersey.

The Farm Bill is a piece of Legislation that affects Food Security, Nutrition, and Public Health in the U.S. The most recent version is entitled The Agriculture Reform, Food and Jobs Act of 2012. It was originally introduced around 50 years ago to help farmers by controlling production and increasing crop prices. It now includes related issues and interests such as nutrition supplementation and education programs.[7] People in the United States are becoming more interested in where their food comes from. In 2009 the United States Department of Agriculture (USDA) launched the "Know Your Farmer Know Your Food"(KYF) initiative. This helps communities scale up local and regional food systems and strengthen their economies. It is also believed that programs such as these will expand marketing opportunities for producers, drive the growth of new local businesses and jobs, and increase healthy food access.[8] Sustainability and the "Farm to Table" movement are very big trends in the Culinary Industry. This topic is explored more in the Culinary Corner of this Chapter.

Culinary Focus on Food

The culinary field has shown a tremendous growth over the past years in providing individuals at restaurants, health spas, resorts, and athletic facilities with healthy alternative cuisine. Menu items such as those seen in Figure 1.1 provide heart-healthy foods. The average consumer, while becoming more aware of the health benefits of proper eating, still values taste as the primary driving force in food selection. The consumer is willing to try "healthy" food at least once, but if the food lacks the taste desired, it will no longer be a choice. The culinary industry has found its niche in

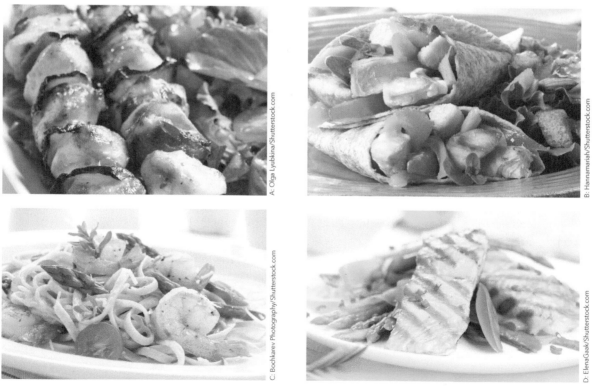

FIGURE 1.1 Examples of Heart-Healthy Menu Items

supplying such offerings. Supermarkets provide a number of specialized food products that are low-fat, reduced-fat, reduced-calorie, salt-free, or low salt. Many products contain creative, healthier flavor enhancers such as herbs and spices to replace the salt. The market is exploding with new products every day. Culinarians involved with research and development share their wisdom of sensory knowledge with health enthusiasts to produce products that the health-conscious consumer can now enjoy. Culinarians can also use their talents in healthcare operations to deliver the proper nutrients to the health impaired. Other areas such as sports nutrition are emerging and are demonstrating the need to combine culinary skills with nutrition knowledge. The "Culinary Corner" at the end of Chapter 1 explores the many avenues available in this field.

Selecting Food: Why Is the Choice So Difficult?

Food selection seems easy! The majority of people know that fruits and vegetables are beneficial, yet they choose to snack on potato chips and candy bars. Fruit juice or water may quench the thirst but a caffeinated soda or coffee seems to provide the extra burst needed. There are many factors that prevent the selection of a good diet. People eat for two basic reasons. The first reason, which is common to all, is **biological**; food and fluids are consumed due to hunger or thirst. The body needs to be nourished to continue functioning, and this need causes it to seek out foods and fluids. When the mouth becomes dry, it is because less saliva is available to moisten the mouth. The signal is a warning to replenish fluids so that the dry mouth feeling is eliminated. This is a simplified version of a complex occurrence. There are other bodily functions as well that are controlled biologically.

Psychological and sociological factors also contribute to reasons for eating. These are external influences concerning food choices, and they vary because of the individual choices made. Unhealthy dietary patterns, developed during childhood and adolescence, may create an increased risk for chronic diseases later in life such as heart disease, osteoporosis, and certain forms of cancer.[9] Think about what influences your food selection. Food selections based on psychological and sociological reasons fall into a variety of categories including availability, cultural and social attitudes, mental status, and economics. Some individuals may be able to shop at a large supermarket that offers a wide range of choices, whereas others may be limited to the selections at the nearest convenience store. Availability is also affected by geographical location. In the Northeast, fruit selections once rose dramatically in the summer months, yet due to advances in agriculture, transportation, and storage, a growing number of offerings are now seen year round.

External factors that influence food selection are cultural and social attitudes. Individuals, because of their ethnic background and traditions, choose certain foods. Food choices may also be based on religious beliefs, such as those of Orthodox Jews who limit their diet to kosher foods. Muslims who practice the Islamic religion do not consume prohibited foods (haram) that include swine, four-footed animals that catch prey with their mouths, and improperly slaughtered animals. Seventh Day Adventists believe in abstaining from flesh foods and widely consume vegetarian diets.[10] People like to share food that reflects their heritage and values. (See Figure 1.2) The consumption of ethnic foods may symbolize not only a culinary acceptance and enjoyment, but also an appreciation of another's heritage. It is important to recognize the link between customs, traditions, and food choices.

Mental status also influences our food selection. Mood can impact not only whether or not one eats, but also what one chooses to eat. Some individuals eat more or less when they are happy, while others eat more or less when they are depressed. Certain foods can bring emotional comfort and feelings of well-being. Ice cream is often the number one comfort food because it is soothing, sweet, and easy to eat. Some individuals state that particular foods make them feel "closer to home." Food choices are also made by habit. Many people eat the same thing for breakfast or lunch every day. Orange juice may be viewed as the only breakfast juice. Take a minute to think of the foods to which you are accustomed and those that you consider to be "comfort foods."

Food selections may be associated with one's economic level as well. Typically, high carbohydrate intakes (pasta, rice, and cereals) are associated with a lower economic level, whereas high-protein items (beef, fish, and pork) are connected with higher economic levels, although not all people in the higher income brackets eat large amounts of meat. Some

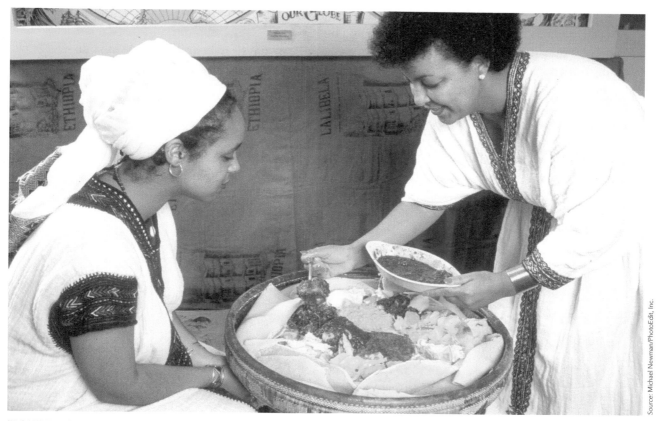

Source: Michael Newman/PhotoEdit, Inc.

FIGURE 1.2 Some individuals like to choose Foods that Reflect their Ethnic Backgrounds.

individuals actually eat for nutritional value and good health. Health-conscious consumers are growing in number due to health-related evidence found in research studies. As previously mentioned, many chronic diseases, including heart disease, hypertension, and strokes, have a diet-related component. Individuals are beginning to make healthier food choices with the goal of living longer and living more productive lives.[11]

Consumers also choose foods based on advertisements. The media provides an abundance of information regarding what should or should not be consumed. Magazines and television ads either focus on health issues or merely attempt to promote the sensory characteristics of the product. A variety of techniques, such as employing well-known sports figures and actors to promote sound and healthy nutrition, is frequently very effective.[12]

Constructing a Good Diet

Information as to what is considered "healthy" changes constantly, leaving consumers confused. It is time-consuming to stay current with all the available information. So how can we maintain a healthy diet? Following a few basic steps can help us to establish a more health-conscious diet.

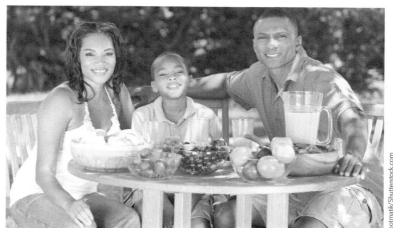

spotmatik/Shutterstock.com

Some individuals choose foods for their nutritional value.

The first step is to determine diet adequacy by assessing whether the diet provides all of the essential nutrients and energy in amounts sufficient to maintain health and body weight. Next, determine whether the nutrients consumed are balanced, not having too much of one nutrient at the expense of another. Individual food items may be high in one nutrient and low in another. For example, calcium is high in dairy products but low in meats. Iron, on the other hand, is high in meats but low in dairy products. It would not be prudent to consume dairy products at the expense of meat items, as this could cause iron deficiency anemia. A balance in nutrient intake must be established to meet complete nutrient needs.

A third consideration in constructing a healthy diet is variety. Foods that offer a variety of nutrients should be selected daily to achieve balance. Calorie control is also an important consideration as all foods contain calories. Some foods are known as **empty-calorie** foods, while others are considered **nutrient-dense** foods. Empty-calorie foods are those that have a high level of calories and a limited amount of nutrients. Food items such as soda and candy are considered empty-calorie food choices. Nutrient-dense foods are those containing a high level of nutrients and a lower number of calories. Foods in this category include most fruits and vegetables. To exhibit calorie control in constructing a good diet, one should select more items from the nutrient-dense category and fewer selections from the empty-calorie food category.

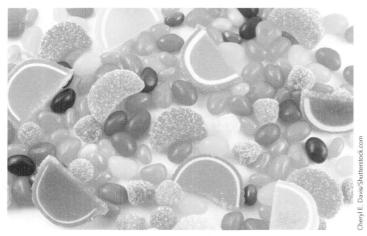

A) Empty-calorie foods such as candy are low in nutrients yet high in calories.

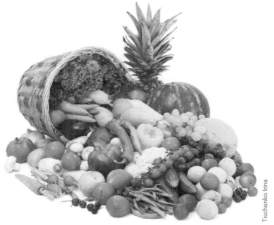

B) Fruits and vegetables are examples of nutrient-dense foods.

The last component in attaining a good diet is moderation. Including the appropriate amount of nutrients in a diet, and not exceeding certain limits, is key in maintaining health. These limits vary depending on the nutrient and the individual's needs. A healthy and sound diet can be maintained when all these factors are taken into consideration. (Figure 1.3)

Who Are the Authorities on Nutrition?

We are constantly bombarded with information on nutrition from a variety of sources: newspapers, magazines, television news and talk shows, doctors, friends, family, health clubs, health food stores, and so on. It is often difficult to sort fact from fiction. In order to obtain

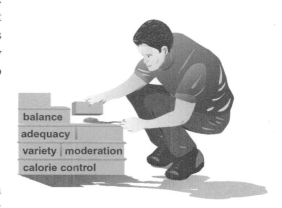

FIGURE 1.3 A healthy, sound diet can be maintained when all these factors are taken into consideration.

sound information on nutrition, it is important to inquire if the person dispensing the advice or information is qualified and/or credentialed in the field of nutrition. Would you take your car to be repaired by a mechanic with no experience? Would you fly in a plane with a pilot who does not have a license? Would you put diesel fuel in a regular car because a friend recommended it?

Who are the experts on nutrition? A qualified professional who is an expert in the area of nutrition is the Registered Dietitian/Nutritionist (RDN). RDN's are accredited by the Commission on Dietetic Registration (CDR) of the Academy of Nutrition and Dietetics (AND). The Academy of Nutrition and Dietetics is the world's largest organization of food and nutrition professionals with over 75,000 members. The process of becoming a RDN involves the following:

1. Complete a bachelor's degree in a college or university program that is accredited by the Accreditation Council for Education in Nutrition and Dietetics (ACEND®) of the AND.

2. Complete an ACEND® -accredited supervised practice program at a healthcare facility or a combined supervised practice program with undergraduate or graduate studies.

3. Upon completion of steps 1 and 2 the individual must then pass a National Examination that is administered by the Commission of Dietetic Registration (CDR).

The average length of the post-graduate programs is 6 months to 2 years. Most states recognize Registered Dietitian/Nutritionists as experts in nutrition and qualified to practice. Many states require licensure of Registered Dietitian/Nutritionists to further protect the consumer from fraudulent professionals and/or practices.[13]

Another qualified nutrition expert is the Dietetic Technician Registered (DTR). Dietetic Technicians must complete an associate's degree from a college or university accredited by the Academy of Nutrition and Dietetics and a supervised practice experience under an approved Dietetic Technician Program, or they must complete a baccalaureate degree from an educational institution accredited by the Academy of Nutrition and Dietetics. Dietetic Technicians work closely with Registered Dietitian/Nutritionists in providing optimal nutritional care.[14] Table 1.2 provides a list of reliable professionals who are qualified to give sound nutritional advice and where and how they might be located.

In addition to certified professionals, reliable sources on nutrition include organizations that disseminate information based on sound scientific facts and consensus, rather than on testimonials or money-based schemes. There are several organizations that can provide reliable nutrition information, including voluntary, scientific, professional, and government organizations. Table 1.3 provides a list of organizations and their websites.

Table 1.4 lists additional sources and websites on food and nutrition that may be useful when discussing material in future chapters of the text.

TABLE 1.2 Nutrition Experts

Qualified Nutrition Experts	How to Locate Them
Registered Dietitian/Nutritionists and Dietetic Technicians Registered	Local hospitals, Yellow Pages, State dietetic associations, National AND Headquarters (web address: www.eatright.org)
Public Health Nutritionists	Local and state public health departments
College Nutrition Instructors/Professors	ACEND accredited colleges and universities (see individual schools for web addresses)
Extension Service Home Economists	State and county USDA Service Offices (general web addresses for USDA: www.usda.gov/fcs)
FDA: Consumer Affairs Staff	National, regional, and state offices (general web address: www.fda.gov)

TABLE 1.3 Sources on Nutrition

Voluntary Organizations	Websites
American Cancer Society	www.cancer.org
American Institute for Cancer Research	www.aicr.org
American Diabetes Association	www.diabetes.org
American Heart Association	www.americanheart.org
Heart Information	www.heartinfo.org
National Dairy Council	www.nationaldairycouncil.org
National Osteoporosis Foundation	www.nof.org
Scientific Organizations	
American Academy for Nutritional Sciences	www.nutrition.org
American Society for Clinical Nutrition	www.faseb.org/ascn
Institute of Food Technologists	www.IFT.org
National Academy of Sciences	www.nas.edu
Professional Organizations	
Academy of Nutrition and Dietetics (AND)	www.eatright.org
American Medical Association	www.ama-assn.org
Society for Nutrition Education and Behavior	www.sneb.org/
Government Organizations/Publications	
Food and Nutrition Information Center	www.nal.usda.gov/fnic/
Healthy People 2010	www.healthypeople.gov
National Institutes of Health	www.nih.gov
National Heart, Lung, and Blood Institute	www.nhlbi.nih.gov
Food and Drug Administration (FDA)	www.fda.gov
Centers for Disease Control (CDC)	www.cdc.gov
U.S. Department of Agriculture (USDA)	www.usda.gov
World Health Organization	www.who.org

TABLE 1.4 Additional Sources and Websites on Food and Nutrition

Ask the Dietitian	www.dietitian.com
About Produce	www.aboutproduce.com
Bio Nutritional Encyclopedia	www.biovalidity.com/notify.cfm
Choose My Plate	www.choosemyplate.gov
Diet and Weight Loss Links	www.diet-i.com/
Five a Day Page	www.5aday.com
Food Terms	www.food.epicurious.com/run/fooddictionary/home
International Food Information Council	www.ific.org
Phytonutrients	www.phytopia.com
The Fruit Newsletter	www.fruitpages.com/nl082002.shtml
Tufts University Navigator	www.navigator.tufts.edu

Career Opportunities in the Dietetics Field

Chefs who have an interest and background in nutrition can use their skills and knowledge base in a variety of career opportunities. These include serving as a chef or foodservice manager in the following areas:

- Healthcare establishments (hospitals, long-term care facilities, assisted living centers)—Chefs may be part of the production or management team in these facilities.
- Sports nutrition—Chefs may become personal chefs for athletes. There are opportunities in collegiate sports programs. Chefs may seek employment with professional sports teams or at Olympic training sites.
- Health spa facilities—Chefs with a sound background and interest in nutrition might seek employment in health and wellness focused spas.
- Home meal replacements—Many supermarkets are promoting meals that are freshly made and ready to eat. A chef with a nutrition background can answer the demand by nutrition-conscious consumers for healthful, prepared foods. Personal chefs are using nutrition as a marketing tool to increase their customer base.
- Research Chefs are now taking active roles in the development of new products. They may work in product development, in quality control, or concentrate on the improvement of nutritional products currently on the market.
- School lunch program- Chefs are working in some school systems to help improve food quality to make it more appealing. Chefs are also training schoolfoodserive workers in basic culinary practices.

Chefs can partner and work with Registered Dietitian/Nutritionists and Dietetic Technicians Registered in numerous areas: creating healthful food choices within the hospitality industry, restaurant consulting and menu development, media communications, culinary nutrition demonstrations, and working in the airline food industry. Chefs who aspire to own their own establishments can use their nutrition background to promote healthful menu choices and to correct the misconception that nutritious food must taste bland.

Opportunities for Registered Dietitian/Nutritionists and Dietetic Technicians Registered include the following:

- Healthcare—RDNs and DTRs are responsible for educating patients about nutrition and administering medical nutrition therapy as part of the healthcare team.
- School Nutrition- RDNs can plan nutritious meals and collaborate with chefs and food service workers on the production of healthy, appealing meals.
- Sports nutrition/corporate wellness programs—In this setting, the Registered Dietitian/Nutritionist is responsible for educating clients about the connection of food, fitness, and health. Employment might be with large or small businesses or with health and fitness organizations.
- Food and nutrition-related industry—Possible involvement might include communications, consumer affairs, marketing, or product development.
- Private practice—A RDN may have a contract with a healthcare provider or food company, or may consult privately.
- Community and public health—RDNs and DTRs in this area may be responsible for educating the public on nutrition-related issues and implementing as well as monitoring public health programs.
- Teaching—RDNs may teach physicians, nurses, and dietetic students at universities or medical centers the science behind foods and nutrition.
- Research—Food companies, pharmaceutical industries, teaching hospitals, and universities offer nutrition research opportunities. RDNs may direct or conduct nutrition-related experimentation that might benefit the overall nutrition of the public at large.

The blend of culinary arts with the science of nutrition is creating exciting new opportunities for chefs and dietetics professionals who are ready to accept the challenge!

Individual Assessment of Nutritional Status

Once the who, what, and why of nutrition have been explored, the status of nutrition can be assessed. Professionals in the area of culinary arts can have a major impact on nutritional status in a variety of settings. Food that is selected and cooked in ways to enhance nutrients can greatly contribute to sound nutritional intake and can help to maintain general health. Cooking vegetables by steaming or stir-frying can increase vitamin and mineral retention. Using a healthy type of fat, such as olive oil in place of butter, reduces saturated fat, adds health promoting polyphenols, and can inprove the overall diet.

Nutritional assessment is the technique of evaluating an individual's or a population's nutritional status by using a comprehensive approach. There are four basic methods used in nutritional assessment:

A. **Anthropometric Assessment**
B. **Biochemical Analysis**
C. **Clinical Methods**
D. **Dietary Methods**

Anthropometry

Anthropometry is the use of measures in studying body composition and development. The measures are calculated and are compared with preset standards to determine a person's nutritional status. Height and weight are examples of measures taken and compared with standard references for a person's sex and age. Other anthropometric techniques include fat-fold measures, body fat percentage, and body mass index. If measurements are above or below set criteria, problems in nutritional status such as malnutrition and growth failure can be detected. Anthropometry such as body fat percentage and muscle mass percentage can assist athletes in achieving maximum performance. Sports nutrition is a growing field that will be mentioned in the Culinary Corner of this chapter.

Biochemical Analysis

Biochemical analysis, which is commonly referred to as laboratory tests, is the use of body tissues or fluids (blood and/or urine) to determine nutritional status. Samples taken are compared with preset values for the age and sex of the individual. Biochemical analysis is used to analyze blood for iron content. Low levels of iron may indicate iron deficiency anemia due to low levels of iron in the diet or to blood loss from a health condition or disease. Biochemical methods are objective means to determine current health and nutrition. Although usually highly accurate, the cost, occasional human error in collecting samples, and poor techniques in analysis are drawbacks that should be considered.

Clinical Methods

Clinical methods of nutritional assessment use historical information and physical examination to determine nutritional status. Historical information can be obtained from four areas: health status, socioeconomic status, medication use, and diet. Health status and illness affect food intake. Family history of health status may predict a person's susceptibility to diseases such as diabetes or heart disease. Socioeconomic history may reflect the ability to purchase a sufficient quantity or quality of food. When examining a person's historical information on medication or drug use, interactions that can alter food absorption and/or utilization may be identified. A diet history may uncover potential nutrient excesses or deficiencies as well as provide clues to the overall nutrient adequacy of a diet.

Dietary Methods

Dietary methods of nutritional assessment involve the use of food intake records and a nutritional analysis of these intakes. There are several methods used in obtaining food intake records. These include the twenty-four-hour recall that records the previous day's intake, the food diary that typically records food intake over a period of three to seven days, and the food frequency questionnaire that looks at food consumption patterns. Food intake records are then analyzed and compared to Dietary Standards that provide information on the amount of nutrients needed to maintain health and prevent disease. Food intake records are analyzed by using food composition tables. There are many computerized programs available that analyze records in a timely and relatively accurate manner.[15]

Population Assessment of Nutritional Status

Nutritional assessment of a population is often used in determining current and future health problems, as well as in determining current and future food trends. The techniques used frequently involve surveys. Governments, as well as private agencies, conduct food surveys. One survey conducted by the U.S. Department of Agriculture is the National Food Consumption Survey (NFCS). Done on two nonconsecutive days, it evaluates the food consumed by an individual. Another study conducted by the Department of Health and Human Services (DHHS) is the National Health and Nutrition Examination Survey (NHANES). This nutrition status survey analyzes anthropometrics, biochemical analysis, clinical, and dietary information obtained from a large number of individuals.

Prior to 1990, the various government agencies assessing nutritional intake did not collaborate. The enactment of the National Nutrition Monitoring and Related Research Act of 1990 brought twenty-two government agencies that were conducting various nutrition-related activities together to coordinate their efforts. The information they generate is important in establishing public policy on nutrition education, food assistance programs, and the regulation of food supply. They also provide vital statistics for scientists to establish research priorities. All nutritional information gathered in the nutritional assessment of individuals as well as of populations, must be analyzed and compared to established standards.[16] Chapter 2 will discuss various nutritional standards that assist in the evaluation of dietary intake for adequacy, deficiency, and/or toxicity.

The Future of the Science of Nutrition

Nutrigenomics

The study of nutrition has evolved considerably through a series of stages that began with the discovery of the contribution of foods to the treatment of common diseases, and evolved to the modern day role of diet in the prevention of disease. The consumption of citrus fruit was found to eliminate scurvy, while a collection of scientific data later revealed the role of particular foods in the prevention of diseases. Folic acid, found in dark leafy greens, for example, has been touted for its role in protecting against various types of cancers by affecting DNA stability. Today nutrition has advanced to the new science of Nutrigenomics.

Nutrigenomics is the study of the effect of the component parts of foods on the expression of genetic information in each individual. Proteins are produced when genes are activated or expressed. Specific genes have been identified that are responsible for the production of proteins including digestive enzymes and transport molecules. Gene expression produces a particular phenotype (observable physical and biochemical characteristics as determined by both genetic makeup and environmental influences), which results in the unique physical traits of an individual, i.e., hair color, skin tone, or even the presence or absence of a disease. Phenotype expression is influenced by nutrition. For example, dietary factors can alter cholesterol levels (including HDL and LDL levels), yet these influences vary among individuals depending on genetic makeup.

There are three primary types of nutrient-gene interactions: direct interactions, epigenetic interactions, and genetic variations. Direct interactions act as transcription factors that bind to DNA and induce gene expression. A short term signal is required to alter gene transportation. This unit consists of a sequence of DNA that occupies a specific location on a chromosome and determines a particular characteristic in an organism. When the nutrient is taken out of the diet, the response is eliminated. Epigenetic interactions actually alter the structure of DNA, and these changes can last throughout a person's lifetime. Lack of nutrients including folate, vitamin B_{12} and vitamin B_6 have been associated with liver tumor genesis in rodents.[17] This is due to lack of methyl groups needed for the biochemical pathways of DNA methylation. The last type of nutrient-gene interaction, genetic variation, involves the alteration in expression or functionality of genes. These three nutrient-gene interactions can result in an alteration of metabolism and the dietary requirements for nutrients.[18]

This science, dedicated to an understanding of how nutrients affect genes, may someday allow healthcare professionals to customize diets to genetic make-up and to manipulate gene expression with the bioactive components found in specific foods. These bioactive agents include a number of nutritive components such as fatty acids, vitamins, minerals, and/or non-nutritive components such as the numerous phytochemicals found in foods. The bioactive components interact with transcription factors, binding to DNA and affecting the transcription of mRNA, and eventually leading to the translation of proteins.[19] Knowing the effect of bioactive food components on gene expression, the metabolic pathways (metabolomics), and the functioning of proteins encoded by the genes (proteomics), provides an abundance of valuable information.[20]

Nutrigenomics may also be able to explain why some people respond better to dietary interventions than others. The possibility of developing specific functional foods to improve the health status of the population and to personalize a diet to prevent the development of a nutrition-related disorder, in individuals who are genetically predisposed, is phenomenal. Clients may someday go to Registered Dietitians to have them examine their genetic profile, and prescribe a diet and lifestyle change that will delay or possibly prevent the development of cancer or heart disease. Table 1.5 provides an example of how nutrients may regulate genes.[21]

TABLE 1.5 How Nutrients May Regulate Genes

Nutrient	Food Source	Gene Impact	Disease Prevention
Folic Acid	Dark Green Leafy Greens	DNA stability	Cancer
Fatty Acids (Omega – 3)	Salmon	Bind to Transcription Factors	Obesity
Theaflavins	Tea	Decrease mRNA synthesis	Arthritis
Flavones	Celery, Sweet Bell Peppers	Decrease mRNA synthesis	Cancer
Genistein	Soy	Inhibit cell growth, increased apoptosis	Prostate Cancer

Culinary Corner
Sustainability and "The Farm to Table Movement"

The popularity of sustainability in the culinary kitchen today is undeniable. According to the National Restaurant Association's Annual Chef Survey, three of the top four culinary trends of 2013 are directly related to sustainability.[22] Chefs around America and their customers have fallen in love with sustainability related initiatives which utilize local, seasonally inspired foods to create dazzling farm-to-table menus. Such practices are believed to be more environmentally friendly as they require less transportation, and are presumed to be healthier because produce is picked closer to the point of ripeness. Though these are some tenets of sustainability, the term can further be used to describe certain farming practices, how product is actually utilized, and how the entire process impacts the environment.

For farmed products to be considered sustainable in the production of food, fiber or other plant or animal products, they must use farming techniques that protect the environment, public health, human communities, animal welfare, and be economically sound. In the marketplace, organic products are often favored over mass-produced, non-organic agribusiness products as being more sustainable choices. While organic products are subject to stricter controls on pesticide use, the environmental impact of transportation must be considered in the sustainability equation. Locally grown products can be considered a more viable option since they don't travel far, are grown in-season, and a customer can see a farm's practices firsthand. In a monetary sense, buying locally also leaves money in a local economy, rather than sending it out to another state or country.[23] This too is considered a sustainable practice.

Other examples of sustainability in a monetary sense include maximum utilization of a product, such as in 'snout-to-tail' cuisine. In this style of cooking and preparation, a chef skillfully utilizes every part of an animal to minimize waste and to bring new and exciting culinary preparations to their diner's table. Another interpretation of maximum utilization is the sourcing of underutilized species of fish on menus. When chefs focus on fish which are abundant and native to a region, overexploited conventional species can be given time to recover and repopulate.[24] Fish such as porgy or sea robin caught in New England, for example, are not only less expensive to source and easier to procure, but they can also be prepared deliciously and in innovative ways.

Perhaps one of the best examples of food sustainability is plant-based cuisine. In plant-based cuisine, animal-based proteins are eliminated or reduced to a supporting role. Vegan and vegetarian cooking, as well as many ethnic cuisine models, are excellent examples of plant-based cuisines. In either scenario, maximizing a variety of nutrient-dense, plant-based foods, while reducing dependency on meat, especially processed red meat, eliminates many big-picture sustainability issues.[25] Through many studies, plant-based cuisine has proven to be healthier for people by reducing the risk of coronary artery disease, type 2 diabetes, hypertension, some cancers, and obesity.[26] Since healthcare costs related to these illnesses are in the billions of dollars for Americans, avoiding them through proper diet is considered the sustainable solution.[27] Plant-based cuisine is also better for the environment due to elimination or reduction of emissions from the growing, processing, refrigeration and transportation of livestock. Further, soil run-off and eutrophication resulting from growing livestock feed, as well as loss of land, habitat and biodiversity are also minimized as a result of a plant-based diet [28, 29].

Whatever a chef's approach or interpretation of sustainability is, he or she must understand that it is more than developing trendy menus. To achieve true sustainability, environmental and economic ramifications, as well as healthfulness of the food served must all be considered.

References

1 F. S. Sizer and E. N. Whitney, *Nutrition Concepts and Controversies*, 9th ed. Belmont, CA: Wadsworth/Thomson Learning, 2003.

2 Durak I, Kavutcu M, Aytac B, Avci A, Devrim E, Ozbek H, Ozturk HS, "Effects of Garlic Extract Consumption on Blood Lipid and Oxidant/Antioxidant Parameters in Humans with High Blood Cholesterol," *Journal of Nutritional Biochemistry* 15 (2004): 373–377.

3 Grassi D, Lippi C, Necozione S, Desideri G, Ferri C, "Short-term Administration of Dark Chocolate is followed by a Significant Increase in Insulin Sensitivity and a Decrease in Blood Pressure in Healthy Persons," *American Journal of Clinical Nutrition* 81 (2005): 611–614.

4   J. N. Variyam and E. Golan, "New Health Information Is Reshaping Food Choices," *Food Review* 25 (2002): 13–18.

5   http://www.fns.usda.gov/fns/regulations.htm

6   http://www.nj.gov/agriculture/divisions/md/prog/wic.html

7   Food and Nutrition Magazine, Mar/Apr 2013 Volume 2 Issue 2: http://FoodandNutritonMag.org

8   http://usda.gov/wps/portal/usda/usdahome?navid=KYF_COMPASS

9   C. Perry, M. Story, and L. A. Lytle, "Promoting Healthy Dietary Behaviors with Children and Adolescents," In *Healthy Children 2001: Strategies to Enhance Social, Emotional and Physical Wellness*, edited by R. P. Weisberg, T. P. Gullotta, G. R. Adams, R. H. Hampden, and B. A. Ryan, 214–250. Thousand Oaks, CA: Sage Publications, 1997.

10 P. Kittler and K. Sucher, *Food and Culture*, 3rd ed. Belmont, CA: Wadsworth/Thomson Learning, 2001.

11 Position of the Academy of Nutrition and Dietetics (AND), "Suffice It to Say, an Individual's Health Is Directly Related to Chronic Disease Development and Quality of Life Issues," *Journal of the Academy of Nutrition and Dietetics (AND)* 96 (1996): 1183–1187.

12 B. G. Galef, Jr., "Food Selection: Problems in Understanding How We Choose Foods to Eat," *Neuroscience and Biobehavioral Reviews* 20 (1996): 67–73.

13 http://www.eatrightacend.org/ACEND/content.aspx?id=6442485467 2015

14 "Check It Out: Careers in Dietetics," Academy of Nutrition and Dietetics (AND) Homepage, Careers in Dietetics, 2003. http://www.eatright.org

15 R. D. Lee and D. C. Nieman, *Nutritional Assessment*, 2nd Ed. New York, NY: McGraw-Hill Publishing, 1996.

16 National Nutrition Monitoring and Related Research Act of 1990. Public Law 101–445.

17 J Steinmetz, K.L., Pogribny, I.P., James, S.J., Pitot, H.C, "Hypomethylation of the Rat Glutathione S-transferase p (GSTP) Promoter Region Isolated from Methyl-deficient Livers and GSTP-positive Liver Neoplasms," *Carcinogenesis* 19 (1998): 1487–1494.

18 Siddique, R.A., Tandon, M., Ambwani, T., Rai, S.N. and Atreja, S.K. "Nutrigenomics: Nutrient-Gene Interactions," *Food Reviews International* 25 (2009): 326–345.

19 B Hirsch, D Evans, "Beyond Nutrition: The Impact of Food on Genes," *Food Technology* 59 (2005): 24–33.

20 RM Debusk, "Nutritional Genomics in Practice: Where Do We Begin," *Journal of the Academy of Nutrition and Dietetics (AND)* 105 (2005): 589–598.

21 EC Marimann, "Nutrigenomics and Nutrigenetics: The "Omics" Revolution in Nutritional Science," *Biotechnology and Applied Biochemistry* 44 (2006): 119–128.

22 National Restaurant Association Forecast for 2013: http://www.restaurant.org/News-Research/Research/What-s-Hot.

23 Mary V. Gold, Sustainable Agriculture Information Access Tools, USDA National Agriculture Library: http://www.nal.usda.gov/afsic/pubs/agnic/susag.shtml.

24 C Jeffrey. et.al., "Encouraging the Use of Underutilized Marine Fishes by Southeastern U.S. Anglers": http://spo.nmfs.noaa.gov/mfr492/mfr49215.pdf

25 D. Pimentel and M. Pimente, American Journal of Clinical Nutrition Supplement (2003): 78660S–3S.

26 Position of the Academy of Nutrition and Dietetics (AND): Vegetarian Diets, *Journal of the Academy of Nutrition and Dietetics (AND)* 109 (2009): 1266-82.

27 E. A. Finkelstein et.al., "Annual Medical Spending Attributable to Obesity: Payer- and Service-Specific Estimates", *Health Affairs* 28 (2009): 822–831.

28 Stec L, Cordero, E, Ph.D. Cool Cuisine, *Taking a Bite Out of Global Warming*, Gibbs Publishing, 2008.

29 An Assessment of Coastal Hypoxia and Eutrophication in U.S. Waters. National Science and Technology Council Committee on Environment and Natural Resources, Washington, D.C. 2003: http://oceanservice.noaa.gov/outreach/pdfs/coastalhypoxia.pdf

Put It into Practice

Define the Term

Review the definitions of **Energy Yielding Nutrients** and **Calorie (kcal)**. Calculate the number of kcal in a serving of food that contains 35 g of carbohydrate, 12 g of fat, and 7 g of protein.

Myth vs. Fact

Determine if the following statement is a myth or fact and support your position with evidence from three research articles on the topic. *Statement: "Skipping meals helps you lose weight."*

For each research article, summarize each component below.
- A. Abstract
- B. Methods
- C. Results
- D. Discussion
- E. Conclusion

The Menu

Review the six essential, energy yielding and organic/inorganic classes of nutrients. Using Table 1.1, The Six Classes of Nutrients as a guide, develop one nutrient dense, creative menu for an upscale restaurant. This menu should consist of an appetizer, an entrée, a vegetable, a starch, and a dessert. It must include all six essential nutrients. From your menu, list the essential nutrients and two foods that contain each of these nutrients. Include the energy value of the energy yielding nutrients and state whether they are organic or inorganic.

Website Review

Navigate three different fast food establishment websites, review and compare the information provided for the following areas: (1) "Menu," (2) "Nutrition Facts," (3) "Careers," (4) "Marketing Promotions," and (5) "Community Outreach." In your opinion, which website is the most user-friendly and interesting? Which of the three establishments provide the most nutrient-dense choices?

Build Your Career Toolbox

Review the textbook section entitled "Career Opportunities in the Dietetics Field."

List two career opportunities for a Chef or a Registered Dietitian/Nutritionist who has a culinary nutrition background in each of the following areas:

- Healthcare
- Sports Nutrition
- Wellness Focused Spa
- Personal Chef
- Product Research and Development
- Food Science
- Community Nutrition
- Private Practice
- Corporate Wellness

Carl's Case Study

Carl is 33-year old a busy construction worker who is short on time and "eats what he likes." His schedule varies day to day—sometimes he eats 2 meals per day, other times he eats 4–5 "meals" per day. On most mornings, he wakes up about 20 minutes before he has to be out the door so breakfast is something quick that he doesn't have to cook. From there, he often will get a snack from the food truck with his friends during his morning break then he will either grab fast food for lunch or, if he's planned ahead, he'll bring a couple of sandwiches from home. Often, after work, he'll stop and have some beer with friends before dinner with his girlfriend.

Carl acknowledges that when he first started his construction job, he gained about 20 pounds, but he reports that his weight hasn't changed in the past 6 months or so. He says that time is his biggest challenge since he doesn't always get time to sit and have a full lunch break; because time is so limited, Carl says that he finds he eats really quickly most of the time. He also says that he and his girlfriend go out to eat with friends about 3 nights per week. When they go out, he says, "I order what I want because it's a party." His favorite restaurants serve things such as steaks, burgers, pulled pork, and macaroni and cheese. Carl also loves desserts, especially anything served a la mode.

After seeing his doctor for a recent check-up, Carl's doctor mentioned that his weight and BMI were in an unhealthy range. Even though Carl doesn't have any current health problems to speak of, Carl's doctor has concerns about his long-term health. Carl was told that if he doesn't make some changes soon, he would be on his way to developing high blood pressure, diabetes, and other medical problems.

Carl met with a dietitian who is helping him identify ways that he can improve his overall dietary habits. She is hoping that a personal chef can work with Carl to come up with foods that he and his girlfriend can prepare so that he can bring healthier foods to work. He's also planning to take some cooking lessons so that he's more comfortable in the kitchen.

Wt: 250 lbs   Ht: 5'10"   BMI: 35.9 kg/m² (obese)
No recent weight change

Dietitian Recommendations:
    Calorie Needs: 2250–2400 (for weight loss)
    Protein Needs: 115–130 g/day
    Fat: 30%–35% of calories, <10% calories from saturated fat
    Fiber: 25–35 g/day
    Sodium: <3 g or <3000 mg/day

Other Recommendations: Avoid sweets and processed meats as much as possible; eliminate soda, minimize alcohol; add fruits and veggies to every meal (at least 5 servings per day); plan for meals and snacks; add omega-3 fatty acids and monounsaturated fats

24-hr recall

Breakfast:
Big bowl of cereal with milk (2½ cups frosted flakes + 1½ cups whole milk), Dunkin Donuts® large hot coffee with extra cream (3 ozs) + extra sugar (8 tsp)

Morning Snack (from the Snack Truck):
3 hotdogs on buns each with 2 tbsp ketchup, 1 tbsp mustard, 1 tbsp sweet relish, 1 tbsp diced onions

Lunch:
2 ham and cheese sandwiches → Each with 2 slices white bread, 2-oz ham, 1 slice of American cheese, 2 tbsp yellow mustard; 24-oz Monster Drink®

Afternoon:
4 bottles of Budweiser®, 1 cup salted peanuts, 1/2 cup salted pretzels

Dinner (out to dinner):
3/4 of a Blooming Onion® with 3 tbsp ranch dressing, 22-oz prime rib + 2 tbsp salted butter + 1 tsp lemon juice, 1½ cups roasted red potatoes with 2 tbsp vegetable oil, a pinch of salt and pepper, 2 dinner rolls (1-oz each) with 1 tbsp butter each, 4 bottles of Budweiser®, caramel apple bread pudding (2-oz bread, 1 tbsp butter, 1/4 cup sugar, 2-oz green apple, 2-oz egg, 3/4 cup whole milk, a dash of cinnamon, 1/4 cup caramel sauce) + 1/2 cup French vanilla ice cream

Preferences: likes meat (especially burgers), cheese, anything fried, ice cream; Dislikes green salad, spicy foods, raw onions, grapefruit, yogurt, whole wheat bread

Study Guide

Student Name _____   **Date** _____

Course Section _____   **Chapter** _____

TERMINOLOGY

National Health and Nutrition Examination Survey (NHANES)_____	A. Looks for trends in a population to establish public policies on food assistance programs
Registered Dietitian/Nutritionist_____	B. Compounds found in carbohydrate, proteins and fats that provide the body with energy to remain active
Nutrition_____	
Clinical methods_____	C. State licensed nutrition professional
Energy yielding nutrient_____	D. Includes food diaries and 24-hr recalls
Anthropometry_____	E. Uses all nutrition assessment techniques to study a population
Licensed Registered Dietitian/Nutritionist_____	F. Includes blood and urine tests
National Nutrition Monitoring and Related Research Act of 1990_____	G. A health professional with a B.S. Degree in Food and Nutrition Science and accredited by the Academy of Nutrition and Dietetics (AND)
Dietary methods_____	H. Includes past medical history and family history
Biochemical analysis_____	I. Includes body measurements (height, weight, BMI)
	J. A science that studies the substances in food and their interactions in the body

Student Name _____   Date _____

Course Section _____   Chapter _____

CALCULATIONS

Show your work to calculate total calories in this meal:

90 gm carbohydrate × _____ calories per gram = _____ **calories from carbohydrates**

30 gm protein × _____ calories per gram = _____ **calories from protein**

28 gm fat × _____ calories per gram = _____ **calories from fat**

Total calories in the meal = _____

Show your work to calculate the percentage of calories from carbohydrate, protein and fat.

_____ calories from carbohydrates ÷ _____ total calories = _____ × 100 = _____%

_____ calories from protein ÷ _____ total calories = _____ × 100 = _____%

_____ calories from fat ÷ _____ total calories = _____ × 100 = _____%

Student Name _____ Date _____

Course Section _____ Chapter _____

Determine the calories of each of the foods listed in the Total Calories column.

Food	CHO	protein	Fat	Total Calories
Example 1 medium Apple	15 grams 15 × 4 calories/gram = 60 calories	1 gram 1 × 4 calories/gram = 4 calories	0 gram 0 × 9 calories/gram = 0 calories	60 + 4 = 64 calories
2 slices of wheat bread	30 grams	4 grams	1 gram	
2oz. of grilled chicken	0 grams	14 grams	5 grams	
2 chocolate chip cookies	20 grams	3 grams	8 grams	
8oz. whole milk	12 grams	8 grams	10 grams	
1/2 cup carrot sticks	5 grams	2 grams	0 grams	
12oz. of soda	38 grams	0 grams	0 grams	
1/8th of a 12" pizza	20 grams	10 grams	7 grams	
1 cup of chocolate Ice Cream	38 grams	6 grams	14 grams	

Student Name _____ **Date** _____

Course Section _____ **Chapter** _____

CASE STUDY DISCUSSION

Carl's Case Study: The Psychology of Eating

Review the biological, psychological and sociological reasons for choosing food that are given in Chapter 1. After reviewing the case study, use this food choice information to answer the following:

1. Explain what is meant by biological reasons for eating.

2. Explain what is meant by psychological and sociological reasons for eating.

3. Using Carl's 24-hr recall, describe each of Carl's food selections and explain whether his choices are based on biological or psychological/sociological factors.

Student Name _____   **Date** _____

Course Section _____   **Chapter** _____

PRACTICE TEST

Select the best answer.

1. The definition of Nutrition is
   a. the study of food
   b. the science of food and its interactions in the body
   c. the composition of food
   d. the relations between food and health

2. An example of an energy-yielding nutrient is
   a. Lipid
   b. Vitamin
   c. Water
   d. Mineral

3. The number of calories in 15 grams of fat is
   a. 30
   b. 60
   c. 75
   d. 135

4. Calculate the number of calories in a meal that consists of 62 grams of carbohydrate, 70 grams of protein and 40 grams of fat.
   a. 538
   b. 688
   c. 748
   d. 888

5. Determine the percentage of calories from carbohydrate, protein and fat in the following meal that consists of 75 grams of carbohydrate, 62 grams of protein and 30 grams of fat.
   a. 30% carbohydrate, 32% protein and 28% fat
   b. 40% carbohydrate, 20% protein and 20% fat
   c. 32% carbohydrate, 38% protein and 30% fat
   d. 37% carbohydrate, 30% protein and 33% fat

Student Name _____   **Date** _____

Course Section _____   **Chapter** _____

TRUE OR FALSE

6. _____ A biological reason to consume food is hunger.

7. _____ Vitamins are organic nutrients.

8. _____ Hypertension is an example of malnutrition.

9. _____ Food energy is measured in grams.

List the 5 components of a healthy diet:

- _____
- _____
- _____
- _____
- _____

List 4 methods of Nutrition Assessment:

- _____
- _____
- _____
- _____

Dietary Standards

2

KEY TERMS

Adequate Intake (AI)
ChooseMyPlate
Dietary Goals
Dietary Guidelines
Dietary Reference
   Intakes (DRIs)
Estimated Average
   Requirement (EAR)

Choose Your Foods Lists for
   Meal Planning
Food Composition Tables
Food Label
Food Guide Pyramid
Healthy People 2020
Mediterranean Food
   Pyramid

Nutrition Facts Panel
Recommended Dietary
   Allowances (RDAs)
Scientific Method
Tolerable Upper Intake (UL)

Introduction

A wide variety of dietary recommendations are made by nutrition professionals. These recommendations are science-based observations that continually undergo changes. In order to study the nutritional needs of the population it is necessary to understand some of the methodology used in making recommendations. An organized, systematic approach known as The Scientific Method is employed to conduct this research. It consists of a series of steps to progressively solve a problem.

These steps include:

1. Identification of the problem

2. Background research

3. The design of the hypothesis

4. Testing the hypothesis

5. Analyzing the results

6. Drawing conclusions

7. Communicating the results

Oftentimes the identification of a problem involves asking a question in a way that evokes a measurable response. Background research obtained from reliable sources is useful in understanding the possible scenarios the question poses as well as the potential outcomes. It is always important to remember any variables. With this information and data drawn from past experiences, a hypothesis can be made. A hypothesis is often referred to as an educated guess that sets the research going in a focused direction. A simple statement is created detailing what is projected to occur. This statement is supported by a previous knowledge of the problem or by the information gathered during the background research. Next the hypothesis must be tested. An experiment is designed and then conducted. At the end of the experimental phase the results are analyzed and conclusions are drawn. The results are then conveyed in the form of a report. Quite often the results raise additional questions that must again be evaluated using the scientific method.

Setting the Standards

Essential nutrients and non-essential nutrients are both necessities in our diets. The amounts needed vary depending upon age, sex, growth status, and genetic traits. Conditions such as pregnancy, breastfeeding, illnesses, and drug use may also increase or decrease nutrient needs. To promote optimal health and to prevent disease, guidelines known as dietary standards have been established to provide information on the essential nutrients necessary to avoid nutritional deficiencies. Dietary standards are merely guidelines that are designed to meet the needs of the majority of healthy persons. These standards vary from one country to another because of national nutritional problems and the interpretations of scientists concerning dietary needs. The overall **dietary goals** for healthy individuals reflect the percentage of calories that should be consumed from each of the three major nutrients. The recommended age-appropriate macronutrient distribution percentages are listed in Table 2.1.[1] The tools that have been developed to determine specific dietary standards are extensive and are discussed in this chapter.

TABLE 2.1 Dietary Goals

Recommended Macronutrient Distribution by Age			
Age	Carbohydrate	Protein	Fat
Young children (1–3 years)	45%–65%	5%–20%	30%–40%
Older children and adolescents (4–18 years)	45%–65%	10%–30%	25%–35%
Adults (19 years and older)	45%–65%	10%–35%	20%–35%

Recommended Dietary Allowances (RDAs)

Since 1941 the Food and Nutrition Board of the Institute of Medicine (IOM) of the National Academy of Sciences has prepared Recommended Dietary Allowances (RDAs) that have set the types and quantities of nutrients that are needed for healthy diets. These values are the basic American standard. They have undergone several revisions that reflect the best scientific judgment on nutrient allowances for the maintenance of good health and the evaluation of diet adequacy for various groups of people. The levels of essential nutrients are determined by the board as adequate in meeting the nutrient needs of practically all healthy persons.

RDAs do not meet the needs of individuals with special nutritional needs resulting from illness, the use of medications, and inherited metabolic disorders. The RDAs for most nutrients are set at levels that exceed the requirements of many individuals. Consumption of less than the required intake is not necessarily inadequate, but as intake falls below recommended levels, the risk of inadequacy increases. The RDA for energy reflects the mean requirement for each category. Consumption of energy at too high a level can lead to obesity in most persons.[2] Similar population nutrient recommendations are set by scientists in other countries as well. The World Health Organization (WHO) is the coordinating health authority for the United Nations system. This organization is responsible for global health matters such as setting norms and standards for dietary recommendations and monitoring and assessing health trends. An important function of the WHO is making global nutrition recommendations, including vitamin and mineral levels for fortification programs.[3]

Dietary Reference Intakes (DRIs)

A set of standards known as the Dietary Reference Intakes or DRIs was developed during the mid-1990s by the IOM. The DRIs are standards determined jointly by American and Canadian scientists to replace the American RDAs and the former Canadian equivalent, the Recommended Nutrient Intakes (RNI). These standards outline the dietary nutrient intakes for healthy individuals in the United States and in Canada.[4] There are over 40 nutrient substance values that are categorized according to the age, gender, and life stage group of individuals. These values are used for planning and assessing diets and include the following tables:

1. Estimated Average Requirements (EAR), Protein, Carbohydrate, Vitamins and Minerals

2. Recommended Dietary Allowances (RDAs) and Adequate Intakes (AI), Vitamins and Minerals

3. Recommended Dietary Allowances (RDAs) and Adequate Intakes (AI), Total Water and Macronutrients

4. Tolerable Upper Intake Levels (UL), Vitamins and Elements

5. Macronutrients Table

6. Doubly Labeled Water Data Set

7. Electrolytes and Water Table.

A description of the most commonly used values is listed in Table 2.2. Complete lists of the updated DRI values are provided in the Appendix of this text.[5]

TABLE 2.2 Nutrient Standards

Dietary Reference Intakes
1. Recommended Dietary Allowances (RDA) Nutrient intake goals for healthy individuals, derived from the Estimated Average Requirements.
2. Adequate Intakes (AI) Nutrient intake goals for healthy individuals, derived from the Estimated Average Requirements. Set when insufficient scientific data is available to establish the RDA value.
3. Tolerable Upper Intake Levels (UL) Suggested upper limits of intakes for nutrients that may be toxic at excessive levels. When consumed at excessive levels, these nutrients are likely to cause illness.
4. Estimated Average Requirements (EAR) An Estimated Average Requirement (EAR) is the average daily nutrient intake level estimated to meet the requirements of half of the healthy individuals in a specific population group.

Dietary Guidelines

The DRIs refer to specific nutrients that are recommended to ensure optimal health and dietary adequacy. **Dietary Guidelines** have been developed by the USDA that translate nutrients into general recommendations about the foods that should be consumed and/or limited. Health officials today are as concerned about overnutrition (excesses of nutrients) as they are about undernutrition. The Dietary Guidelines emphasize that sensible choices in the diet can promote health and reduce the risk for chronic diseases such as heart disease, certain cancers, diabetes, stroke, and osteoporosis, which are some of the leading causes of death and disability among Americans. Although many guidelines have stressed the importance of variety in the diet, a shift to also include fitness reflects the results of recent research conducted on the problem of overweight and obese individuals in the United States.[6] The Dietary Guidelines for Americans were first released in 1980, jointly published by the U.S. Department of Agriculture (USDA) and the U.S. Department of Health and Human Services (HHS). Secretaries of the USDA and HHS are required to jointly publish a report on the Dietary Guidelines for Americans at least every five years.

The recently released 2015 Dietary Guidelines for Americans continue to make recommendations utilizing the most recent scientific knowledge in promoting health and preventing chronic diseases for current and future generations. A focus of the current guidelines is on the importance of healthy eating patterns as a whole and the way that an array of foods and beverages act together to affect health. The guidelines recognize that the U.S population is now faced with the cumulative effects of poor eating and physical activity patterns. As a result of these unhealthy practices, approximately 117 million Americans have one or more preventable chronic diseases such as cardiovascular disease, hypertension, type 2 diabetes, some cancers, and poor bone health. The high rates of overweight and obesity in more than two thirds of adults and approximately one third of children and youth have contributed to many of these health risks and diseases.

The five general 2015 Dietary Guidelines and Key Recommendations are included in Table 2.3. A picture of the 2015 Dietary Guidelines brochure is found in Figure 2.1.[7]

TABLE 2.3 The 2015-2020 Dietary Guidelines and Key Recommendations

The Guidelines
1. Follow a healthy eating pattern across the lifespan. All food and beverage choices matter. Choose a healthy eating pattern at an appropriate calorie level to help achieve and maintain a healthy body weight, support nutrient adequacy, and reduce the risk of chronic disease.
2. Focus on variety, nutrient density, and amount. To meet nutrient needs within calorie limits, choose a variety of nutrient-dense foods across and within all food groups in recommended amounts.

(Continued)

TABLE 2.3 The 2015-2020 Dietary Guidelines and Key Recommendations (*continued*)

3. Limit calories from added sugars and saturated fats and reduce sodium intake. Consume an eating pattern low in added sugars, saturated fats, and sodium. Cut back on foods and beverages higher in these components to amounts that fit within healthy eating patterns.

4. Shift to healthier food and beverage choices. Choose nutrient-dense foods and beverages across and within all food groups in place of less healthy choices. Consider cultural and personal preferences to make these shifts easier to accomplish and maintain.

5. Support healthy eating patterns for all. Everyone has a role in helping to create and support healthy eating patterns in multiple settings nationwide, from home to school to work to communities.

Key Recommendations

The Dietary Guidelines' Key Recommendations for healthy eating patterns should be applied in their entirety, given the interconnected relationship that each dietary component can have with others.

Consume a healthy eating pattern that accounts for all foods and beverages within an appropriate calorie level.

A healthy eating pattern includes:[1]

- A variety of vegetables from all of the subgroups—dark green, red and orange, legumes (beans and peas), starchy, and other

- Fruits, especially whole fruits

- Grains, at least half of which are whole grains

- Fat-free or low-fat dairy, including milk, yogurt, cheese, and/or fortified soy beverages

- A variety of protein foods, including seafood, lean meats and poultry, eggs, legumes (beans and peas), and nuts, seeds, and soy products

- Oils

A healthy eating pattern limits:

- Saturated fats and trans fats, added sugars, and sodium

Key Recommendations that are quantitative are provided for several components of the diet that should be limited. These components are of particular public health concern in the United States, and the specified limits can help individuals achieve healthy eating patterns within calorie limits:

- Consume less than 10 percent of calories per day from added sugars[2]

- Consume less than 10 percent of calories per day from saturated fats[3]

- Consume less than 2,300 milligrams (mg) per day of sodium[4]

- If alcohol is consumed, it should be consumed in moderation—up to one drink per day for women and up to two drinks per day for men—and only by adults of legal drinking age.[5]

In tandem with the recommendations above, Americans of all ages—children, adolescents, adults, and older adults—should meet the *Physical Activity Guidelines for Americans* to help promote health and reduce the risk of chronic disease. Americans should aim to achieve and maintain a healthy body weight. The relationship between diet and physical activity contributes to calorie balance and managing body weight. As such, the *Dietary Guidelines* includes a Key Recommendation to meet the *Physical Activity Guidelines for Americans*.[6]

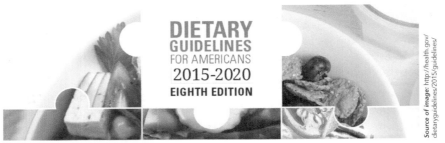

FIGURE 2.1 2015–2020 Dietary Guidelines Brochure

Source of image: http://health.gov/dietaryguidelines/2015/guidelines/

Overall Nutrition Goals for the Nation

As discussed in chapter one, the nutritional status of the U.S. population is determined by evaluating information received from government surveys under the auspices of the National Nutrition Monitoring and Related Research Act of 1990. The data obtained is being used to measure the Nation's progress in implementing the recommendations of the Dietary Guidelines for Americans and to determine if the objectives of the Healthy People 2010 were met. This 10-year plan was developed by the United States Department of Health and Human Services (HHS) to establish healthy objectives for the nation. The initiative addresses the proportion of the population that consumes a specified level of particular foods and/or nutrients, and the average amount of food eaten by population groups. Objectives may target areas such as undernutrition, including iron deficiency, growth retardation, and food security.[8] The Healthy People 2020 document presents new objectives based on strong science that supports the health benefits of eating a healthful diet and maintaining a healthy body weight. The goals encompass the importance of increasing household food security and eliminating hunger. Table 2.4 provides a sample list of nutrition objectives outlined in the Healthy People 2020 document.[9, 10]

TABLE 2.4 Sample Nutrition Objectives from the Healthy People 2020

- Increase the number of states with nutrition standards for foods and beverages provided to preschool-aged children in child care.
- Increase the proportion of schools that offer nutritious foods and beverages outside of school meals.
- Increase the proportion of schools that do not sell or offer calorically sweetened beverages to students.
- Increase the number of states that have state-level policies that incentivize food retail outlets to provide foods that are encouraged by the Dietary Guidelines.
- Increase the proportion of school districts that require schools to make fruits or vegetables available whenever other food is offered or sold.
- Increase the proportion of primary care physicians who regularly assess body mass index (BMI) for age and sex in their child or adolescent patients.
- Increase the proportion of Americans who have access to a food retail outlet that sells a variety of foods that are encouraged by the Dietary Guidelines for Americans.
- Increase the proportion of worksites that offer nutrition or weight management classes or counseling.
- Increase the proportion of physician office visits that include counseling or education related to nutrition or weight.
- Reduce the proportion of children and adolescents who are considered obese.
- Reduce the proportion of adults who are obese.
- Increase the contribution of total vegetables to the diets of the population aged 2 years and older.

- Increase the variety and contribution of vegetables to the diets of the population aged 2 years and older.

- Increase the contribution of fruits to the diets of the population aged 2 years and older.

- Reduce household food insecurity and, in so doing, reduce hunger.

- Reduce consumption of calories from solid fats and added sugars in the population aged 2 years and older.

- Increase the contribution of whole grains to the diets of the population aged 2 years and older.

- Reduce consumption of saturated fat in the population aged 2 years and older.

- Reduce iron deficiency among young children and females of childbearing age.

- Reduce consumption of sodium in the population aged 2 years and older.

- Increase consumption of calcium in the population aged 2 years and older.

http://health.gov/dietaryguidelines/2015/guidelines/

Obtaining Nutrition Information

In order to make recommendations for the population, or for an individual, it is necessary to gather data. Methods that may be employed include: administering surveys, conducting interviews and gathering medical records. One of the most effective means of gathering information is the use of the National Health and Nutrition Examination Survey (NHANES), conducted by Center of Disease Control's National Center for Health Statistics. The NHANES process is designed to assess the health and nutritional status of adults and children in the United States. This comprehensive survey combines personal interviews with standardized physical examinations, diagnostic procedures, and lab tests on approximately 5,000 persons each year. Fifteen counties across the country are visited each year to assess and interview individuals. They are interviewed on the following topics; demographics, socioeconomics, dietary, and health-related questions. The examination component is administered by highly trained medical personnel and includes medical, dental, physiological measurement, and lab tests.

Additional questions address health history and food intake. The diseases, medical conditions, and health indicators studied include:

- Respiratory disease
- Obesity
- Anemia
- Oral health
- Diabetes
- Osteoporosis
- Eye diseases
- Physical fitness and physical functioning
- Hearing loss
- Kidney disease
- Nutrition
- Vision
- Cardiovascular Disease
- Environmental Exposures
- Infectious Diseases
- Reproductive History and Sexual Behavior
- Sexually Transmitted Diseases

This compilation of information is an extremely comprehensive analysis of the health and well-being of the American population. The data is then reviewed and a list of recommendations is submitted. Examples of the data collected from the NHANES 1999-2016 resulted in the following conclusions:

- Overweight prevalence data has led to the proliferation of programs in emphasizing diet and exercise. It has also stimulated additional research and a means to track trends in obesity.

- Data continues to indicate undiagnosed diabetes. As a result this has stimulated government and private agencies to increase public awareness especially among minority populations.

- Information in the survey will help the Food and Drug Administration decide if there is a need to change the vitamin and mineral fortification regulations of the Nation's Food supply.

- NHANES data continues to steer education and prevention programs to reduce hypertension and cholesterol levels, and to measure the success in curtailing risk factors with the Nations' number one cause of death, cardiovascular disease.

The importance of gathering data, and carefully reviewing it, is imperative to the future health and wellness of the Nation. Gathering this data is not often easy. One of the main obstacles in this process is the reliability of the individuals who are recording the information.[11]

Food Composition Tables

Nutrient Composition Tables, also known as Food Composition Tables, provide numerical data on nutrients found in foods. Laboratory analysis must be completed on each food to derive this data. The USDA has compiled data on a large number and variety of foods, which is published through the USDA in Agriculture Handbook 8, Composition of Foods: Raw, Processed, Prepared. The USDA Nutrient Data Base for Standard Reference also provides this information. Approximate nutrient components such as energy value, proteins, carbohydrates, fats, minerals, and vitamins are included.[12] Numerous other computer programs on nutrient data also exist. Nutrition Composition Tables are useful in analyzing dietary intakes to determine if the consumption of nutrients is adequate. Chefs can utilize these tables to gain information on the approximate nutritional analysis of the recipes and menus they serve. A sampling of this database can be seen in Table 2.4A.

Table 2.4A Nutritive Value of the Edible Part of Food

Food No.	Food Description	Measure of Edible Portion	Weight (g)	Water (%)	Calories (kcal)	Protein (g)	Total Fat (g)	Fatty Acids Saturated (g)	Fatty Acids Mono-unsaturated (g)	Fatty Acids Poly-unsaturated (g)
Dairy Products (continued)										
	Yogurt (continued)									
	Without added milk solids									
138	Made with whole milk, plain..	8-oz ....227 container	88	139	8	7	4.8	2.0	0.2
139	Made with nonfat milk, low calorie sweetener, vanilla or lemon flavor.......	8-oz ....227 container	87	98	9	Tr	0.3	0.1	Tr
Eggs										
	Egg									
	Raw									
140	Whole	1 medium.........44	75	66	5	4	1.4	1.7	0.6
141		1 large.............50	75	75	6	5	1.6	1.9	0.7

No.	Description	Amount	Weight	Water	Calories	Protein	Fat	Sat	Mono	Poly
142		1 extra large	58	75	86	7	6	1.8	2.2	0.8
143	White	1 large	33	88	17	4	0	0.0	0.0	0.0
144	Yolk	1 large	17	49	59	3	5	1.6	1.9	0.7
	Cooked, whole									
145	Fried, in margarine, with salt	1 large	46	69	92	6	7	1.9	2.7	1.3
146	Hard cooked, shell removed	1 large	50	75	78	6	5	1.6	2.0	0.7
147		1 cup, chopped	136	75	211	17	14	4.4	5.5	1.9
148	Poached, with salt	1 large	50	75	75	6	5	1.5	1.9	0.7
149	Scrambled, in margarine, with whole milk, salt	1 large	61	73	101	7	7	2.2	2.9	1.3
150	Egg substitute, liquid	¼ cup	63	83	53	8	2	0.4	0.6	1.0
Fats and Oils										
	Butter (4 sticks per lb)									
151	Salted	1 stick	113	16	813	1	92	57.3	26.6	3.4
152		1 tbsp	14	16	102	Tr	12	7.2	3.3	0.4
153		1 tsp	5	16	36	Tr	4	2.5	1.2	0.2
154	Unsalted	1 stick	113	18	813	1	92	57.3	26.6	3.4
155	Lard	1 cup	205	0	1,849	0	205	80.4	92.5	23.0
156		1 tbsp	13	0	115	0	13	5.0	5.8	1.4
	Margarine, vitamin A-fortified, salt added									
	Regular (about 80% fat)									
157	Hard (4 sticks per lb)	1 stick	113	16	815	1	91	17.9	40.6	28.8
158		1 tbsp	14	16	101	Tr	11	2.2	5.0	3.6
159		1 tsp	5	16	34	Tr	4	0.7	1.7	1.2
160	Soft	1 cup	227	16	1,626	2	183	31.3	64.7	78.5
161		1 tsp	5	16	34	Tr	4	0.6	1.3	1.6
	Spread (about 60% fat)									
162	Hard (4 sticks per lb)	1 stick	115	37	621	1	70	16.2	29.9	20.8
163		1 tbsp	14	37	76	Tr	9	2.0	3.6	2.5
164		1 tsp	5	37	26	Tr	3	0.7	1.2	0.9
165	Soft	1 cup	229	37	1,236	1	139	29.3	72.1	31.6
166		1 tsp	5	37	26	Tr	3	0.6	1.5	0.7
167	Spread (about 40% fat)	1 cup	232	58	801	1	90	17.9	36.4	32.0
168		1 tsp	5	58	17	Tr	2	0.4	0.8	0.7

Food Labels

Another tool or standard used to assist both members of the public and health professionals in meeting dietary guidelines and recommendations is the Food Label. Food labels offer complete, useful, and accurate information that can assist consumers in choosing the nutrients to include or limit in their diet. The Nutrition Labeling and Education Act of 1990 (NLEA), which was implemented by the Food and Drug Administration of the Department of Health and Human Services, requires labeling of most foods (except meat, fish and and poultry), and authorizes the use of nutrient claims and appropriate FDA-approved claims. Nutrition information is available for many raw foods including the 20 most eaten raw fruits, vegetables, fish, and the 45 best-selling cuts of meat. A 1996 survey by the FDA found that more than 70% of U.S. stores were in compliance with this law. Restaurant menu items may require nutrition labeling if a health or nutrient-content claim is made. The NLEA does not require nutrition labeling in the following cases:

- Food served for immediate consumption (for example cafeteria food and food vendor products)
- Ready to eat food prepared on site (for example bakery and deli items)
- Food shipped in bulk
- Plain coffee, tea, and spices

Requirements on the Food Label

Food labels must be uniform in the United States and contain the following information:

- The usual or common name of the product
- The name and address of the manufacturer, and the date "to be sold by"
- The net contents or weight, and quantities of specified nutrients and food constituents
- The ingredients in descending order by weight
- The serving size and number of servings per container

Nutrition Information

Under the label's "Nutrition Facts" panel, which appears in bold black letters, manufacturers are required to provide information on certain nutrients that are in their product. The panel provides an easy-to-read format that allows consumers to quickly find the information they need to make healthy food choices. When looking at the Nutrition Facts it is helpful to read the label in the order listed below to determine the nutritional content of the product.

1. Serving Size/Servings per container
   When looking at the Nutrition Facts label, start by looking at the serving size and number of servings per container. These are listed in standardized familiar units such as cups and ounces followed by the metric amount in grams.

2. Calories and Calories from fat
   Examine how many calories are provided in one serving of the product, as well as the calories that are derived from fat.

3. The Nutrients
   The Nutrient section on the label includes some of the key nutrients that may have an impact on your health.
   Limit these nutrients:
   > Total Fat
   > Saturated Fat
   > Trans Fat
   > Cholesterol
   > Sodium

   Get enough of these nutrients:
   > Dietary fiber
   > Vitamin A
   > Vitamin C
   > Calcium
   > Iron

4. The Percent Daily Value
   The * symbol is used after the heading % Daily Value. This refers to the Footnote in the lower part of the nutrition label and includes the % Daily Values. The Percent Daily Values are based on the daily value recommendations for key nutrients for a 2000 calorie diet. The % Daily Value helps to determine if a serving of food is high or low in a nutrient. 5% DV or less is low for nutrients, and 20% DV or more is high.

Figure 2.2 provides a sample panel that highlights and explains the information on the Original Nutrition Facts panel of the food label.[13]

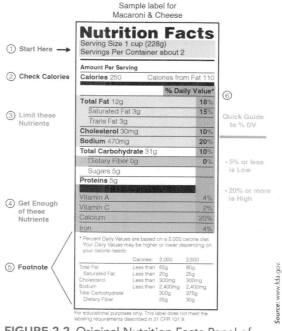

FIGURE 2.2. Original Nutrition Facts Panel of the Food Label

New Rules for Updating the Nutrition Facts Label

In March of 2014, July of 2015, and then most recently May 2016, The Food and Drug Administration issued supplemental new rules for updating the Nutrition Facts Label. Manufacturers will have until 2018 to comply with the changes. A summary of the changes include the following:

1. A greater understanding of Nutrition Science
    – Required information about added sugars
    – Updated daily values for nutrients like sodium, dietary fiber and Vitamin D
    – Require manufacturers to declare the gram amount of Potassium and Vitamin D on the label in addition to the existing %Daily Value(DV)
    – Calcium and iron continue to be required, Vitamins A and C can be included on a voluntary basis
    – "Total Fat", "Saturated Fat", and "Trans Fat", will continue to be required but "Calories from Fat" will be removed since research shows the type of fat is more important than the amount

2. Updated Serving Size Requirement
    – Serving size requirements are changed to reflect how people eat and drink today not what they "should" eat
    – Packaged foods, including drinks that are typically eaten in one sitting, must be labeled as a single serving and the calorie and nutrient information must be declared for the entire package
    – Packages that are larger and could be consumed in one sitting or multiple sittings must provide dual column labels which indicate "per serving" and "per package" calories and nutrient information

3. Refreshed Design
    – Make Serving sizes and Calories more prominent to emphasize parts of the label that are important in addressing current public health issues
    – The Percent Daily Value (%DV) is shifted to the left so it comes first

Figure 2.2A shows a comparison of the current Nutrition Facts Panel to the new one. Figure 2.2B illustrates the need to educate on serving sizes.[14]

Nutrition Facts

Serving Size 2/3 cup (55g)
Servings Per Container About 8

Amount Per Serving

Calories 230	Calories from Fat 72

	% Daily Value*
Total Fat 8g	**12%**
Saturated Fat 1g	**5%**
Trans Fat 0g	
Cholesterol 0mg	**0%**
Sodium 160mg	**7%**
Total Carbohydrate 37g	**12%**
Dietary Fiber 4g	**16%**
Sugars 1g	
Protein 3g	

Vitamin A	10%
Vitamin C	8%
Calcium	20%
Iron	45%

* Percent Daily Values are based on a 2,000 calorie diet.
 Your daily value may be higher or lower depending on
 your calorie needs.

	Calories:	2,000	2,500
Total Fat	Less than	65g	80g
Sat Fat	Less than	20g	25g
Cholesterol	Less than	300mg	300mg
Sodium	Less than	2,400mg	2,400mg
Total Carbohydrate		300g	375g
Dietary Fiber		25g	30g

Nutrition Facts

8 servings per container

Serving size	2/3 cup (55g)

Amount per 2/3 cup

Calories	**230**

% DV*	
12%	**Total Fat** 8g
5%	**Saturated Fat** 1g
	Trans Fat 0g
0%	**Cholesterol** 0mg
7%	**Sodium** 160mg
12%	**Total Carbs** 37g
14%	**Dietary Fiber** 4g
	Sugars 1g
	Added Sugars 0g
	Protein 3g

10%	**Vitamin D** 2mcg
20%	**Calcium** 260mg
45%	**Iron** 8mg
5%	**Potassium** 235mg

* Footnote on Daily Values (DV) and calories
 reference to be inserted here.

FIGURE 2.2A Original Nutrition Facts Panel vs New

Source: http://www.fda.gov/Food/GuidanceRegulation/GuidanceDocumentsRegulatoryInformation/
LabelingNutrition/ucm385663.htm

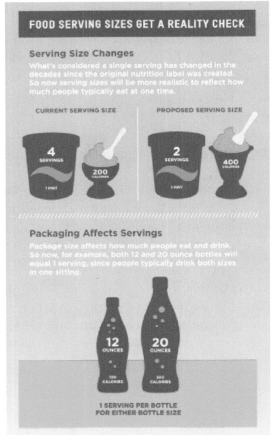

FIGURE 2.2B Serving sizes get a reality check

Source: http://www.fda.gov/Food/GuidanceRegulation/GuidanceDocumentsRegulatoryInformation/LabelingNutrition/ucm385663.htm

Health Claims on Food Labels

The FDA has identified the relationship between some nutrients and their positive impact on health. These claims may often be seen on food packages. There are three different categories of claims that can be used on food and dietary supplement labels. The categories are nutrient content claims, health claims and structure/function claims. The FDA and the Federal Trade Commission are responsible for ensuring the validity of these claims. The nutrient content claim describes the level of a nutrient or dietary substance in the product. Terms such as free, low, reduced, lite, more, and high are used when comparing the level of a nutrient in a food to that of another food. The terms must meet requirements that are consistent for all types of foods. Calorie-free products for example, must always be less than 5 calories/serving, while a product that is high in fiber must be 5 grams or more/serving. Health claims on a food label describe the relationship between a food, food component, or dietary supplement ingredient, and their potential for reducing the risk of a disease or health-related condition. Examples of approved health claims and their requirements can be seen in Table 2.5. The final claim refers to the structure/function, and is found on the labels of conventional foods, dietary supplements, and some drugs, to describe the role of a nutrient or dietary ingredient intended to affect normal structure or function in humans. Examples of structure function claims include; "calcium builds strong bones" and "antioxidants maintain cell integrity." The manufacturer is responsible for the validity of such a claim, and a disclaimer must be included on the label stating that the FDA has not evaluated the claim.[15, 16]

TABLE 2.5 Examples of Claims on Food Labels

Health Claim	Nutrient Claim	Label Claim
Calcium and Osteoporosis	High in calcium (20% or more of Daily Value)	Regular exercise and a healthy diet with enough calcium helps teens and young adult white and Asian women maintain good bone health and may reduce their high risk of osteoporosis later in life.
Sodium and Hypertension	Low sodium (140 milligrams or less)	Diets low in sodium may reduce the risk of high blood pressure, a disease associated with many factors.
Dietary Fat and Cancer	Low fat (3 grams of fat or less)	Development of cancer depends on many factors. A diet low in total fat may reduce the risk of some cancers.
Folate and Neural Tube Defects	Good source of folate (at least 40 micrograms) delete	Healthful diets with adequate folate may reduce a woman's risk of having a child with a brain or spinal cord defect.
Soy Protein and Risk of Coronary Heart Disease	At least 6.25 grams of soy protein. Low saturated fat (1 gram or less-no more than 15% of calories) Low cholesterol (10 milligrams or less) Low fat (3 grams or less)	25 grams of soy protein, as part of a diet low in saturated fat and cholesterol, may reduce the risk of heart disease. A serving of (name of food) supplies _____ grams of soy protein.

Food Allergies and the Food Label

The Food and Drug Administration (FDA) in the United States requires food manufacturers to list the most common food allergens. These include: milk, eggs, peanuts, tree nuts, fish, shellfish, soy, and wheat. The Food Allergen Labeling and Consumer Protection Act of 2004 (FALCPA) is a law that applies to all foods whose labeling is regulated by

FDA, both domestic and imported. The labeling must be in a simplified form so older children are able to understand the information. The food label must list the type of allergen as well as any ingredient in the product that contains a protein derived from one of the above listed food allergens. This also includes allergens that can be found in additives including flavorings and colors. A food manufacturer only needs to state the food allergen in that product. FALCPA's labeling requirements do not apply to the potential or unintentional presence of major food allergens in foods resulting from cross-contamination from a manufacturing plant that processes other products that contain a food allergen. Cross-contamination may be problematic for individuals who exhibit severe allergic reactions to an allergen. Most manufacturers will voluntarily include an advisory statement such as "this product was manufactured in a plant that also processes wheat."[17]

Organic Products and the Food Label

There are a variety of reasons consumers purchase organic foods. These include concerns about the effects of conventional farming practices on the environment, animal welfare and the belief that organic products taste better and are more healthful than conventional foods. A review of the current literature suggests that organic foods are not more nutritious than conventional foods. It has been found that organic foods may reduce exposure to pesticide residues and antibiotic-resistant bacteria.[18]

In order for a food or other agricultural product to be labeled organic it must have been produced through approved methods. The methods used must involve the integration of biological, cultural and mechanical practices that promote cycling of resources and ecological balance, and conserve biodiversity. Additional requirements by the USDA include prohibiting the use of synthetic fertilizers, sewerage sludge, irradiation, and genetic engineering.

In the United States the National Organic Program regulates all organic crops, livestock, and agricultural products. They are certified to the United States Department of Agriculture (USDA) organic standards. The USDA organic seal as shown in Figure 2.3 ensures that the product is certified organic and has 95% or more organic content.

There are additional voluntary labels for livestock products which include meat and eggs. The use of animal raising claims must be truthful and not misleading. Examples include:

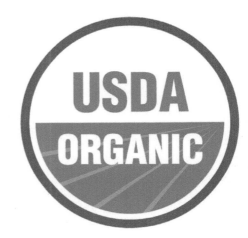

FIGURE 2.3 The UDSA Organic Seal

- Cage-free: In order for this label to be used the flock must be able to freely roam a building, room or enclosed area. They must have unlimited access to food and fresh water during their production cycle.
- Free-range: This label may be used when the flock was provided with shelter in a building, room, or area. They must have unlimited access to food and fresh water during their production cycle and have continuous access to the outdoors.
- Natural: Meat, poultry, and egg products that are labeled "natural" must be minimally processed and contain no artificial ingredients. This does not pertain to any standards regarding the farm practices.
- Grass-fed: The use of this label requires that grass-fed animals receive a majority of their nutrients from grass throughout their life. This is different from animals that may have their diets supplemented with grain. Meat products that are labeled as grass-fed organic may also add the "natural" label if they contain no artificial ingredients.[19]

Food Guide Pyramid

It is often difficult to assess the recommended nutrient amounts of actual foods and meals that one should consume. Standards are developed to help make the transition between recommendations and that which should actually be consumed in a healthy diet.

The Food Guide Pyramid, which was developed by the USDA is widely used to make good food choices. The original food guide pyramid was developed in 1992 as an educational tool used to help Americans select healthful diets. The 6th edition of the pyramid, entitled MyPyramid, was released in 2005 by the U.S. Department of Agriculture. MyPyramid translates the concepts of the 2005 Dietary Guidelines for Americans to assist consumers in making healthier food and physical activity choices. The pyramid includes a motivational symbol and slogan, "Steps to a Healthier You" as seen in Figure 2.4. In the MyPyramid graphic the color bands represent the various food groups needed each day for health. As illustrated in Figure 2.4. the orange band represents grains, the green for vegetables, the red for fruit, blue for milk, purple for meat and beans, and yellow for oils. The width of

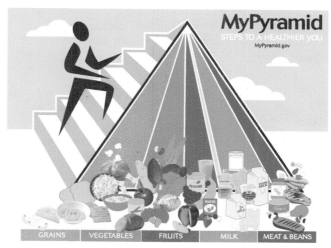

FIGURE 2.4 The U.S. Food Guide Pyramid

the colored bands also varies to suggest the quantity of food that should be eaten from each group. The pyramid also reminds consumers to include physical activity choices every day.

Data from the Dietary Reference Intakes and from the USDA's Agricultural Research Service, on the nutritional content of foods and on food consumption patterns, was used to update food intake patterns used in the MyPyramid plan. The daily food intake patterns identify the amount of product to consume from each group and subgroup at a variety of energy levels.[20]

ChooseMyPlate

In June of 2011 the U.S. Department of Agriculture unveiled "ChooseMyPlate" the most simplified and user-friendly chart of dietary guidelines developed to date. This newly designed icon was created to appeal to a more extensive audience and to encourage greater participation in healthy eating in order to reduce the ever-increasing obesity rate in the U.S.

The new symbol consists of a circular plate accompanied by a smaller circle (representing a glass), found on the top right hand side of the plate. The plate is divided into 4 sections representing 4 food groups: (1) Vegetables (in green) make up the largest sector of the plate; (2) Fruits (in red); (3) Grains (in orange) made up of whole grains, refined grains and other carbohydrates; and (4) Proteins (in purple) consisting of meats, fish, poultry, eggs, beans, peas, nuts, and seeds. Together fruits and vegetables represent half of the plate. The fifth group (5) in the small blue circle is the dairy group, which may include a glass of fat-free or low-fat milk or a cup of yogurt.

The ChooseMyPlate icon can be seen in Figure 2.4a. The plate visual is easy to understand and includes fruit, vegetable, grains, and protein and dairy groups. Figure 2.5 identifies sample portion sizes for each of these food groups.

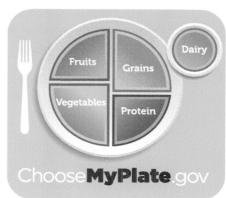

FIGURE 2.4A The USDA ChooseMyPlate icon

FIGURE 2.5 Sample portion sizes used in ChooseMyPlate Food Groups

Grains

What is the quantity needed of each item shown in the grains group to ultimately provide 1 ounce of grains?

In general, 1 slice of bread, 1 cup of ready-to-eat cereal, or ½ cup of cooked rice, cooked pasta, or cooked cereal can be considered a 1 ounce equivalent from the grains group.

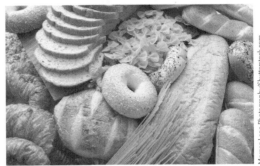

Morgan Lane Photography/Shutterstock.com

Dairy

What quantity of the items shown in the dairy group is needed to equal 1 cup of dairy product?

In general, 1 cup of milk or yogurt, 1½ ounces of natural cheese, or 2 ounces of processed cheese can be considered as 1 cup from the dairy group.

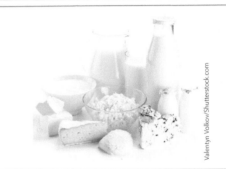

Valentyn Volkov/Shutterstock.com

Vegetables

What is the quantity of each vegetable needed to equal a cup of vegetables?

In general, 1 cup of raw or cooked vegetables or vegetable juice, or 2 cups of raw leafy greens can be considered as 1 cup from the vegetable group.

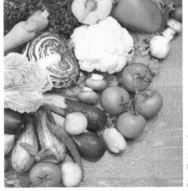

Taiga/Shutterstock.com

Proteins

What is the quantity needed of the foods in this food group to produce an ounce of protein?

In general, 1 ounce of meat, poultry or fish, ¼ cup cooked dry beans, 1 egg, 1 tablespoon of peanut butter, or ½ ounce of nuts or seeds can be considered as 1 ounce equivalent from the protein foods group.

Gabriela Duran/Shutterstock.com

Fruits

Which foods in the fruit group can provide the equivalent of 1 cup of fruit?

In general, 1 cup of fruit or 100% fruit juice, or ½ cup of dried fruit can be considered as 1 cup from the fruit group.

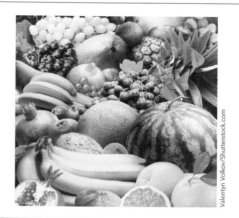

Valentyn Volkov/Shutterstock.com

Oils

How does one assess oil intake?

A teaspoon of oil is a serving. A person's allowance for oils depends on their age, sex, and level of physical activity.

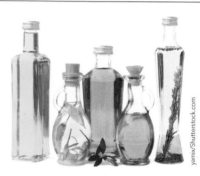

yamix/Shutterstock.com

Selected consumer messages focus on 3 key categories. The first category consists of balancing calories. This message encourages enjoying food but eating less and avoiding oversized portions. The second consumer message involves the foods to increase. Recommendations in this area include filling half your plate with fruits and vegetables, consuming half the prescribed quantity of grains in the form of whole grains and drinking fat-free or low-fat milk. The last consumer message deals with reducing certain nutrients. It encourages comparing food labels to identify lower sodium items and drink water in place of sugary drinks.

Information on ChooseMyPlate can be found at www.ChooseMyPlate.gov. This web-based interactive tool allows consumers to receive a personalized set of appropriate recommendations based on age, sex, and physical activity levels. Information and tips to help follow the recommendations are also provided.[21]

The development of the Healthy U.S.-Style Pattern is based on type and proportion of food Americans typically consume, but included are the more nutrient-dense forms and appropriate amounts. The pattern is designed to meet a person's nutrient needs yet not exceeding caloric requirements. The use of current food consumption data is used to determine the mix and proportions of foods to include in each group. The most current food composition data is also used to select a nutrient-dense sampling for each food.

The amounts of each food group (and subgroup) are adjusted when needed to meet nutrient and Dietary Guidelines standards while staying within the limits for calories and over-consumed dietary components. Standards for nutrient adequacy aim to meet the Recommended Dietary Allowances (RDA), which are designed to cover the needs of 97 percent of the population, and Adequate Intakes (AI), which are used when an average nutrient requirement cannot be determined. The Healthy US-Style Patterns meet these standards for most nutrients, exceptions being Vitamin D and E, potassium and choline. In most cases, an intake of these particular nutrients below the RDA or AI is not considered to be of public health concern.

The Healthy U.S.-Style Pattern includes 12 calorie levels to meet the needs of individuals across the lifespan. To follow this Pattern, first identify the appropriate calorie level, then choose a variety of foods in each group and subgroup in the recommended amounts, and, lastly, limit the choices that are not in nutrient-dense forms so that the overall calorie limit is not exceeded. The recommended amounts from each group for a 2000 calorie level can be found in Figure 2.6.[22]

TABLE 2.6 Samples of the Healthy Mediterranean-Style and Vegetarian Eating Patterns		
Food Group	Healthy Mediterranean-Style Eating Pattern	Healthy Vegetarian Eating Pattern
Vegetables	2½ c-eq/day	2½ c-eq/day
Dark green	1½ c-eq/week	1½ c-eq/week
Red and orange	5½ c-eq/week	5½ c-eq/week
Legumes (beans and peas)	1½ c-eq/week	3 c-eq/week[c]
Starchy	5 c-eq/week	5 c-eq/week
Other	4 c-eq/week	4 c-eq/week
Fruits	2½ c-eq/day	2 c-eq/day
Grains	6 oz-eq/day	6½ oz-eq/day
Whole grains	≥3 oz-eq/day	≥3½ oz-eq/day
Refined grains	≤3 oz-eq/day	≤3 oz-eq/day
Dairy	2 c-eq/day	3 c-eq/day
Protein Foods	6½ oz-eq/day	3½ oz-eq/day[c]
Seafood	15 oz-eq/week[d]	-
Meats, poultry, eggs	26 oz-eq/week	3 oz-eq/week (eggs)
Nuts, seeds, soy products	5 oz-eq/week	14 oz-eq/week
Oils	27 g/day	27 g/day
Limit on Calories for Other Uses (% of calories)	260 kcal/day (13%)	290 kcal/day (15%)

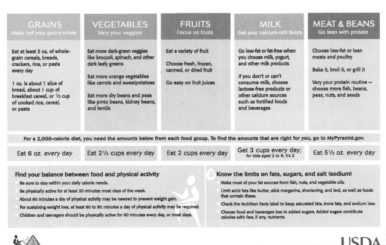

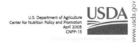

FIGURE 2.6 Sample 2000 Calorie Plan from ChooseMyPlate.gov

Cultural Adaptations to the Food Guide Pyramid

Cultural Adaptations may be made to the Food Guide Pyramid to reflect cultural and ethnic food choices. These can include influences such as Asian, Mexican, and Latino foods. One of the more popular adaptations to the Food Guide Pyramid is the **Mediterranean Pyramid.**

The Mediterranean region encompasses a large geographical area that includes the countries of Spain, Portugal, Southern France, Syria, Israel and many other nations as well. Although the cuisine in these regions varies, many characteristics in their composition are similar. Foods from this region are commonly low in saturated fats and high in monounsaturated fats, in particular their olive oil content. Dishes are low in meat and meat products, while high in fruits, vegetables, legumes, and grains (including bread). There is also moderate consumption of milk, milk products, and alcohol. Figure 2.7 explains how to follow the Mediterranean diet.

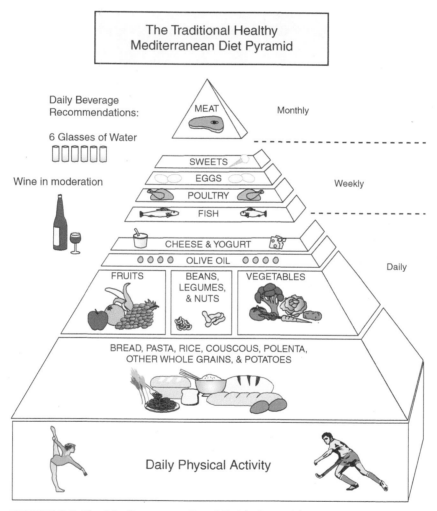

FIGURE 2.7 The Mediterranean Food Guide Pyramid

The Healthy Mediterranean-Style Pattern has been adapted from the Mediterranean Pyramid and the Healthy US-Style Pattern to better reflect dietary habits in the US and the health benefits associated with the Mediterranean Diet. The Healthy Mediterranean-Style Pattern contains more fruits and seafood and less dairy than does the Healthy U.S.-Style Pattern. The amounts of oils in the Pattern were not changed since the Healthy U.S.-Style Pattern already contains an amount that is similar to the amount associated with positive health outcomes, and are also higher than typical intakes in the United States. The amount of meat and poultry in the Healthy U.S.-Style Pattern are lower than the typical intake in the United States and yet similar to amounts associated with positive health outcomes. Nutrient content is comparable to the Healthy US-Style Pattern with the exception of calcium and vitamin D because of the lower dairy intake in the Healthy Mediterranean-Style pattern.

Another variation of the U.S. Food Guide Pyramid is the Vegetarian Pyramid, which assists vegetarians in obtaining a healthy, balanced diet. The sections of the pyramid include at the base; fruits and vegetables, whole grains, legumes and beans; in the middle nuts and seeds, eggs, soy milk and dairy, and plant oils; and at the top eggs and sweets. Dietary data from vegetarians across the world that enjoyed the lowest recorded rates of chronic diseases and the highest adult life expectancy show a pattern similar to the one illustrated in the list below:

1. Multiple daily servings of foods from fruits, vegetables, whole grains, legumes, and beans.
2. Daily servings from nuts, seeds, plant oils, soy milk, and dairy.
3. Occasional or small quantity servings from eggs and sweets.
4. Attention to consuming a variety of foods from all sections of the pyramid.
5. Daily consumption of enough water throughout the day to assure good health.
6. Regular physical activity at a level which promotes healthy weight, fitness, and well-being.
7. Reliance upon whole foods and minimally processed foods in preference to highly-processed foods.
8. Moderate regular intake of alcoholic beverages such as wine, beer, or spirits (optional).
9. Daily consumption of unrefined plant oils.
10. Dietary supplements as necessary, based upon factors such as age, sex, and lifestyle, with special attention to those avoiding dairy and/or eggs.

The Healthy Vegetarian Pattern is derived from the Healthy U.S.-Style Pattern, yet modifies the amount recommended from some of the food groups to more closely reflect eating patterns that have been reported by vegetarians in the National Health and Nutrition Examination Survey (NHANES). The development of the Healthy Vegetarian Pattern is therefore based on evidence of the foods and amounts consumed by vegetarians, with the addition of meeting the same nutrient and Dietary Guidelines standards as the Healthy U.S.-Style Pattern. Based on a comparison of the food choices of these vegetarians to non-vegetarians in NHANES, amounts of soy products (particularly tofu and other processed soy products), legumes, nuts and seeds, and whole grains were increased, and meat, poultry, and seafood were eliminated. Dairy and eggs were included because they were consumed by the majority of the vegetarians. To adjust the Pattern to be vegan all dairy choices would be comprised of fortified soy beverages, such as soymilk, or other plant-based dairy substitutes. The Pattern is similar in meeting nutrient standards to the Healthy U.S.-Style Pattern, but somewhat higher in calcium and fiber and lower in vitamin D due to differences in the foods included. Samples of the Healthy Mediterranean-Style and Vegetarian Eating Patterns can be seen in Table 2.6.[23,24,25]

Choose Your Foods: Food Lists for Diabetes

The Choose Your Foods system was designed by a committee made up of the American Diabetes Association and the Academy of Nutrition and Dietetics.[26] Initially designed to assist diabetics needing special diets, the system is based on the principles of good nutrition that apply to everyone. The Choose Your Foods Lists provide estimates of macronutrients (carbohydrate, protein, fat), for each food group. The six Choose Your Foods Lists are Milk, Starch, Fruit, Non-starchy vegetables, Proteins, and Fat. Food amounts that are listed are equal to one choice for that group. The selection of a variety of offerings that are both appealing and diverse can also be made to develop sample daily menus. The Choose Your Foods List menu planning system is used to plan meals for people requiring a nutritionally balanced diet and a specific number of calories. In practice, The Choose Your Foods Lists are used to plan meals for people needing to gain or to lose weight, for athletes who require a high calorie level and for people with diabetes. The Choose Your Foods Lists are found in Appendix B.

Go Ahead and Eat!

Eating is one of life's pleasures that need not be a rigorous exercise in decision-making. Food is meant to be enjoyed, a concept with which chefs are familiar. The wide array of nutritious foods available to consumers allows the choice of healthy foods that taste good. Chefs can have a major impact on the promotion of healthy menus by incorporating ingredients that have sensory qualities. By using health-conscious guides such as ChooseMyPlate, and by incorporating fresh ingredients to prepare healthy nutrient dense meals, chefs can make eating healthy a greater possibility than ever before!

Culinary Corner

Using the Mediterranean Pyramid for Menu Planning

Chefs can utilize a variety of Food Guide Pyramids from around the world when planning menus. A popular trend in today's restaurants is Mediterranean cuisine. Chefs may select the Mediterranean Pyramid as a guide in preparing exciting, healthy menus. Traditional Mediterranean diets are similar in many characteristics. Most are high in fruits and vegetables, and high in grains, potatoes, beans, nuts, and seeds. Olive oil is a primary fat that is included in the daily diet, while low to moderate amounts of dairy are recommended. Fish and poultry are consumed in low to moderate amounts, a few times per week, while the amount of red meat is limited to a few times a month. Eggs, sweets and wine should be consumed in moderate amounts. An abundance of fresh plant food and minimally processed food is also suggested. Physical activity also adds to the effectiveness of this diet.

The Mediterranean diet is higher in fat percentage than that recommended in the U.S. It is important to provide the proper information on the consumption of excess calories in any form to prevent over-consumption of calories leading to weight gain and potential obesity. Although the Mediterranean diet is higher in fat than the American diet, the type of fat is primarily in the form of olive oil, which has been proven to help in preventing and treating heart disease.[27] The merits of olive oil are discussed in greater detail in the Culinary Corner of Chapter 5. As long as the calories in the diet are controlled, the Mediterranean diet, although not low fat, may contribute to the prevention and treatment of obesity because of its variety and palatability. The traditional Mediterranean diet reflects dietary patterns found in olive growing areas of the Mediterranean region more than 30 years ago.[28] Table 2.7 offers sample menu items from a variety of countries that use the Mediterranean diet.[29]

TABLE 2.7 Sample Mediterranean Menu Items	
Egypt	Falafel (Broad Bean Patties)
Spain	Gazpacho (Cold tomato and vegetable soup)
Tunisia	Oumek Houria (Spicy hot carrots)
Greece	Horiatiki Salata (Greek salad)
Morocco	Tajine Dial Hout (Grouper stew)
France	Fougasse (Fruit Loaf)

(Continued)

Egypt	Koftit Ferakh (Chicken Meatballs)
Cyprus	Salata Pantzaria (Beetroot salad)
Yugoslavia	Rolada Od Spinata (Spinach Roll)
Italy	Risotto Nero (Black Rice)
Algeria	Chorba Loubia Marhiya (Cream of Haricot Bean soup)
Israel	Levivot (Potato Cakes)
Portugal	Carne De Parco Com Ameijoas (Pork with Clams)
Turkey	Paticalnli Pilav (Rice with Aubergines)

References

1   *Dietary Reference intakes for energy, carbohydrate, fiber, fat, fatty acids, cholesterol, protein, and amino acids.* A report of the Panel on Macronutrients, Subcommittees on Upper Reference Levels of Nutrients and Interpretation and Uses of Dietary Reference Intakes, and the Standing Committee on the Scientific Evaluation of Dietary Reference Intakes, National Academy of Sciences Institute of Medicine; 2002, 2005. http://www.iom.edu/Activities/Nutrition/SummaryDRIs/DRI-Tables.aspx

2   *Recommended Dietary Allowances: 10th Edition* (1989) Food and Nutrition Board, National Academy of Sciences-National Research Council, Washington, D.C.

3   Report of the WHO Meeting on Estimating Appropriate Levels of Vitamins and Minerals for Food Fortification Programs: The WHO Intake Monitoring, Assessment and Planning Program (IMAPP) Geneva, Switzerland, 22 July 2009. http://www.who.int/nutrition/en/

4   *Dietary Reference Intakes Series*, National Academy Press, Copyright 1997, 1998, 2000, 2001, 2005 by the National Academy of Sciences, National Academy Press, Washington, D.C.

5   Dietary Reference Intake Tables and Applications, National Academy of Sciences, 2011. http://www.iom.edu/Activities/Nutrition/SummaryDRIs/DRI-Tables.aspx

6   United States Department of Agriculture Press Release: USDA and HHS Announce New Dietary Guidelines to Help Americans Make Healthier Food Choices and Confront Obesity Epidemic, Office of Communications SW Washington, Jan. 31, 2011. oc.news@USDA.gov

7   http://health.gov/dietaryguidelines/2015/guidelines/

8   U.S. Department of Health and Human Services, *Healthy People 2010, 2nd Ed. With Understanding and Improving Health and Objectives for Improving Health,* 2 vols. Washington, DD: U. S., Government Printing Office, November 2000.

9   HHS Announces the Nation's New Health Promotion and Disease Prevention Agenda, *Healthy People 2020,* HHS News U.S. Department of Health and Human Services, December 2010. www.hhs.gov/news

10 *Healthy People 2020,* Nutrition and Weight Status Objectives, U.S. Department of Health and Human Services, December 2010. http://www.healthypeople.gov/2020/topicsobjectives2020/default.aspx

11 About the National Health and Nutrition Examination Survey (NHANES), http://www.cdc.gov/nchs/nhanes/about_nhanes.htm 11/2015

12 DB Haytowitz, "Information From USDA's Nutrient Data Bank," *Journal of Nutrition* 125 (1995): 1952–1955.

13 U.S. Food and Drug Administration, Center for Food Safety and Applied Nutrition, *How to Understand and Use the Nutrition Facts Label,* 2004. www.cfsan.fda.gov

14 http://www.fda.gov/Food/GuidanceRegulation/GuidanceDocumentsRegulatoryInformation/LabelingNutrition/ucm385663.htm

15 U.S. Food and Drug Administration, Center for Food Safety and Applied Nutrition, *Claims That Can be made for Conventional Foods and Dietary Supplements,* CFSAN/Office of Nutritional Products, Labeling, andDietarySupplements,2003. http://www.fda.gov/Food/LabelingNutrition/LabelClaims/ucm111447.htm

16 U.S. Food and Drug Administration Center for Food Safety and Applied Nutrition, *A Food Labeling Guide,* September 1994 (Editorial revisions June 1999 and November 2000, October 2009). http://www.fda.gov/Food/LabelingNutrition/default.htm

17   Food Allergies: What you need to know. http://www.fda.gov/food/resourcesforyou/consumers/ucm079311.htm

18   Spangler-Smith, Crystal et.al, "Are Organic Foods Safer or Healthier Than Conventional Alternatives? A Systematic Review", *Annals of Internal Medicine* 157 (2012): 348–366.

19   http://www.ams.usda.gov/AMSv1.0/nop

20   *MyPyramid, USDA's New Food Guidance System, 2005*, U.S. Department of Agriculture, Center for Nutrition Policy & Promotion. www.mypyramid.gov/professionals/index.html (Website modified February 2011)

21   ChooseMyPlate, USDA's New Food Guidance System, 2011. U.S. Department of Agriculture, Center for Nutrition Policy & Promotion. www.choosemyplate.gov

22   *http://health.gov/dietaryguidelines/2015/guidelines/appendix-3/*

23   *http://health.gov/dietaryguidelines/2015/guidelines/appendix-4/*

24   W. C. Willet et al. "Mediterranean Diet Pyramid: A Cultural Model of Healthy Eating," *American Journal of Clinical Nutrition* 61 (1995): 1329–1337.

25   http://oldwayspt.org/resources/health-studies?tid_1=1324&tid=All

26   *Wheeler, ML, et al., Choose Your Foods: Food Lists for Diabetes. American Diabetes Association and The Academy of Nutrition and Dietetics. 2014*

27   Ramon Estruch, MD, PhD. et.al,, "Primary Prevention of Cardiovascular Disease with a Medterranean Diet", *The New England Journal of Medicine* 368 (2013): 1279–1290.

28   2000 International Conference on The Mediterranean Diet. 2000 Consensus Statement Dietary Fat, The Mediterranean Diet and Lifelong Good Health, Royal College of Physicians, London England, January 13–14, 2000. http://www.chd-taskforce.com/2000consesusstament/index_e.htm

29   International Olive Oil Council, Mediterranean Cooking with Olive Oil, Iberica GraŁc,S.¨L., Madrid, Spain, 1996.

Put It into Practice

Define the Term

Review Figure 2.7, The Mediterranean Food Pyramid, The Culinary Corner "Using the Mediterranean Pyramid for Menu Planning" and Table 2.6, Sample Mediterranean Menu Items. Choose at least five menu items from the Table and place the main ingredients into the correct food group categories on the Mediterranean Diet Pyramid.

Myth vs. Fact

Determine if the following statement is a myth or fact and support your position with evidence from three research articles on the topic. *Statement: "Organic foods are more nutritious than conventional foods."*

   For each research article, summarize each component below.
   A. Abstract
   B. Methods
   C. Results
   D. Discussion
   E. Conclusion

The Menu

Using the "Choose Your Foods Lists for Meal Planning" in Appendix B, design a 1-day meal plan (including portion sizes) for the following:

Breakfast

   1 fruit choice
   1 meat choice
   1 milk choice
   2 starch choices
   2 fat choices

Lunch

   1 fruit choice
   2 meat choices
   2 vegetable choices
   2 starch choices
   2 fat choices

Dinner

   2 fruit choices
   4 meat choices
   2 vegetable choices
   1 milk choice
   3 starch choices
   2 fat choices

Website Review

Navigate the website for "Healthy People 2020" www.healthypeople.gov. Provide the mission, vision, and overarching goals for this initiative. Using Table 2.4 in the textbook, "Sample Nutrition Objectives" from Healthy People 2020, choose five objectives and list three specific steps for each that food professionals can take to help meet the objective. The steps must be measurable. Include the resources and the educational tools needed to achieve these objectives.

Build Your Career Toolbox

Review the textbook section entitled "Cultural Adaptations to the Food Guide Pyramid." A public health nutritionist is an expert in both food and nutrition. These professionals may work in health clinics, non-profit organizations, super markets or state health departments. They advise people in at risk communities about how they can better lead a healthy way of life.

Many public health nutritionists will give customized health information to individuals and specific groups. For instance, some nutritionists could teach patients in poor communities about high blood pressure, and how to prepare more healthy foods with less sodium. Other public health nutritionists could work with at risk communities with health problems about how to plan a diet for their families that has less sugar and fat.

Create a job description in the public health area for a Chef or a Registered Dietitian/Nutritionist for the following diverse cultures: Asian, Mexican, Latino and Mediterranean. Include cultural challenges, culinary experience, educational background and salary range for each.

Ally's Case Study

Ally is a 35-year-old mother of three who tries to make appropriate food choices while grocery shopping. She and her husband have a 14-year-old boy who plays football year round, a 12-year-old daughter who is a competitive gymnast, and a 2-year-old son who is still in diapers. Her husband works long hours and is a truck driver so he eats most of his meals on the road. Ally tries to prepare well-balanced meals for her family and her personal goal is to eat a healthy vegetarian diet due her my family history of heart disease and breast cancer. Ally needs help understanding the difference between marketing terms, FDA approved nutrient claims, health claims, and structure function claims.

When she enters the supermarket, she heads directly toward the produce department where it is pretty easy to make healthy choices. Unfortunately, her budget does not allow her to purchase all organic fruits and vegetables. She looks around and next to the bananas there is a sign that reads "Great Source of Potassium," so she purchases a big bunch of bananas. Near the tomatoes a placard states "Contains Antioxidants such as Lycopene," so in her cart they go. She chooses some leafy greens such as spinach and romaine lettuce, as well as some cucumbers and carrots. In the cold case, there are various flavored pomegranate juices with labels that announce that they are "Fat Free" and "Can Prevent Cancer." These juices are on sale so she decides to buy three large 32-oz bottles.

Ally also wants her family to consume more whole grains, so she makes her way to the pasta isle. She chooses spaghetti that has claims on the box stating: "Made with Natural Goodness," "Kid Approved," and "Doctor Recommended." These "buzz terms" lead her to believe that this product must be the best choice for my entire family. She chooses the low sodium spaghetti sauce because she reads on the label a claim that states "diets low in sodium may reduce the risk of high blood pressure." As she looks at the crackers, she notices that there is a brand that claims that their product is "A good source of fiber." Unfortunately, the label does not include the words whole wheat, but rather the words isolated fiber made from chicory root. The Nutrition Facts panel lists 3 g of fiber per serving, so she assumes that this must be a good choice.

Ally makes a few more food selections including cranberry juice and canned green beans. Both of these items have claims that state: "*Strengthen your immune system.*" She needs a snack for her 2-year old child, so she finds the perfect product: Fruit Juice Treats that contain "real fruit." The packaging is decorated with pictures of fresh oranges and pineapple even though the main ingredients are corn syrup, sugar, and white grape juice concentrate. Last on her list are dairy products such as cheese, milk, and yogurt. Milk is another perfect choice for the entire family because she reads that it is "High in calcium; 20% Daily Value," and "Calcium builds strong bones." Ally feels that her shopping trip is a success and she made good choices today.

Study Guide

Student Name _____ **Date** _____

Course Section _____ **Chapter** _____

TERMINOLOGY

Dietary Reference Intakes (DRI)_____	A. 10-35%
Scientific Method_____	B. A set of guidelines developed by the USDA to convert nutrients into general recommendations about foods that should be consumed and/or avoided
The dietary goal for carbohydrate recommended range for adults_____	
Mediterranean Food Pyramid_____	C. 20-35%
The dietary goal for protein recommended range for adults_____	D. An organized, systematic approach to conduct research. Consists of a series of steps to progressively solve a problem
Dietary Guidelines_____	E. A set of dietary standards determined jointly by American and Canadian scientists designed to meet the needs of healthy individuals
Healthy People 2020_____	F. A plan developed to establish healthy objectives for the nation
Food Label_____	G. A tool used to assist the public and health professionals in choosing nutrients to include or avoid in their diet
The dietary goal for fat recommended range for adults_____	H. 45-65%
	I. A food guide plan which reflects the food intakes in Spain, Portugal, Southern France, Syria and Israel

Student Name _____   Date _____

Course Section _____   Chapter _____

"FOOD CHOICE" MENU PLANNING

Use Appendix B "Choose Your Foods Lists for Meal Planning"

1. **Identify which Food Choice the following foods belong in:**

   White bread: _____

   Chicken breast: _____

   Mayonnaise: _____

   Grapes: _____

   Corn: _____

   Almonds: _____

   Carrots: _____

2. **How many choices do the following foods contain?**

   1 cup pasta: _____

   8oz orange juice: _____

   3oz salmon: _____

3. **Fill in food choices that the following meal represents (place an "X" in the appropriate box, and indicate the number of choices).**

Food	Starch	#	Fruit	#	Veg	#	Milk	#	Protein	#	Fat	#
1 cup rice and 4 tsp butter												
4oz grilled flank steak												
2 cups mixed raw greens with 2 tsp olive oil												
3 slices Italian bread (1oz each)												

Student Name _____   Date _____

Course Section _____   Chapter _____

CASE STUDY DISCUSSION

Ally's Case Study: Claims on a Food Label

Review the section in Chapter 2: Claims on a label including health claims, nutrition content claims, and structure/function claims. After reviewing the case study, use this information to answer the following:

1. **Explain and provide an example of a Health Claim.**

2. **Explain and provide an example of a Nutrient claim.**

3. **Explain and provide an example of a Structure/ Function claim.**

4. **Describe each claim that Ally finds while shopping and determine if each is an approved health claim, nutrient content claim, a structure/function claim or a marketing term.**

Student Name _____   Date _____

Course Section _____   Chapter _____

PRACTICE TEST

Select the best answer.

1. The Dietary Goal for adults for protein intake is
   a. 10-15%
   b. 10-25%
   c. 10-35%
   d. 10-45%

2. The Dietary Goal for adults for fat intake is
   a. 0-10%
   b. 10-15%
   c. 15-30%
   d. 20-35%

3. The Dietary Goal for adults for carbohydrate intake is
   a. 0-10%
   b. 30-55%
   c. 45-66%
   d. 50-60%

4. The RDA
   a. is set at levels that exceed requirements for most individuals
   b. meets the needs of individuals with special nutritional needs
   c. is set by the USDA
   d. is not a useful tool

5. The Dietary Guidelines
   a. were developed by the FDA
   b. translate specific nutrient values into general recommendations
   c. can increase the risk of chronic disease
   d. are used only by manufacturers on food labels

Student Name _____   Date _____

Course Section _____   Chapter _____

TRUE OR FALSE

_____ The DRIs outline the dietary nutrient intakes for healthy individuals in the U.S. and Canada.

_____ UL represents tolerable upper intake level.

_____ The Mediterranean Diet contains a higher level of animal products than the American diet.

_____ Food Composition Tables can be used by chefs to analyze menu recipes.

_____ Dietary Standards are based on age, gender and growth stages

1. Other than the shape, provide 3 ways the Mediterranean Food Guide Pyramid differs from the USDA ChooseMyPlate.

2. List 3 benefits derived from the Mediterranean Diet to help in the reduction of heart disease.

Carbohydrates

3

KEY TERMS

Amylopectin	Complex carbohydrates	Fructose
Amylose	Diabetes	Galactose
Carbohydrate	Disaccharide	Glucagon
Carbohydrate loading	Fasting hypoglycemia	Gluconeogenesis
Celiac disease	Fiber	Glucose

Introduction

Carbohydrates are the body's preferred fuels for energy. They are organic nutrients that consist of the elements carbon, hydrogen, and oxygen. Plants capture the energy from the sun and, through the process of photosynthesis, form carbohydrates. Although most carbohydrates are derivedfrom plants, dairy products do provide animal-derived forms of carbohydrates. The common abbreviation for a carbohydrate is CHO (an acronym formed from the first letter of each of its elements). Carbohydrates, particularly in the form of whole grains, are universally recommended as part of a healthful diet. Despite the knowledge and scientific findings about whole grains as essential components of the diet, surveys reveal that Americans eat far less than the recommended amount, averaging a mere one or fewer servings per day.[1]

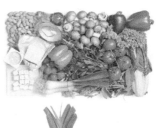
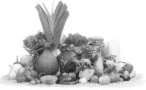
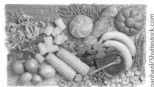

Healthy choices of carbohydrates include grains, vegetables, and fruits.

Healthy food sources of carbohydrates include fruits, vegetables, and grains. Additional sources are found in dairy products and legumes. Carbohydrates that provide little nutritive value, or empty calories, come from such sources as candy, soda, fruit drinks, and nutritive sweeteners. A government survey shows that only 50% of Americans consume the recommended number of servings for vegetables and a mere 22% choose the daily recommended number of fruit servings. Ninety percent meet the daily recommendations for grain servings.[2] A more recent survey showed that Americans are consuming an average of 6.7 ounces of grain per day, or 106% of the recommendation. Despite the fact that Americans are consuming the majority of the grains they need, the source is from refined products.[3]

The consumption and offerings of empty-calorie carbohydrate foods such as table sugar and high-fructose corn syrup have risen dramatically in the past decade. A considerable increase in the consumption of sweetened soft drinks such as soda, sports drinks, and fruit drinks contribute to this growth. On average an individual in the United States consumes about 64 pounds of sugar each year.[4] Assuming that each ounce of a sweetened beverage has approximately 1 teaspoon of sugar, an estimated 90 pounds of sugar is consumed per person per year by drinking 24 ounces of a sweetened beverage (such as soda) daily! The restaurant business contributes considerably to this figure. Soft drink sizes usually range from 20–48 ounces each, which is the equivalent of 1/3 to 1 cup of sugar. Chefs can promote moderation in the intake of sugars by encouraging alternative beverage

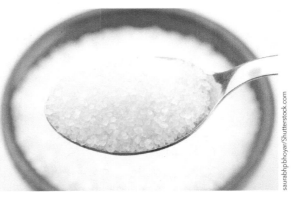

An estimated 64 pounds of sugar is consumed per person every year.

choices such as vegetable and fruit juices, flavored waters, and sparkling waters. The types, functions, and sources of the various types of carbohydrates are discussed next.

Types of Carbohydrates

Carbohydrates can be classified into two general categories. The first category is that of the **simple sugars** comprised of **monosaccharides** and **disaccharides**. The second category consists of the **polysaccharides** (commonly referred to as **complex carbohydrates**). There are three general types of polysaccharides: **starch**, **glycogen**, and **fiber**. A fourth type of carbohydrate known as **sugar alcohols** is a close relative of the polysaccharides. Carbohydrates contain approximately 4 calories per gram. Sugar alcohols range from approximately 1–3 calories per gram. The type of carbohydrate consumed and the meal composition determine the rate at which it is used by the body for energy.

Simple Sugars: Monosaccharides

Simple sugars are easily digested and absorbed by the body, and are quickly used as energy. Six sugars are classified as simple sugars. Three of these are made of one molecule and are called monosaccharides (prefix mono = 1, saccharide = sugar). (Figure 3.1) These are the simplest of all carbohydrates and require little or no digestion. They can be directly absorbed by the absorbed into the intestine and transported into the blood. The first monosaccharide is **glucose**, a sugar that is used by both plants and animals for quick energy. This sugar is made by photosynthesis in plants, and is commonly known as blood sugar in animals. Glucose circulates in our blood to provide needed energy to the cells.

The second single sugar unit is called **fructose**, derived from the prefix "fruct" meaning fruit, and the suffix "ose," meaning sugar. The major sources of fructose (a sugar with a very intense sweetness) are fruits and honey. Although fructose and glucose are the most common monosaccharides, there is a third monosaccharide, **galactose**, which is found in milk. It occurs only in combination with another molecule of glucose.

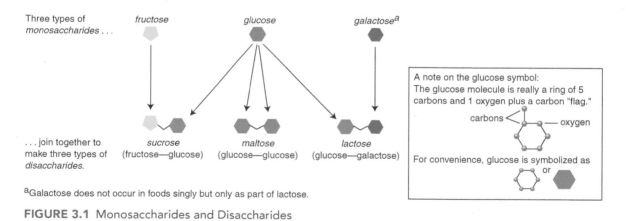

FIGURE 3.1 Monosaccharides and Disaccharides

Simple Sugars: Disaccharides

Disaccharides comprise the three remaining simple sugars that consist of two molecules. Unlike monosaccharides, they require a small amount of digestion before they are absorbed into the blood, and then the body quickly uses them for energy. The disaccharide **sucrose** is formed when a molecule of glucose and a molecule of fructose are combined. (See Figure 3.1) Common "table sugar," is made up of sucrose. **Maltose**, more commonly referred to as "malt sugar," is another disaccharide. Maltose consists of two molecules of glucose. It is formed when starch is broken down, as in germinating seeds, and during the digestion of starch in the intestine. The last disaccharide is **lactose**. Lactose is made up of one molecule of glucose and one molecule of galactose. It is referred to as "milk sugar." A person who is lactose intolerant has difficulty digesting the lactose sugar that is found in milk. Lactose intolerance varies in individuals.

Some people are able to tolerate small amounts of milk, while others cannot have any milk products whatsoever without symptoms of bloating, cramping, gas, and diarrhea. Treatment of lactose intolerance includes consuming lactase enzyme supplements or lactose-reduced products, or simply avoiding lactose-containing products.[5] Dairy products are the major source of Vitamin D and calcium in the US diet. If these are avoided, supplements may be necessary.

Complex Carbohydrates: Polysaccharides

Long chains of glucose molecules are called *polysaccharides*, or complex carbohydrates. The prefix "poly" means many, and saccharides refer to sugars. These carbohydrates also provide energy to the body, however at a slower rate than the simple sugars, as they require increased digestion before they are absorbed into the blood. Complex carbohydrates provide more long-term energy and are popular in the diet of athletes. Chefs who prepare meals for athletes include whole grains (in the forms of rice, pasta, and bread), potatoes, and vegetables, to supply complex carbohydrates. These foods are often central to the diets of athletes who are in training or in competition. There are three basic types of polysaccharides: starch, glycogen, and fiber.

Polysaccharides: Starch

Starch consists of long strands of glucose that are found in plants. Plants store their glucose for future energy in their granules and seeds, and use it to provide energy for the growth of new plants. Humans consume plant starch for energy by digesting long strands of glucose and breaking them down into individual units. There are two types of starches found in plants: **amylose** and **amylopectin**. Amylose consists of straight chains of glucose molecules and has gel-like properties. A large amount of this starch is found in corn. Amylopectin, on the other hand, is made of branched chains of glucose, and has a waxy, maize consistency. Arrowroot and tapioca contain large quantities of this starch. (See Figure 3.2) Every plant species has a distinct proportion of amylose and amylopectin that determines the nature of the starch.

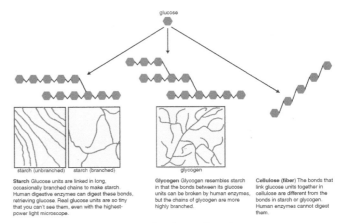

Starch Glucose units are linked in long, occasionally branched chains to make starch. Human digestive enzymes can digest these bonds, retrieving glucose. Real glucose units are so tiny that you can't see them, even with the highest-power light microscope.

Glycogen Glycogen resembles starch in that the bonds between its glucose units can be broken by human enzymes, but the chains of glycogen are more highly branched.

Cellulose (fiber) The bonds that link glucose units together in cellulose are different from the bonds in starch or glycogen. Human enzymes cannot digest them.

FIGURE 3.2 Formation of Polysaccharides

Chefs use starch as a thickening agent. It is actually the swelling and gelling of starch when heated that causes the thickening properties of a roux. Fat is used to separate the granules so that they do not clump. Slurry is made from an equal mixture of liquid, such as water, and a starch, such as cornstarch, flour, or arrowroot. Food starch in commercial food products is modified to retain thickening properties that are lost in ordinary starch after cooling and storage. Puddings, gravies, soups, and salad dressings often contain modified food starch. Modified food starch can be used in lieu of oil, for example, to reduce the fat content in prepared foods, such as low-fat salad dressings.

Polysaccharides: Glycogen

Humans and animals store carbohydrates in the form of glycogen. Glycogen is not consumed directly from foods. When glucose obtained from foods is stored in the body, it is called glycogen. Glycogen consists of branch chains of glucose molecules similar to those found in plant starch. Glycogen is the body's most readily available source of energy, and can quickly be broken down to glucose. Approximately three-fourths of a pound of glycogen is usually stored in the muscles and liver. The amount of glycogen stored can be altered through diet. Endurance athletes, who engage in **carbohydrate loading**, first deplete the body's glycogen stores by routine training exercise and a low-carbohydrate diet. A high-carbohydrate diet is then consumed to improve glycogen storage and to increase athletic endurance.[6] Some studies show that even without a glycogen-depleting period of exercise and diet, athletes can store maximum amounts of muscle glycogen when consuming a high carbohydrate diet for one day and abstaining from physical activity.[7] Chefs who specialize in the area of sports nutrition must develop menu plans that are both appealing and specific to the needs of athletes.

Polysaccharides: Fiber

Plant fiber (leaves, stems, skins, and seeds) provides the plant's structure and consists mainly of long chains of sugars or polysaccharides. Humans cannot digest plant fiber as they lack the specific enzymes needed to hydrolyze these carbohydrates. Fiber passes through the digestive tract without providing energy. Foods containing fiber do have positive health effects that include a delay in the absorption of cholesterol, the binding of bile for excretion, the stimulation of bacterial fermentation in the colon, and the increase of stool weight. Terms regarding the definition and classification of fiber are found in the Dietary Reference Intakes.[8] Three definitions concerning nondigestible carbohydrates in the food supply follow:

1. Dietary fiber refers to the nondigestible carbohydrates and lignin found in plants.

2. Functional fiber refers to the isolated nondigestible carbohydrates that have beneficial physiological effects in humans.

3. Total fiber is the sum of dietary fiber and functional fiber.

Fiber can also be classified by its water solubility. Certain plant fiber is soluble in water (water-soluble fiber), while other plant fiber is not soluble in water (water-insoluble fiber). Each category of fiber has potential positive effects on health as outlined in Table 3.1. In addition to these benefits, a fiber-rich meal is processed more slowly and promotes satiety that may be helpful in treating and preventing obesity. A diet that is rich in fiber is also rich in micronutrients and nonnutritive ingredients that may contribute positively to one's health. Table 3.1 provides an explanation of water-soluble and water-insoluble fiber.[9] Table 3.2 supplies examples of the types of carbohydrates, their composition, special issues involved, and foods in which they are found.

TABLE 3.1 Water-Soluble and Water-Insoluble Fibers

Types	Food Sources	Potential Health Effects
Soluble		
Gums, mucilages, pectins	Barley, fruits, legumes, oats, vegetables	May lower blood cholesterol (LDL) and slow glucose absorption.
Insoluble		
Cellulose, lignin	Legumes, vegetables, seeds, whole grains	Regulate bowel movements. Increase fecal weight and reduce transit time of fecal passage through the colon. May reduce the risk of diverticular disease.

TABLE 3.2 Types of Carbohydrates, their Composition, Examples, Special Issues, and Sources

Name/Type	Composition	Examples	Special Issues	Sources
Monosaccharides	1 sugar unit	Glucose Fructose Galactose	Rarely found separate from their companion molecules except for fructose	Apples (fructose) Pears (fructose) Honey (fructose)

(Continued)

TABLE 3.2 Types of Carbohydrates, their Composition, Examples, Special Issues, and Sources (Continued)

Name/Type	Composition	Examples	Special Issues	Sources
Disaccharides	2 linked sugar units	Sucrose (50% glucose, 50% fructose) Lactose (50% galactose, 50% glucose) Maltose (100% glucose-glucose bond) High fructose corn syrup (HFCS) (generally 55% fructose–sometimes 42% fructose–varies)	Occurs naturally in foods (sucrose, lactose) Produced by starch digestion (maltose) Hydrolysis of corn (High-Fructose Corn Syrup)	Fruit Milk Vegetables
Oligosaccharides (OS)	3–10 linked sugar units	Raffinose Stachyose	May cause intestinal gas	Dry beans and peas Onions Breast milk Added to food as inulin and other OS
STARCHES				
Polysaccharides	Many linked glucose units	Starch Glycogen–animal starch	Most are broken down to glucose for absorption	Starchy vegetables Grains Dry beans and peas Nuts and seeds
Resistant Starch (Resistant starch does undergo digestion in the small intestine)				Dry beans, peas, pasta Refrigerated cooked potatoes
FIBERS				
Polysaccharides/ Lignin	Many linked sugar units	Dietary Fiber, i.e., nondigestible carbohydrates and lignin that are intrinsic and intact in plants Functional Fiber, i.e., isolated nondigestible carbohydrates that have beneficial physiological effects in human beings Total Fiber = Dietary Fiber + Functional Fiber	Different chemical bonding; human enzymes cannot break bonds; pass relatively intact through upper digestive tract Can be fermented by colonic microflora to gases and short-chain fatty acids	Vegetables Fruits Whole grains Dry beans and peas Nuts and seeds

Carbohydrate Requirements

Glucose from carbohydrate is the preferred energy source for the body and most of its functions. Proteins and fats can be broken down and converted to fuel by the body but are not as efficient in their metabolism as are carbohydrates. A good rule of thumb is that vegetables, fruits, and starches should make up one-half of an individual's total diet. Chefs do not usually follow this recommendation, serving a meal consisting of three-fourths protein and fat with small amounts of starch and vegetables as an accompaniment.

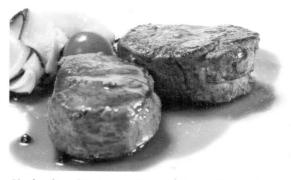

Chefs often fill plates with protein and fat with small amounts of starch and/or vegetables.

The Dietary Reference Intakes recommendations of The Institute of Medicine (IOM, 2002) established a minimum Recommended Dietary Allowance for carbohydrates of 130 grams per day for adults and children 1 year of age and older. This amount is required to provide the brain with an adequate supply of glucose. The acceptable macronutrient distribution range (AMDR) for carbohydrate is 45%–65% of total calories. A caloric intake of 2000 kcal per day that provides 50% of calories as carbohydrate, would be equal to 1000 kcal from carbohydrates, and would yield 250 grams of carbohydrate. This intake is well above the RDA requirement for brain function.

As a result of the increasing evidence on the negative effects of the consumption of excessive "added sugars", the 2015-2020 Dietary Guidelines for Americans has recommended reducing the consumption of added sugars to 10% or less of total calories. People with diets that are at or above this recommendation have been found to have poorer intakes of essential nutrients.[10] The basic definition of "added sugars" is sugars and syrups that are added to foods or beverages when they are processed or prepared. The naturally occurring sugars which include those found in milk and fruits are not included in this group. Regular soft drinks, energy drinks and sports drinks are some of the major sources of added sugars for Americans. In addition the following foods also contribute to added sugars intake: candy, cakes, cookies, pies, pastries and donuts, fruit drinks, and dairy desserts.[11]

The IOM set an Adequate Intake in its 2002 report of 14 grams of fiber per 1000 kcal consumed. The IOM's fiber recommendations are highest for populations who consume the most calories (mainly young males). Women and the elderly, consequently, have lower recommendations. Table 3.3 outlines the acceptable carbohydrate distribution ranges.[12]

TABLE 3.3 Acceptable Carbohydrate Distribution Ranges
Acceptable Total Carbohydrate Intake
▪ 45%–65% of total Calories
Acceptable Fiber Intake
▪ 14 grams per 1000 kcal of Intake

Carbohydrate Digestion

All carbohydrates must be broken down into monosaccharides by the digestive system to be absorbed by the small intestine. The digestion of starch, a polysaccharide, begins in the mouth with the help of an enzyme, salivary amylase, found in saliva that splits the molecule into smaller units. Carbohydrate digestion temporarily ceases in the stomach due to the presence of hydrochloric acid. Once the material enters the small intestine, carbohydrates are broken down to disaccharides by carbohydrate enzymes from the pancreas. Final digestion to the monosaccharides occurs in the mucosal lining of the small intestine. The polysaccharide fiber is not broken down by human enzymes, but rather by bacteria in the lower section of the digestive tract that allows it to be absorbed in very small amounts for energy. Since the amounts are insignificant, fiber is not considered to provide the body with energy value. Fiber does play an important function in the digestion and in the elimination of wastes and in the promotion of growth of helpful colonic bacteria. Monosaccharides do not require digestion and can be directly absorbed by the small intestine and also through the mucosal lining of the mouth. All monosaccharides are transported into the blood and brought to the liver for metabolism.

Carbohydrate Metabolism: How the Body Uses Glucose

Once carbohydrates are broken down and absorbed as glucose, fructose, and galactose, they travel through the blood to the liver. The liver converts fructose and galactose to glucose, which is then transported by the blood to the cells, or converted to other products such as fats. The liver can also convert glucose to a storage form called glycogen. Glycogen can be stored in the liver or may be sent to the muscles for later use. When needed, glycogen can be converted into glucose and sent to the blood. Glucose must then enter the cell to be transformed into energy. For this to occur, the pancreas must secrete the hormones **insulin** and **glucagon** which assist in glucose metabolism.

Glucose is converted to pyruvate releasing initial ATP (adenosine triphosphate) through an anaerobic process. ATP then enters the Krebs Cycle for aerobic respiration to produce additional ATP that is used as an energy source for the body. Further discussion of this process is found in chapter 8.

The Role of Insulin

When glucose levels rise in the blood, a message is sent to the pancreas to release the hormone insulin. Insulin signals the body's cells to take up the glucose, which is converted in the cell to energy for the body. Excess glucose that is not used for energy is stored as glycogen or as fat. The liver stores about one-third of the glycogen, and the remaining two-thirds is retained by the muscles.

The Role of Glucagon

The body must always have an adequate supply of glucose in the blood to feed the cells. When glucose levels drop, the pancreas produces the hormone glucagon, which stimulates the liver to break down glycogen into glucose. Glucose can then be sent to the blood so that blood sugar levels can return to normal. Hormones that promote the conversion of protein to glucose are also released. If inadequate levels of glucose are released from glycogen, glucose can be made from noncarbohydrate sources such as protein. This process is called **gluconeogenesis** and may occur when an individual is fasting or has high energy expenditure. When a sufficient amount of carbohydrates are consumed to store adequate glycogen, the body need not convert significant amounts of protein to glucose for energy. This optimal situation is termed **protein sparing**. When there are adequate carbohydrates in the diet, fats can also be broken down into glucose and contribute to energy. These reserve energy sources are more difficult to metabolize than other nutrients. During prolonged fasting or when certain diseases are present, fats may be improperly broken down for energy into compounds called **ketone** bodies that are used by the heart and muscle tissues. The brain, however, must continue to rely on glucose.

The Glycemic Index

When discussing carbohydrates, a measure of carbohydrate metabolism should be examined. Certain carbohydrates are said to increase blood glucose and insulin levels faster than others. **Glycemic index** is the ranking of how carbohydrate foods affect blood sugar levels and elicits an insulin response relative to the consumption of pure glucose. Foods that have a low glycemic index include basmati rice, bran cereals, lentils, and milk. White bread, white rice, mashed potatoes, and sugar-sweetened soft drinks have a high glycemic index. When there is disruption in the production or utilization of the hormones that help regulate glucose metabolism, abnormal glucose metabolism may result.

Glycemic Load

Both the quality and quantity of carbohydrates determine an individual's glycemic response to food. Glycemic Index (GI) compares equal quantities of available carbohydrate in a food to the carbohydrates found in white bread or glucose to provide a measure of carbohydrate quality. The Glycemic Load (GL) is evaluated by taking the food's GI and its total available carbohydrate content: GL = [GI × carbohydrate (g)]/100, which further allows for a measure of the glycemic impact of a typical serving of food. Foods with a GL value equal or less than 10 are low GL foods, while those with a GL value that is equal or greater than 20 are considered high. Increases in GL show increases in postprandial blood glucose and/or insulin levels. Low GL can result from high carbohydrate/low GI foods or from low carbohydrate/high GI foods. It is always best to compare the GI of Foods of similar composition within a food group.[13]

Health Issues Related to Carbohydrate Digestion and Metabolism

If the body is not able to effectively handle carbohydrates, health consequences may occur. Too much sugar in the blood, known as hyperglycemia, is a cause for concern because it may indicate diabetes. Hypoglycemia, a condition that occurs when the blood sugar is too low, may also be dangerous.

Diabetes

Diabetes is a chronic disease of abnormal carbohydrate metabolism. It is technically called diabetes mellitus (DM) and is characterized by elevated blood glucose levels and inadequate or ineffective insulin production or action. Diabetes and uncontrolled blood glucose levels can lead to other serious diseases and complications such as amputations, blindness, heart disease, kidney disease, and premature death. A discussion of the various types of diabetes follows.

Type 1 Diabetes

Type 1 diabetes previously called Insulin Dependent Diabetes Mellitus (IDDM), is the more severe form of diabetes. It is the least common form of the two types and accounts for approximately 10%–20% of all cases. This type of diabetes typically occurs during childhood or young adulthood. Type 1 diabetes attacks certain cells in the pancreas that are responsible for producing insulin. Blood-glucose levels remain elevated after a meal (hyperglycemia) because glucose is unable to reach the cells where it is needed.

Genetics, viral infections and other diseases, toxins, and immune disorders may all contribute to type 1 diabetes. Individuals with type 1 diabetes must receive insulin, typically by injections or via an insulin pump, for the cells to use the glucose. Insulin that is ingested is digested as protein and cannot reach the blood. Newer methods such as inhalers and nasal sprays that deliver insulin are now being researched. A list of some of the initial warning signs of diabetes is found in Table 3.4.

TABLE 3.4 Potential Warning Signs of Diabetes (These signs are frequently seen in type 1 diabetes and occur in the later stages in type 2 diabetes.)
Abnormally high glucose in the blood
Constant hunger
Drowsiness, fatigue, irritability

(Continued)

TABLE 3.4 Potential Warning Signs of Diabetes (These signs are frequently seen in type 1 diabetes and occur in the later stages in type 2 diabetes.) (*Continued*)

Dry skin, itchiness
Excessive urination and thirst
Frequent infections, particularly of the skin, gums, and urinary tract
Glucose in the urine
Pain in the legs, feet, and/or fingers
Poor healing of cuts and bruises
Visual disturbances, blurred vision
Unexplained weight loss

Treatment of type 1 diabetes focuses on three main areas: insulin delivery, diet, and physical activity. Diet focuses on controlling the type and the amount of carbohydrates consumed, providing adequate protein, moderating fat intake, and consumption of a variety of nutritious foods. The typical range of calories for each of the nutrients is as follows: carbohydrates 45%–60%, proteins 10%–20%, and fats 20%–40% (10% or less from saturated, less than 300 mg cholesterol/day). The exchange lists for meal planning were discussed in Chapter 2 and are found in Appendix B. These are helpful in planning meals for persons with diabetes. In type 1 diabetes, insulin must be given multiple times daily. A system of meal planning where the amount of insulin administered is matched with the amount of CHO consumed is most often used in type 1 diabetes. This system is known as CHO Counting. Exercise also helps to lower blood sugar and is believed to improve cell receptiveness to insulin. People with Type 1 diabetes are best treated when their healthcare teams include physicians, diabetes nurses, educators, and dietitians who provide them with the necessary tools to control the disease and prevent complications.[14]

Type 2 Diabetes

Type 2 diabetes is the more common form of diabetes and accounts for approximately 80%–90% of all cases. Known previously as Non-Insulin Dependent Diabetes Mellitus (NIDDM), or adult-onset diabetes, it is associated with the resistance of the body's cells to insulin. Type 2 diabetes is characterized by high levels of glucose as well as high levels of insulin. When glucose approaches the entry points to the cells the cells respond with less sensitivity (insulin resistance) than normal. People who are obese appear to have a higher risk for insulin resistance and a greater susceptibility for type 2 diabetes. Until recently, type 2 diabetes was viewed as a disease of older adults. With an increasing rate of obesity among children, type 2 diabetes is no longer restricted to an older population. Figure 3.3 shows this alarming diabetes/obesity trend.

Individuals who have insulin resistance and are obese, especially those with abdominal adiposity, have a risk for metabolic syndrome. Metabolic syndrome is the name for a group of risk factors that occur

OBESITY

Overeating → Enlarged Fat Cells

Increased Appetite → Insulin Resistance

TYPE 2 DIABETES

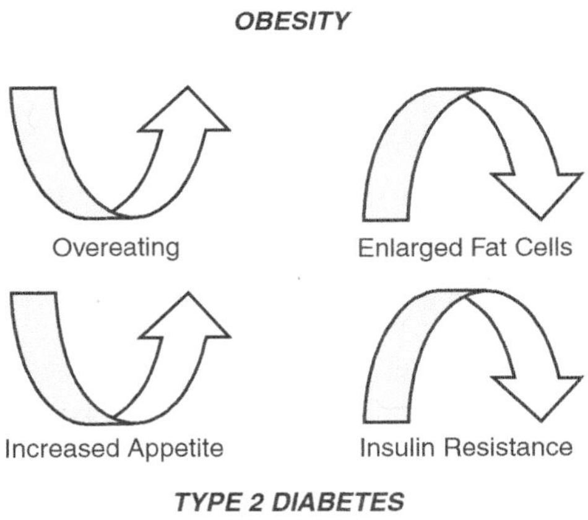

FIGURE 3.3 Type 2 Diabetes/ Obesity Trend

together and increase the risk for type 2 diabetes, coronary artery disease, and stroke. The diagnosis of metabolic syndrome includes elevated blood pressure, elevated blood glucose levels, and elevated blood cholesterol and triglyceride levels. Recent studies have shown that interactions between genetic and environmental factors promote the progression of Type 2 DM and Metabolic Syndrome. There are many important environmental factors that modulate expression of genes that are involved in these metabolic pathways but it appears nutrition may be the most important. One example of a diet that may have potential to modify the genetic predisposition of these conditions is consumption of foods that are rich in monounsaturated fatty acids and low in saturated fatty acids. This would suggest that the incorporation of nutrigenetics in personalized nutrition counseling for Type 2 DM and Metabolic Syndrome will have the potential to change diet-related disease prevention and therapy.[15]

A recent meta-analysis reviewed the consumption of sugar-sweetened beverages (SSBs) and their connection to weight gain, the risk of being overweight and obesity, and the development of related chronic metabolic diseases such as metabolic syndrome and type 2 diabetes. Sugar-sweetened beverages include soft drinks, fruit drinks, iced tea, and energy and vitamin drinks. It is believed that SSBs lead to weight gain due to their high added sugar content, low satiety value, and lack of reduction in energy intake after consumption at subsequent meals. The relationship of consumption of SSBs to metabolic syndrome and type 2 diabetes is thought to cause weight gain because of the high levels of rapidly-absorbable carbohydrates in the form of added sugars, which are used to flavor these beverages. It is believed that limiting the consumption of these beverages, and replacing them with healthy alternatives such as water will help to reduce obesity-related chronic disease risk.[16]

As with type 1 diabetes, type 2 diabetes treatment involves dietary considerations as well as physical activity. Weight reduction is encouraged for overweight individuals because any decrease in weight may help control blood-sugar levels and improve insulin resistance. Medications that lower blood-sugar levels may also be prescribed to improve the tissue's ability to take up glucose, or to stimulate the pancreas to produce more insulin. If blood-sugar levels cannot be controlled with diet, exercise, and/or medication, people with type 2 diabetes may require insulin treatment. In younger individuals the management of type 2 diabetes may present several challenges. A focus on both the family and the individual's lifestyle is needed for successful treatment.[17]

A third type of diabetes occurs during pregnancy and is called gestational diabetes. This form of diabetes occurs in approximately 3%–8% of all pregnancies and is characterized by abnormally high blood sugar, caused by the stress of pregnancy. The condition is closely monitored during pregnancy to prevent any complications for both the mother and baby. Gestational diabetes is known to increase the risk for developing type 2 diabetes. Recent studies suggest that up to 50% of women with gestational diabetes may develop type 2 diabetes over 20–30 years. Women who experience gestational diabetes should be monitored so that early lifestyle changes can be implemented.[18]

Hypoglycemia: Fasting vs. Postprandial

Hypoglycemia refers to abnormally low fasting blood glucose. The postprandial form of hypoglycemia is a medical condition of abnormally low blood glucose levels after the consumption of a meal. Some of the symptoms include fatigue, dizziness, irritability, a rapid heart rate, anxiety, sweating, trembling, hunger, and headaches. Postprandial hypoglycemia is diagnosed by a specific blood test, as similar symptoms can be associated with other conditions and diseases as well. Another type of hypoglycemia is termed fasting hypoglycemia and is often the result of another illness such as cancer of the pancreas or liver. In this form of hypoglycemia blood-sugar levels remain dangerously low after 8 to 14 hours of fasting. In addition to medical treatment, a diet that consists of frequent, balanced, small protein containing meals, and the avoidance of concentrated sweets and alcohol is recommended.

Celiac Disease

Another disorder involving carbohydrates is celiac disease. Celiac disease is a disorder of the gastrointestinal tract that is characterized by inflammation and injury of the mucosal lining of the small intestine. The incidence of celiac disease is on the rise, possibly due to improvements in diagnostic techniques. Inflammation is caused by insensitivity to gluten, a protein found in wheat, rye, and barley. The inflammatory reaction causes the flattening of the villi in the small intestines, which increases the risk of malabsorption of both micronutrients and macronutrients. Initial symptoms of celiac disease are typically gastrointestinal in nature, for example, abdominal pain, bloating, alternating constipation with diarrhea, and anorexia. Additional long-term problems may include anemia, fatigue, neuropathy, and weight loss. The risk of celiac disease increases by 10%–20% when another family member also has the disease. It is typically more common in individuals with Type 1 diabetes and in females. Additional individuals at risk include those with a history of thyroid disease, irritable bowel syndrome, anemia, chronic diarrhea, chronic fatigue, unexplained weight loss, short stature, epilepsy, infertility, and unexplained elevations of transaminase levels. In addition to blood tests, a biopsy of the duodenum is used to confirm the presence of celiac disease.[19]

Once the diagnosis is made, the treatment recommended for the disease is a gluten-free diet. The inflammation of the bowel lining subsides and healing begins when the gluten consumption is avoided. It may take some patients several months or even years on this diet for maximal recovery. A gluten-free diet involves the elimination of not only wheat products but also products containing rye and barley. Alternative starches that can be included in the diet are rice, corn, flax, quinoa, tapioca, millet, amaranth, buckwheat, bean flour, and potato starches. Other food groups, such as meats, vegetables, fruits, legumes, and dairy are also permitted. Food labels must be carefully checked for the presence of wheat products.[20]

The Culinary Corner at the end of the Chapter explores celiac disease and the area of gluten-free cooking in greater detail.

Sugar and Sugar Alternatives

Americans have an affinity for sweet-tasting foods. Americans are consuming more and more sugar—up to 100 pounds of added sugar per year. This is approximately 32 teaspoons per day, on average, in the 1990s as compared with 7 teaspoons per day in 1890.[21] Health-conscious individuals are now turning to alternative forms of **nutritive** and **nonnutritive sweeteners**. The highest category among alternative nonnutritive sweeteners is the high-intensity sweeteners. The demand in the US for alternative sweeteners is projected to increase 3.4% per year to more than 1.3 billion dollars in 2013.[22]

Nutritive Sweeteners

Nutritive sweeteners by definition are those that provide energy value. They include refined sugars, high-fructose corn syrup, crystalline fructose, glucose, dextrose, corn sweeteners, honey, lactose, maltose, various syrups, and invert sugars. Nutritive sweeteners have approximately the same energy and nutritive value. Individual preference, cooking quality, and sensory qualities, rather than nutrition, should be the deciding factors in choosing a sweetener. Stevia is a natural sweetener that has little energy value, but is not "artificial."

Stevia

Stevia is a genus of plants belonging to the Asteraceae (sunflower) family, tribe Eupatoriae. It consists of 150–300 species, perhaps the best known and most commercially important of which is *S. rebaudiana* Bertoni. In the United States and other English-speaking countries, the plant is also known as candy leaf, sweet honey leaf, sweetleaf, sugarleaf, or simply stevia. *S. rebaudiana* is valued for its sweet taste, which is said to be about 300 times as intense as that of sucrose, common table sugar. The Guarani Indians of Paraguay and Brazil are said to have used stevia leaves for centuries as a sweetener and a treatment for a variety of medical problems. They added stevia leaves (which they called "kaa he-he," or "sweet her") to the bitter mate tea they drank or simply chewed the leaves to enjoy their unusually sweet taste. They also used the plant to treat obesity, hypertension, heart problems, heartburn, diabetes, dental caries, infections, fatigue, and depression.

By far the most important modern application of stevia, however, is as a sweetener. Stevia is not artificial, but rather a natural product. Research has shown that it appears to have no harmful effects on humans. On the contrary, evidence exists to suggest that stevia may actually enhance glucose tolerance in humans, making it a logical choice as a sweetener for diabetics. The herb is now widely used as a sweetener in most parts of East Asia, especially in Japan, where it accounts for more than half of the sweetener market since 2008. It is also popular as a sweetener throughout South America and the Caribbean.

Due to FDA regulations in the United States today, stevia cannot be advertised or sold as a food or a food additive, although it can be advertised and sold as a dietary supplement. There are no reports of side effects from using stevia at the amounts normally used for sweetening purposes.[23]

Sugar Alcohols

Sugar alcohols such as sorbitol, mannitol, and xylitol contain one molecule of sugar and one of alcohol. They are nutritive in the sense that they provide calories; however, they are metabolized differently by the body than regular sugar. They also provide less energy and a reduced glycemic response, and do not contribute to dental caries. These sweeteners are found naturally in fruits and berries, and are also commercially synthesized and used in lieu of sugar. Sugar alcohols are not completely broken down by the intestine, and consumption of large quantities of these may cause diarrhea. Sugar alcohols are commonly used in chewing gums, candies, jams and jellies, and baked goods.

Nonnutritive Sweeteners

Nonnutritive sweeteners provide no energy or nutritive value. Artificial sweeteners can help consumers cut down on calories and control weight. They can help to manage chronic conditions such as diabetes, and potentially prevent cavities, according to the Academy of Nutrition and Dietetics. They are chemically synthesized, sweeten with little volume, and are referred to as high-intensity sweeteners. The United States is responsible for approximately 50% of the consumption of high-intensity sweeteners. This group of compounds is also called macronutrient substitutes, sugar substitutes, sugar replacers, or alternative sweeteners. The nonnutritive sweeteners that are currently approved by the Food and Drug Administration for use in the United States include aspartame, saccharin, acesulfame-K, neotame, and sucralose. The agency regulates artificial sweeteners as food additives, which must be approved as safe before they can be marketed.

Table 3.5 describes the common nonnutritive sweeteners and their relative sweetness in relation to pure sucrose. Nutrition professionals believe that nutritive and nonnutritive sweeteners are safe to consume, if consumed in moderation and within the context of a diet that is consistent with the dietary guidelines.[24]

TABLE 3.5 Nonnutritive Sweeteners			
Nonnutritive Sweetener	Brand Name	Relative Sweetness	Uses/Comments
Saccharin	Sweet and Low Sugar Twin	200–700 times	Not reduced with heat. Tabletop sweetener used in baked goods and pharmaceutical products.
Aspartame	Nutrasweet Equal	160–220 times	General purpose sweetener in food and beverages.
Acesulfame-K	Sunette One Sweet One	200 times	Tabletop sweetener used in pudding, gelatins, candies, baked goods, desserts, alcoholic beverages.
Sucralose	Splenda	600 times	Used in carbonated drinks, dairy products, baked goods, coffees, teas, syrups, tabletop sweeteners, frozen desserts, and salad dressings.
Neotame		7000–13000 times	General purpose sweetener

Aspartame

Aspartame was first approved by the FDA in 1981 as a tabletop sweetener, and for use in gum, breakfast cereal, and other dry products. The use of aspartame was expanded to sodas in 1983, and then for use as a general-purpose sweetener in all foods and drinks in 1996. When ingested, aspartame is converted in the body to methanol and two amino acids—aspartic acid and phenylalanine. Because of the phenylalanine component, aspartame does carry a risk for individuals who have the rare genetic disorder phenylketonuria. People who have this disorder should avoid or restrict the use of aspartame because of their difficulty in metabolizing phenylalanine. The use of aspartame can cause phenylalanine build-up in the blood at higher levels than normal. The aspartame regulation requires that a statement be placed on the label of all products containing aspartame specifically to alert phenylketonurics of the presence of phenylalanine.

Saccharin

Saccharin was discovered in 1879 and was generally recognized as safe (GRAS) until 1972, when it was removed from the GRAS list by the FDA. In 1977, the FDA proposed a ban on saccharin, based on laboratory experiments with rats which developed bladder cancer after receiving high doses of saccharin. In response, Congress passed the Saccharin Study and Labeling Act. This legislation put a moratorium on the use while more safety studies were under way. Foods containing saccharin were required to carry a label warning that the sweetener could be a health hazard and that it was found to cause cancer in laboratory animals. According to the National Cancer Institute, further studies showed that saccharin did not cause cancer in humans, and that the bladder tumors in rats were triggered by a mechanism that is not relevant for humans. In 2000, the National Toxicology Program determined that saccharin should no longer be listed as a potential cancer-causing agent. Federal legislation followed in 2001, removing the requirement for a saccharin warning label. Saccharin is used in tabletop sweeteners, baked goods, soft drinks, jams, and chewing gum.

Acesulfame-K (Potassium)

Acesulfame-K was first approved by the FDA in 1988 for specific uses, including as a tabletop sweetener. The FDA approved the sweetener in 1998 for use in beverages. In December 2003, it was approved for general use in foods, but not in meat or poultry. Acesulfame-K can be found in baked goods, frozen desserts, candies, beverages, cough drops, and breath mints. The FDA and the Food and Agriculture Organization/World Health Organization (FAO/WHO) Joint Expert Committee on Food Additives have evaluated the sweetener's safety. More than 90 studies support the safety of acesulfame-K.

Neotame

Neotame can be 7,000 to 13,000 times sweeter than sugar, depending on how it's used in food. It does not contain calories. The FDA approved neotame in 2002, as a general-purpose sweetener in a wide variety of food products other than meat or poultry. It has been approved for use in baked goods, soft drinks, chewing gum, frosting, frozen desserts, jams, jellies, gelatins, puddings, processed fruit and fruit juices, toppings, and syrups. Data compiled from more than 100 animal and human studies on neotame, found no adverse effects when neotame is ingested at the levels used in foods.

Sucralose

Sucralose, known under the brand name Splenda, is 600 times sweeter than sugar, on average, and has no calories. Although sucralose is made from table sugar, it adds no calories because it isn't digested in the body. After reviewing data compiled from more than 110 studies conducted on animals and humans, the FDA approved sucralose in 1998 for use in 15 food categories, including tabletop sweeteners, beverages, chewing gum, frozen desserts, fruit juices, and gelatins. In 1999, the FDA allowed sucralose as a general-purpose sweetener in all foods.[25]

Creative Ways of Increasing Complex Carbohydrates

Carbohydrates are found in an array of foods and provide the body with its preferred fuel source as well as with countless vitamins, minerals, and phytochemicals. Chefs may capitalize on their colors, textures, and flavors to educate the public on the healthy choices available from this nutrient. In many restaurants, the entrée or protein on the plate is the center of the meal as well as the largest portion of food served. The starch and vegetable accoutrements are frequently small in portion size and lack creativity. Chefs may introduce the customer to a variety of carbohydrates to improve the healthfulness of the meal and to reduce food cost. Carbohydrates are derived mainly from plant foods such as cereal grains, fruits, vegetables, and legumes. White rice, white bread, and instant mashed potatoes are carbohydrates that are quickly broken down to sugars and rapidly raise the blood sugar. These are considered high-glycemic-index foods. Chefs might encourage the consumption of foods that have a lower glycemic index by offering them more frequently. These carbohydrate choices are often much more flavorful, and offer more texture and color than other carbohydrate choices. Dense breads that contain a lot of whole grain, stone ground flour breads, long-grain basmati rice, whole-grain cereals (oatmeal, semolina, muesli, all bran), and legumes (including soybean, kidney beans, lentils, chickpeas, black beans) have a low glycemic index.[26]

A variety of grains, with descriptive copy about their qualities, may be introduced on menus. Grains can be used as single dishes or combined with other grains, fruits, or vegetables. Often subtle in flavor, grains can carry other flavors. They serve as a good base for pungent flavors found in such dishes as spicy stews or Mexican dishes. Grains may be enhanced with a variety of flavors such as herbs, spices, stocks, wines, vinegars, and oils. A sample list of grains and how they may be paired with foods is provided in Table 3.6.[27, 28]

TABLE 3.6 Examples of Whole Grains		
Whole Grains	**Description**	**Uses**
Basmati Rice	Long-grain rice with a nutty flavor	Asian, Middle Eastern cuisine side dish
Brown Rice	Whole-grain rice without the outer husk, mild in flavor	Side dishes, soups, pudding
Buckwheat	A seed to make buckwheat flour, hulled buckwheat groats are crushed kernels used to make kasha	Kasha, breads
Bulgur	Wheat kernels steamed, dried, crushed	Breakfast cereal, pilafs, salads
Jasmine Rice	Fragrant rice similar to basmati	Side dish, salads
Kamut	High-protein wheat	Pastas, puffed cereal, crackers, salads, grain dishes
Millet	High-protein, small, yellow grain	Cereals, grain dishes, breads
Pearled Barley	Barley grain, with lots of flavor and texture	Cereals, breads, pilafs
Quinoa	High-protein grain	Replacement for rice
Triticale	Hybrid of wheat and rye, nutty flavor, low in gluten	Good in cereals, grain dishes
Wheat Berries	Unprocessed grain	Cereals, salads, baked into breads

Culinary Corner
Cooking the Gluten-Free Way

Celiac disease is recognized as a fairly common multi-system disorder, occurring in one in 133 people.[29] The treatment for celiac disease is adherence to a gluten-free meal pattern including strict avoidance of proteins from wheat, rye, and barley. Although not everyone suffering from celiac disease exhibits symptoms, the most notable characteristics associated with celiac disease are diarrhea, wasting, malabsorption, failure to grow, bloating, and abdominal cramps. Recent studies have shown that many individuals with celiac disease don't experience typical symptoms of the condition and are only diagnosed when seeking medical care for other issues such as anemia, osteoporosis, peripheral neuropathy, infertility, and fatigue.[30, 31]

The only treatment for celiac disease is lifelong adherence to a gluten-free diet. The elimination of wheat, rye and barley, and products containing these ingredients, is considered crucial. Cross-contamination with wheat, rye, and barley during food processing, preparation, and handling must also be avoided. Ingestion of even a small amount of gluten can cause intestinal damage. Careful monitoring of ingredients and processing is a vital part of the gluten-free diet.

Several studies have reported that individuals with celiac disease (treated and untreated) are more likely to experience gastrointestinal symptoms such as diarrhea, constipation, abdominal pain and bloating, nausea or vomiting, reduced gut motility, and delayed gastric emptying. Compliance with a gluten-free diet reduces the prevalence of these symptoms.[32]

Studies also report that compliance with a gluten-free dietary pattern results in significant improvements in nutritional laboratory values, such as serum hemoglobin, iron, zinc and calcium, as a result of intestinal healing and improved absorption. Adherence to a gluten-free dietary pattern may result in a diet that is high in fat and low in carbohydrates and fiber, as well as low in calcium and iron.[33, 34, 35, 36]

The gluten-free diet requires careful planning and medical nutrition therapy by a Registered Dietitian to ensure consumption of adequate fiber and nutrients. Individuals with celiac disease are advised to consume whole or enriched gluten-free grains and products such as brown rice, wild rice, buckwheat, quinoa, amaranth, millet, and sorghum. The Registered Dietitian should advise individuals with celiac disease to consume a daily gluten-free multivitamin and mineral supplement that is age and sex specific, if the intake of these nutrients is marginal.

A gluten-free diet can be challenging to follow. Aside from the dietary restrictions placed on an individual with celiac disease, specially manufactured whole and enriched most gluten free, refined grains are not enriched but they are still costly.[37] It is especially important that individuals with celiac disease carefully read the ingredient list on food labels. A list designed to help individuals with celiac disease adhere to a gluten-free diet follows:

- Do not eat anything that contains wheat, rye and barley.
- Because oats are sometimes processed in machines that also process wheat products, cross-contamination can be a concern. It is prudent to contact the manufacturer by mail, email or phone to ensure that this is not the case.
- Corn, potato, rice, soybeans, tapioca, arrowroot, carob, buckwheat, millet, amaranth and quinoa may be eaten in any amount.
- Malt vinegar does contain gluten, whereas distilled white vinegar does not.

If the following terms are found on food labels, there may be gluten in the product:

- Hydrolyzed Vegetable Protein (HVP), unless made from soy or corn
- Flour or Cereal products, unless made with pure rice flour, corn flour, potato flour or soy flour
- Vegetable Protein, unless made from soy or corn
- Malt or Malt Flavoring, unless derived from corn
- Modified Starch or Modified Food Starch, unless arrowroot, corn, potato, tapioca, waxy maize, or maize is used
- Vegetable Gum, unless made from carob bean, locust bean, cellulose, guar, gum arabic, gum aracia, gum tragacanth, xantham or vegetable starch
- Soy Sauce or Soy Sauce Solids, unless you know they do not contain wheat
- Stabilizers
- Starch
- Flavoring
- Emulsifier
- Hydrolyzed Plant Protein

Removing gluten from the diet is not easy. Grains are used in the preparation of so many foods. However, staying on a strict gluten-free diet can dramatically improve the condition of someone suffering from celiac disease. Recent research has focused on alternative ways to treat celiac disease other than diet alone. One of the new prospects for therapy includes having infants at high risk avoid gluten-containing foods for the first year of life. This allows for full maturity of the immune system. It is believed that this approach may delay or prevent the onset of celiac disease entirely. Other studies focus on medications that help in the breakdown of gluten and the use of vaccines to make T cells tolerate and not react to gluten.[38]

References

1   J. Slavin, "The Role of Whole Grains in Disease Prevention," *Journal of the Academy of Nutrition and Dietetics* 101 (2001): 780–785.

2   Results from USDA's 1994–1996 Diet and Health Knowledge Survey: Table Set 19. Agricultural Research Service, 2000.

3   B. Ling and S. Yen, "The U.S. Grain Consumption Landscape: Who Eats Grain, in What Form, Where, and How Much?" ERS Summary Report November 2007, Economic Research Services USDA. www.ers.usda.gov

4   B. Leibaman, National Health Newsletter, CSPI, April 1999.

5   D. L. Swagerty Jr., "Lactose Intolerance," *American Family Physician* 65 (2002): 1845–50.

6   D. E. Greydanus, "Sports Doping in the Adolescent Athlete, the Hope, Hype, and Hyperbole," *Pediatric Clinics of North America* 49 (2002): 829–55.

7   V. A. Buusau, "Carbohydrate Loading in Human Muscle: An Improved 1-Day Protocol," *European Journal of Applied Physiology* 87 (2002): 290–290.

8   Food and Nutrition Board Institute of Medicine, Dietary Reference Intakes Proposed Definition of Dietary Fiber, A Report of the Panel on the Definition of Dietary Fiber and the Standing Committee on the Scientific Evaluation of Dietary Reference Intakes, Washington, D.C.: National Academy Press, 2005.

9   "Health Implications of Dietary Fiber-Position of ADA," *Journal of The Academy of Nutrition and Dietetics* 102 (2002): 993–1000.

10 http://health.gov/dietaryguidelines/2015/guidelines/executive-summary/

11 http://www.choosemyplate.gov/what-are-added-sugars

12 Report of the Dietary Guidelines Advisory Committee on the Dietary Guidelines submitted by the DGAC to the Secretaries of USDA and HHS - June 14, 2010. http://www.cnpp.usda.gov/Publications/DietaryGuidelines/2010/DGAC/Report/D-5-Carbohydrates.pdf

13   A. W. Barclay, "Glycemic Index, Glycemic Load, and Glycemic Response Are Not The Same," *Diabetes Care* 28 (2004): 1839.

14   S. J. Brink, "Education and Multidisciplinary Team Care Concepts in Pediatric and Adolescent Diabetes Mellitus," *Journal of Pediatric Endocrinology and Metabolism* 15 (2002): 1113–1130.

15   C. Phillips, "Nutrigenetics and Metabolic Disease: Current Status and Implications for Personalized Nutrition," *Nutrients* 2013 (1): 32–57.

16   V. S. Malik, et al., "Sugar-Sweetened Beverages and Risk of Metabolic Syndrome and Type 2 Diabetes," *Diabetes Care* 33 (2010): 2477–2483.

17   The International Diabetes Federation Consensus Workshop, "Type 2 Diabetes in the Young: The Evolving Epidemic," *Diabetes Care* 27 (2004): 1798–1811.

18   A. J. Lee and R. J. Hiscock, "Gestational Diabetes Mellitus: Clinical Predictors and Long-Term Risk of Developing Type 2 Diabetes," *Diabetes Care* 30 (2007): 878–883.

19   D. A. Nelsen, "Gluten-Sensitive Enteropathy (Celiac Disease): More Common Than You Think," *American Family Physician* 66 (2002): 2259–2266.

20   L. K. Mahan and S. Escott-Stump, Krause's *Food Nutrition & Diet Therapy*, 12th ed. Philadelphia, PA: WB Saunders Company, 2008.

21   U.S. Department of Agriculture, Economic Research Service; *A Dietary Assessment of the US Food Supply; Comparing Per Capita Food Consumption with the Food Guide Pyramid Serving Recommendations*, Washington, D.C. AER no.772.

22   Beverage World, August 15, 2009, 128 (8), pg. 110.

23   "Stevia," David Edward Newton, Ed.D. The Gale Encyclopedia of Alternative Medicine. Ed. Laurie Fundukian, 3rd ed. Detroit: Gale Publishing, 2009.

24   "Use of Nutritive and Nonnutritive Sweeteners-Position of ADA," *Journal of The Academy of Nutrition and Dietetics* 98 (1998): 580–587.

25   Department of Health and Human Services, Food and Drug Administration, "*Food Additives Permitted for Direct Addition to Food for Human Consumption; Sucralose*," 21 CFR, Part 172, Docket No. 99F-0001, 1999. www.fda.gov/OHRMS/DOCKETS/98fr/cf9947.pdf

26   J. Miller, J. Burani, and K. Powell, *The Glucose Revolution*, New York, N.Y.: Marlow and Company, 2001.

27   P. Berton, *The Whole Foods Diabetic Cookbook*, Summertown TN: The Publishing Company, 2002.

28   S. Kapoor, *Professional Healthy Cooking*, New York, NY: John Wiley and Sons Inc., 1995.

29   P. H. Green, "The Many facès of Celiac disease: Clinical Presentation of Celiac disease in the Adult population," *Gastroenterology* 128 (2005): 74–78.

30   G. Brandimarte and A. Tursi, "Changing Trends in Clinical form of Celiac disease. Which is Now The Main Form of Celiac disease in Clinical Practice?," *Minerva Gastroenterology Dietology* 48 (2002): 121–30.

31   National Institutes of Health Consensus Development Program, Consensus Development Conference Statement, NIH Consensus Conference on Celiac Disease, June 28–30, 2004. http://consensus.nih.gov/2004/2004CeliacDisease118html.htm.

32   J.A. Murray and T. Watson, "Effect of a Gluten-free diet on Gastrointestinal Symptoms in Celiac Disease," *American Journal Clinical Nutrition* 79 (2004): 669–673.

33   M. T. Bardella, and C. Fredella, "Body Composition and Dietary Intakes in Adult Celiac disease Patients Consuming a Strict Gluten-free Diet," *American Journal Clinical Nutrition* 72 (2000): 937–939.

34   C. Hallert, "Evidence of Poor Vitamin Status in Celiac Patients on a Gluten-free Diet for 10 years," *Alimentary Pharmacology Therapeutics* 16 (2002): 1333–1339.

35   E. G. D. Hopman, "Nutritional Management of the Gluten-free Diet in Young People with Celiac disease in the Netherlands," *Journal Pediatric Gastroenterology Nutrition* 43 (2006): 102–108.

36   T. Thompson and M. Dennis, "Gluten-free Diet Survey: Are Americans with Celiac Disease Consuming Recommended Amounts of Fiber, Iron, Calcium, and Grain Foods?," *Journal of Human Nutrition and Dietetics* 18 (2005): 163–169.

37   A. R. Lee, D. L. Ng, J. Zivin, and P. Green, "Economic Burden of a Gluten-free Diet," *Journal of Human Nutrition and Dietetics* 20 (2007): 423–430.

38   A. Fasano, "Surprise from Celiac Disease: Study of a Potentially Fatal Food-Triggered Disease has Uncovered a Process that May Contribute to Many Autoimmune Disorders," *Scientific American*, August 2009.

Put It into Practice

Define the Term

Provide the definitions of fiber, water-insoluble fiber, and water-soluble fiber and review Table 3.1 "Water-Soluble and Water-Insoluble Fibers." Conduct an Internet search for the dietary fiber content of common foods. List the dietary fiber amount per serving of five foods from your search and determine if they are sources of soluble or insoluble fiber.

Myth vs. Fact

Determine if the following statement is a myth or fact and support your position with evidence from three research articles on the topic. *Statement: "Honey is more healthful than table sugar."*

For each research article, summarize each component below.

A. Abstract
B. Methods
C. Results
D. Discussion
E. Conclusion

The Menu

Develop four dinner meals for an upscale restaurant that contain at least two of the whole grains outlined in Table 3.6 "Examples of Whole Grains." Each meal must include an appetizer, entrée, starch, vegetable, and dessert. List the two whole grains found in each meal and include a description of each.

Website Review

Navigate the Center for Celiac Research website: www.celiac.com. Review the consumer information available on each of the tabs indicating: recipes, reviews, and research. Conduct a website search and review three additional gluten free websites. List the website addresses and summarize the recipe, review, and research information provided on each site.

Build Your Career Toolbox

Review the textbook section entitled "Culinary Corner: Cooking the Gluten Free Way." List ten terms on a food label that indicate there might be gluten in a particular product. Provide a 1-day gluten free menu including at least three breakfast, lunch, and dinner choices. Each lunch and dinner meal must include an appetizer, entrée, starch, vegetable, and dessert. Develop a job description for a "Gluten Free Chef."

Cecilia's Case Study

Cecilia is a 42-year-old woman who was recently diagnosed with Celiac disease. Her symptoms began about a year and a half ago, when she started experiencing abdominal pain, bloating, and severe constipation. She also experienced recurrent iron-deficiency anemia during this time, which did not improve with medication. Over the course of the past 8 months, she has had a 31 lb weight loss.

She recently saw a dietitian who educated her on avoiding gluten-containing foods, cross-contamination, and food label reading. The dietitian has asked you to prepare a higher calorie gluten-free sample menu for Cecilia which is as close to her usual intake as possible.

Anthropometric Data

Wt: 93 lbs   Ht: 5'4"   BMI: 16 kg/m^2
Usual Wt: 124 lbs (with a BMI of 21.3 kg/m^2)

Recommendations

Calorie needs: 2000–2200 (for weight gain)
Protein: 75–85 g
Fiber: >25 g
Vitamin B12: >2.4 mcg
Iron: 18–22 mg
Calcium: 1000–1200 mg

24-hr Recall

Breakfast: 1½ cup oatmeal (1/2 cup instant oatmeal cooked with 1 cup 1% milk) with 1/2 sliced banana, 1-oz walnuts; 6-oz coffee with 1 tsp sugar and 2 tbsp light cream

Lunch: Ham and cheese sandwich on wheat bread (2 slices bread, 2 slices honey ham and 1 slice American cheese, 2 tsp mustard, 1 lettuce leaf, 1 slice tomato), 1-oz pretzels, 2 tbsp hummus

Dinner: Chicken parmesan (4-oz chicken breast, 1 tbsp egg wash, 2 tbsp Italian breadcrumbs, 1 slice mozzarella cheese) shallow fried in canola oil, 1 cup spaghetti, and 1/2 cup tomato sauce

Snack: 2 chocolate chip cookies, 12 oz 1% milk

Preferences: Loves pasta and bread; dislikes quinoa, spaghetti squash, red meat, and most salads.

Daniel's Case Study

Daniel is a 7-year-old boy who was very active in sports, enjoys playing with friends after school, and is average weight for his height. Over the past month, he has been going to the bathroom much more frequently. His family assumed that he was just probably drinking more water than usual. As time went on, Daniel began to look very tired and had no ambition to play his favorite sports. Soon after, Daniel was always thirsty and began to wet the bed. He began to feel very sick with an upset stomach and vomiting. He slept all day and could not get out of bed to go to school. His mother took him to the doctors for testing and the doctor diagnosed him with type 1 diabetes. He then began an insulin regimen and needed to see a dietitian for meal planning.

Wt: 53 lbs Ht: 48" BMI: 17 kg/m^2 (normal weight)
Recent weight change: 8 pound weight loss in 2 months

Dietitian Recommendations:
 Calorie Needs: 1800–2000
 Protein Needs: 80–100 g
 Carbohydrate Needs: 200–250 g

Other recommendations: Meals and snacks should be eaten at the same times each day. Use the "Choose My Foods" Exchange System for meal planning. Limit sugary, refined carbohydrates, fruit juices, and dried fruit. Do not skip meals and snacks. Keep the amount and types of food (carbohydrates, fats, and proteins) consistent from day to day.

24-hr Recall

Breakfast: 2 eggs scrambled, 2 slices white toast and butter, 4 slices of bacon, 10-oz orange juice

Lunch: peanut butter and jelly sandwich on white bread, 1 cup pretzel sticks, 16-oz whole milk

Snack: 1 orange

Dinner: 6-oz meatloaf, 1 cup mashed potato with butter and gravy, 3/4 cup canned corn, 20-oz sweetened lemonade

Snack: 3 cups microwave popcorn with butter and salt

Preferences

Likes: sugary cereal such as frosted .akes and cinnamon toast crunch, whole milk, pop tarts, eggs and bacon, pasta with meatballs, steak, white bread, chocolate chip cookies, oranges, bananas, pomegranate, corn, raw carrots, and celery

Dislikes: beans, spinach, salad, most fruits, and vegetables.

Study Guide

Student Name _____   Date _____

Course Section _____   Chapter _____

TERMINOLOGY

Diabetes_____		A.	A form of polysaccharide that is non-digestible by humans
Glycemic Index_____		B.	A hormone produced by the pancreas that stimulates the liver to break down glycogen into glucose
Fiber_____		C.	A chronic disease of abnormal carbohydrate metabolism
Ketones_____		D.	A measurement used to evaluate the rise in blood sugar levels in response to carbohydrate intake
Insulin_____		E.	The synthesis of glucose from a non-carbohydrate source such as protein
Celiac disease_____		F.	High blood sugar levels
Hyperglycemia_____		G.	A form of polysaccharide that is stored in the liver and muscles of the body
Glucagon_____		H.	A hormone produced by the pancreas that signals the body's cells to take up glucose
Gluconeogenesis_____		I.	A substance formed when fat is used as an energy source
Hypoglycemia_____		J.	A disorder of the gastrointestinal tract characterized by inflammation and injury of the lining of the small intestine
Glycogen_____		K.	Low blood sugar levels

Student Name _____   Date _____

Course Section _____   Chapter _____

"FOOD CHOICE" MEAL PLANNING

Use Appendix B "Choose Your Foods Lists for Meal Planning"

2 slices whole wheat bread	1 small apple	2 slices tomato (1/4 cup)
2oz turkey breast	8oz low fat milk	2 large lettuce leaves (3/4 cup)
1 tablespoon mayonnaise		

Directions:

1. Using the meal above, write the food item where it belongs in column (b) based on the corresponding food group listed in (a). List the number of choices in (c) for each of the food items.

2. Record the Carbohydrate (d), Protein (e), and the Fat (f) for each item.

3. Calculate the total grams of Carb, Protein, and Fat (g) in the meal.

4. Calculate the caloric content of the nutrients (h) using the appropriate factor

5. Total the sum of calories in the meal (i).

6. Calculate the percentage of calories from carbs, protein, and fat in the meal (j).

Food Group (a)	Food Item (b)	# Food Choices (c)	Carb grams (d)	Protein grams (e)	Fat grams (f)	
Starch						
Fruit						
Milk						
Vegetables						
Lean Protein						
Medium Fat Protein						
High Fat Protein						
Fat						
Total Grams (g)			g	g	g	
Calories per Gram (h)			X _____	X _____	X _____	
Total Calories						= (i)
(j)			%	%	%	

Student Name _____   Date _____

Course Section _____   Chapter _____

CASE STUDY DISCUSSION

Cecilia's Case Study: Discovering Gluten Free Choices

Review the sections on Celiac Disease and "Culinary Corner: Cooking the Gluten Free Way". After reviewing the case study, use this information to answer the following:

1. Explain what Celiac disease is and how gluten affects the small intestine.

2. List the 3 grains which contain gluten.

3. Using the list of gluten free alternatives in the textbook, develop a one day gluten free menu including breakfast, lunch, dinner and one snack. The lunch and dinner meal must include an appetizer, entrée, starch, vegetable and dessert.

Student Name _____   Date _____

Course Section _____   Chapter _____

CASE STUDY DISCUSSION

Daniel's Case Study: Diabetes Diagnosis

Review the sections "Health Issues Related to Carbohydrate Digestion and Metabolism". After reviewing the material, use this information to answer the following:

1. What is the difference between Type 1 and Type 2 Diabetes?

2. Using Table 3.4 "Potential Warning Signs of Diabetes" explain the warning signs that Daniel experienced in his diagnosis of diabetes.

Student Name _____   **Date** _____

Course Section _____   **Chapter** _____

PRACTICE TEST

1. The body's preferred energy source is
   a. carbohydrates
   b. fats
   c. proteins
   d. vitamins

2. Carbohydrates are found mainly in
   a. plant products
   b. animal products
   c. plant and animal products equally
   d. organ meats

3. Fruit sugar is known as
   a. fructose
   b. sucrose
   c. maltose
   d. galactose

4. Sucrose is made up of
   a. glucose and glucose
   b. glucose and galactose
   c. glucose and fructose
   d. glucose and maltose

5. Type 2 diabetes is
   a. caused by a cell's resistance to insulin
   b. treated by insulin injections
   c. rare
   d. the most severe form of diabetes

Student Name _____ Date _____

Course Section _____ Chapter _____

TRUE OR FALSE

_____Table sugar is made up of maltose.

_____Fructose is a complex carbohydrate.

_____Fiber is indigestible by humans.

_____Hypoglycemia is a condition that refers to low blood sugar levels.

_____Sugar alcohols are nonnutritive sweeteners.

List the type of carbohydrates found in the following:

- Fruit_____
- Blood_____
- Table sugar_____
- Milk_____

Calculate the total calories from carbohydrates in this meal._____

3 oz turkey (0 grams)

2 slices of whole wheat bread (15 grams per slice)

4 oz. of 1 % milk (12 grams per one cup)

lettuce and tomato (5 grams)

1 small apple (15 grams)

Lipids

4

Adipose tissue	Hidden fats	Oxidation
Antioxidant	Hydrogenated	Phospholipid
Atherosclerosis	Hydrophilic	Polyunsaturated
Autoimmune	Lipid peroxidation	Rancidity
Bile	Lipoprotein	Reactive oxygen species
Cholecystokinin	Lymphatic	Saturated
Chylomicrons	Macronutrient	Steroid hormones
Emulsifier	Microparticulated	Sterols
Essential fatty acids	Monounsaturated	Trans-Fatty Acids
Free radicals	Nonessential fatty acids	Triglycerides
Gastric lipase	Omega-3 and 6 fatty acids	Unsaturated

Introduction

Fats are often thought of as culprits in the American diet, and they are the major nutrient on which individuals try to cut back. But fats also provide many benefits that should not be ignored. Fats are found in both plant and animal foods and are able to supply calories and essential fatty acids to help in the absorption of the fat-soluble vitamins A, D, E, and K. There are many different types of fats. In this chapter the term lipids (fats) is used to describe a range of organic compounds that do not dissolve in water. Lipids are composed of the same elements that make up carbohydrates; carbon, hydrogen, and oxygen. These lipids are present both in a pat of butter and in a slice of bread, but the differing number of each of these three elements and their arrangement make these foods very different in nutritive value. Fats have many more carbon and hydrogen atoms and fewer oxygen atoms than those found in carbohydrates.

Current dietary habits in the United States show a daily intake of fats that exceeds the recommended level. This high intake is due to both the consumption of fats and the **hidden** fats in foods. It is simple to understand that butter, mayonnaise, and oils contribute to fat intake, but the hidden fat found in foods such as donuts, whole milk, and in the marbling in meats is often ignored. Unseen fats can increase total fat consumption considerably. (Table 4.1)

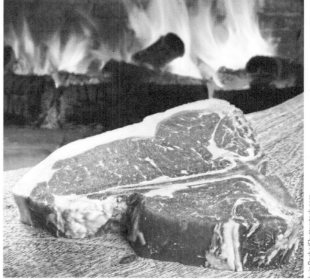

Hidden fats are found within foods as shown by fat marbling in this steak.

Luiz Rocha/Shutterstock.com

TABLE 4.1 Unseen fats can increase total fat consumption considerably

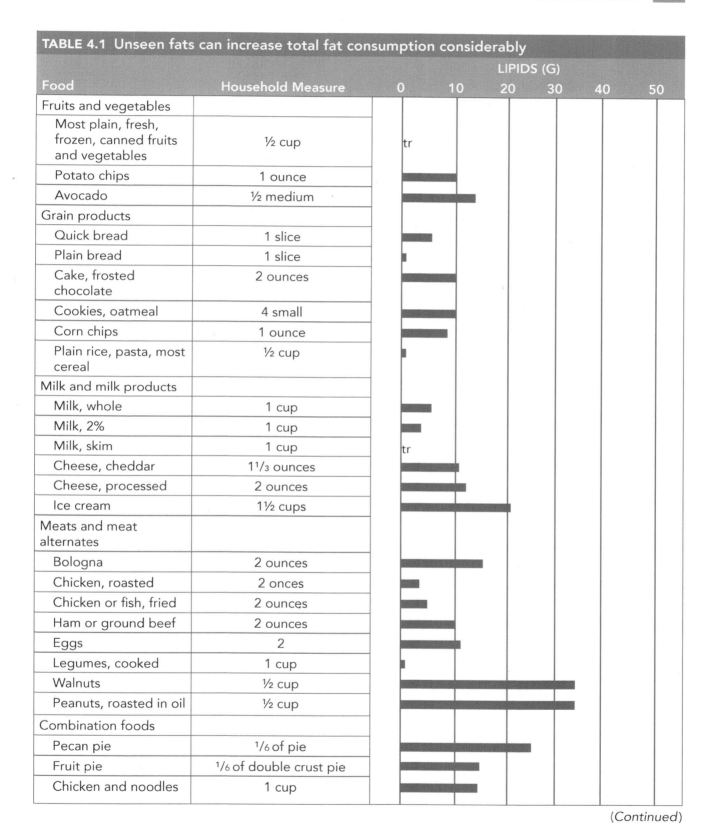

Food	Household Measure	LIPIDS (G)					
		0	10	20	30	40	50
Fruits and vegetables							
Most plain, fresh, frozen, canned fruits and vegetables	½ cup	tr					
Potato chips	1 ounce						
Avocado	½ medium						
Grain products							
Quick bread	1 slice						
Plain bread	1 slice						
Cake, frosted chocolate	2 ounces						
Cookies, oatmeal	4 small						
Corn chips	1 ounce						
Plain rice, pasta, most cereal	½ cup						
Milk and milk products							
Milk, whole	1 cup						
Milk, 2%	1 cup						
Milk, skim	1 cup	tr					
Cheese, cheddar	1⅓ ounces						
Cheese, processed	2 ounces						
Ice cream	1½ cups						
Meats and meat alternates							
Bologna	2 ounces						
Chicken, roasted	2 onces						
Chicken or fish, fried	2 ounces						
Ham or ground beef	2 ounces						
Eggs	2						
Legumes, cooked	1 cup						
Walnuts	½ cup						
Peanuts, roasted in oil	½ cup						
Combination foods							
Pecan pie	⅙ of pie						
Fruit pie	⅙ of double crust pie						
Chicken and noodles	1 cup						

(Continued)

Food	Household Measure	LIPIDS (G)					
		0	10	20	30	40	50
Pizza	1/8 of 15" cheese	▮▮					
Beef soup with noodles	1 cup	▮					
Assorted extras							
Oil, butter, margarine, mayonnaise	1 teaspoon	▮					
Cream cheese	1 1/3 ounces	▮▮					
Italian salad dressing	1 ounce	▮▮▮					
French salad dressing	1 ounce	▮▮▮					
Bacon	3 slices	▮▮					
Sour cream	2 tablespoons	▮					

TABLE 4.1 Unseen fats can increase total fat consumption considerably (*Continued*)

Classifications of Lipids

Lipids are divided into three classes:

- **Triglycerides**
- **Phospholipids**
- **Sterols**

These classes are distinguished by their unique configurations and properties, and each is responsible for a wide range of functions in the body. Although they are all made up of carbon, hydrogen, and oxygen, each has a different number and arrangement of these elements.

Triglycerides

Triglycerides are the most common lipids in both our food supply and our bodies. They comprise about 95% of all lipids. Phospholipids and sterols make up the remaining 5%. Triglycerides are the fats that the body is able to utilize for energy and to store when not needed. Triglycerides are what we commonly classify as fats or oils in foods. Fats are solid at room temperature while oils are liquid at room temperature. All triglycerides are composed of three (tri) fatty acids and one glycerol molecule. The glycerol molecule is considered the backbone of the triglyceride to which the fatty-acid chain (composed of a carbon chain with varying amounts of hydrogen atoms) is attached. (Figure 4.1) Fatty acids that make up these chains may be essential fatty acids or nonessential fatty acids. The fatty-acid chain determines whether the triglyceride is liquid or solid at room temperature, and the length of this chain and its degree of saturation determine whether the triglyceride has fat or oil properties.

Essential Fatty Acids

Essential fatty acids are necessary in the diet because the body cannot make them in sufficient quantities. There are two essential fatty acids: linoleic acid and linolenic acid. Essential fatty acids help to maintain the structural parts of cell membranes and to create hormone-like substances that help regulate blood pressure, blood clotting, and immune response.[1]

Chain Length

The chain length of the fatty acid can be anywhere from 4 to 24 carbons. The chain is composed of carbons set up in multiples of two, that is, 4, 8, 12, 18, etc., so that energy usage from the triglyceride is more efficient.

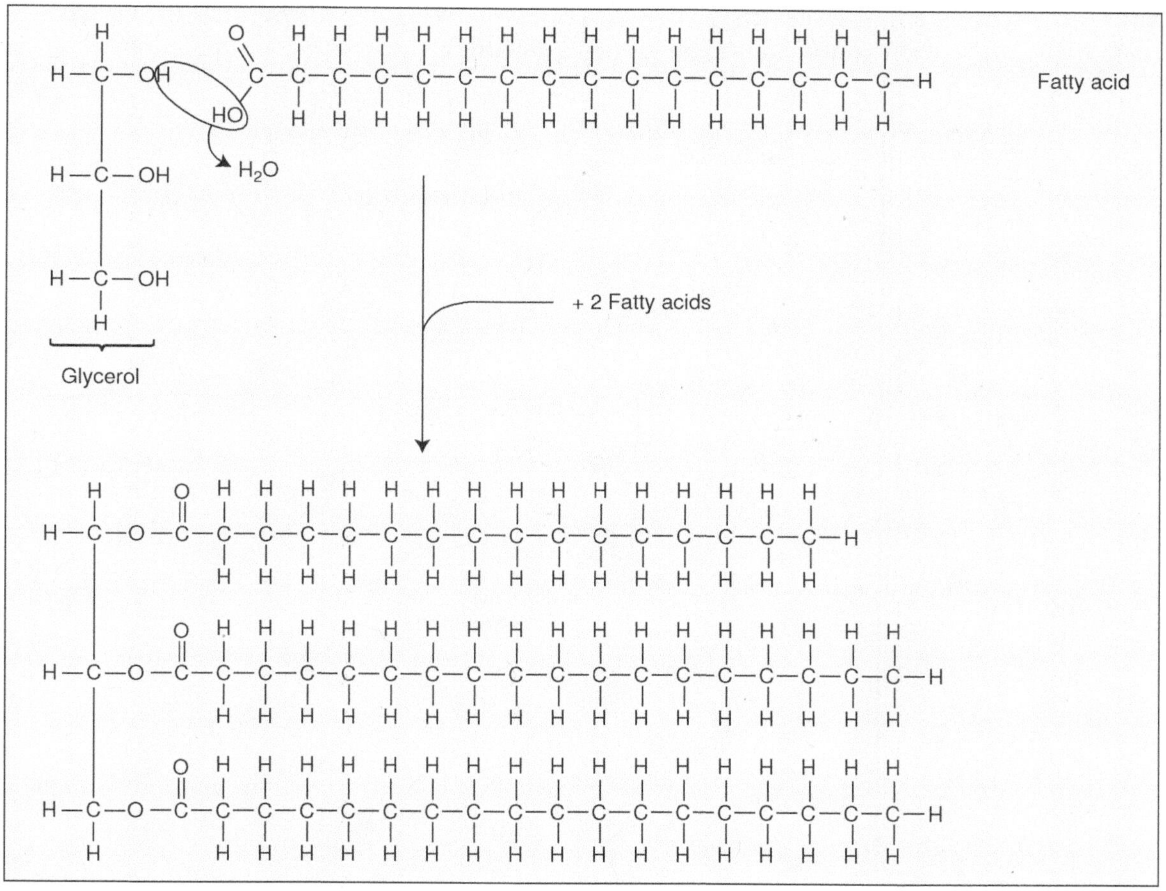

FIGURE 4.1 Triglycerides are composed of three fatty acids and a glycerol.

The 18-carbon chain fatty acids are the most common in foods and are also those associated with health issues such as blood clotting and cardiovascular disease. Long-chain fatty acids, composed of 12 to 24 carbons are found in meat and fish. Dairy products contain 6 to 10-carbon medium-chain fatty acids and also contain short-chain fatty acids of less than 6 carbons. Chain length helps to determine whether the lipid is classified as a fat (solid) or oil (liquid). In general, the longer the carbon chain, the more solid the fat is at room temperature.

Degree of Saturation

The degree of saturation affects the solid or liquid characteristics of the lipid. **Saturated** fats have hydrogen atoms attached to every available position on the carbon atom of the fatty-acid chain, which allows them to be completely saturated. **Unsaturated** fats, on the other hand, lack some hydrogen atoms that allow for points where saturation cannot occur. At these points of omission a double bond forms between the carbon atoms involved. (Figure 4.2) When there is only one double bond, or point of unsaturation, the fat is referred to as **monounsaturated**. When two or more double bonds exist, the fat is known as **polyunsaturated**. Saturated fats are typically solid at room temperature while unsaturated fats are liquid at room temperature. Each type of fat is derived from different sources. Saturated fats typically come from animal products, from **hydrogenated** products (see next section), or from a group of fats known as tropical oils, which include palm and coconut oils. Unsaturated fats come in both monounsaturated (canola, olive, and peanut oils), and polyunsaturated (corn, sunflower, and soybean oils) forms. Fat is a mixture of saturated, monounsaturated, and polyunsaturated fatty acids. The type of fat that predominates generally characterizes the fat. Olive oil, for example, is characterized as a monounsaturated fat although it contains small amounts of saturated and polyunsaturated fatty acids. Figure 4.3 depicts the fatty-acid composition of some common fats and oils. A discussion of the health implications of olive oil and other unsaturated fatty acids follows.

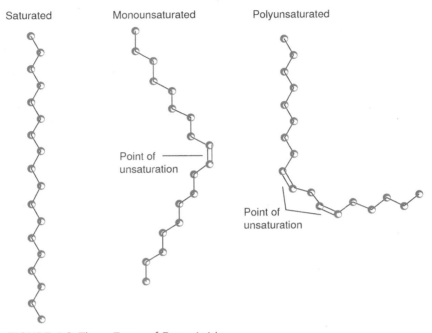

FIGURE 4.2 Three Types of Fatty Acids

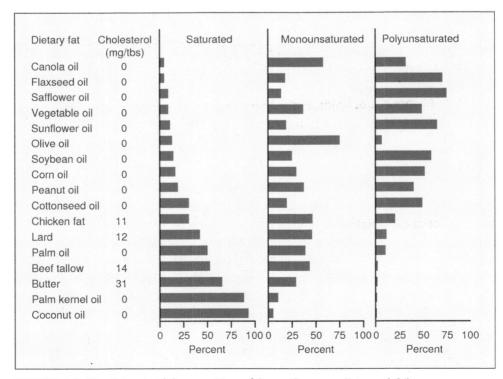

FIGURE 4.3 The Fatty Acid Composition of Some Common Fats and Oils

Hydrogenated Fats

Fats that are unsaturated are susceptible to oxidation, which occurs when a substance combines with oxygen. This can lead to problems of rancidity in fats and oils. To increase the stability of a fat, a chemical process referred to as hydrogenation is carried out on the unsaturated fat. Hydrogenation is a process that adds hydrogen to unsaturated fats to make them more saturated and consequently more stable and more solid in nature. Typically the shelf life, cooking properties, and the taste of vegetable oils are improved through hydrogenation. Examples of hydrogenated fats include margarine and shortening.

An unsaturated liquid vegetable oil undergoes hydrogenation to become a hydrogenated solid margarine. Although this process appears to offer tremendous benefits, it also yields a more saturated fat. Corn oil has only 6% saturated fat while corn oil margarine has 17% saturated fat.[2] During the hydrogenation process, some of the fatty acids change their arrangement from the cis form to the trans form of the fatty acid. (Figure 4.4) The trans form has been associated with the development of heart disease. Both saturated fats and trans-fatty acids are discussed in detail later in the chapter.

Phospholipids

A phospholipid is a compound that is similar to a triglyceride. Phospholipids, however, contain a phosphorous molecule that replaces one of the fatty acids attached to the glycerol. (Figure 4.5) This substitution enables a phospholipid to be both soluble and insoluble in water. The phosphorus-containing chain is soluble in water while the fatty-acid chain is insoluble. This property gives phospholipids the characteristics of an emulsifier. The most widely known of the phospholipids are the lecithins. Lecithins have the same configuration as other phospholipids (i.e., two fatty acids attached to the glycerol backbone), but the third leg of the compound contains not only a molecule containing phosphorus but also one containing choline (a nitrogen-containing compound found in plant and animal tissues). (Figure 4.6) Emulsifying ability is an important feature in certain foods. Naturally occurring emulsifiers are used in the production of mayonnaise. The lecithin found in the egg yolks used in mayonnaise allows emulsification of the oil and water (vinegar) components. Chefs use egg yolks in foods such as hollandaise sauce because of their emulsification properties. Lecithin is also found in liver, soybeans, wheat germ, and peanuts. Lecithin is widely used in food manufacturing and can be found in such items as crackers, breads, puddings, ice creams, pastries, salad dressings, etc. Most of the lecithin in processed foods is derived from soy.

Phospholipids also play important roles in the body. Phospholipids are an integral part of each cell membrane. The ability of

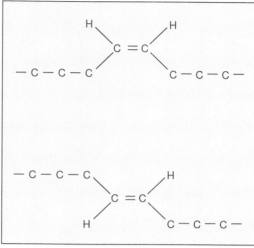

FIGURE 4.4 The Formation of Trans-Fatty Acids

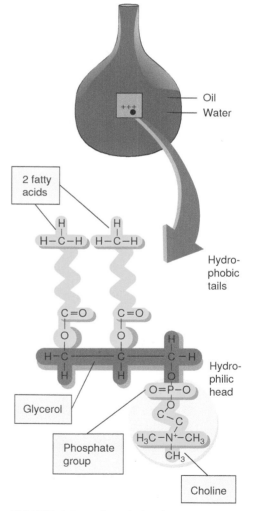

FIGURE 4.5 A phospholipid contains a phosphoric molecule, two fatty acids, and a glycerol molecule.

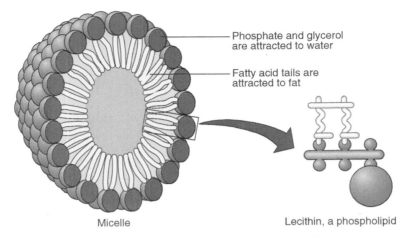

Phosphate and glycerol are attracted to water

Fatty acid tails are attracted to fat

Micelle

Lecithin, a phospholipid

FIGURE 4.6 Lecithin, a phospholipid, acts as an emulsifier.

the phospholipid to act as an emulsifier enables fat-soluble substances, such as vitamins and hormones, to travel back and forth through the lipid-containing cell membranes to the watery fluids on both sides. Phospholipids also transport fat-soluble substances in the blood. A part of the phospholipid attaches itself to the fat-soluble substance, while the water-soluble fraction of the phospholipid transports the fat-soluble substance in the watery fluid, the blood, through the body. The third role of phospholipids is the synthesis of the neurotransmitter acetylcholine, which is involved with memory. Health food promoters recommend the use of lecithin supplements because lecithin contains a choline, which is an essential component of acetylcholine. Studies have been done with Alzheimer's patients using lecithin, however results are inconclusive.[3]

Sterols

The third class of lipids consists of sterols, which are lipids with multiple ring structures. They vary considerably from the two lipid classifications previously mentioned. The most well-known sterol is cholesterol. (Figure 4.7) Although sterols can be found in both plants and animals, cholesterol is found only in animal sources because it is produced in the liver of animals. The greatest amounts of cholesterol can be found in organ meats, such as liver and kidneys, and in egg yolks. Table 4.2 lists the cholesterol content of some commonly consumed foods.

Cholesterol is often associated with health issues and is frequently perceived as a negative substance in food, although 800 to 1500 milligrams of cholesterol are produced in the liver each day. Would the body make so much of a substance if it were completely harmful? Of course not! Cholesterol takes on many important roles as a starting point for many compounds. It serves

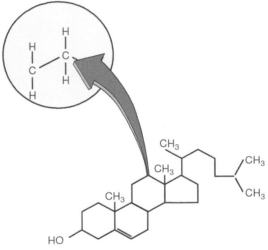

Cholesterol

FIGURE 4.7 The most common sterol is cholesterol.

The more carbon atoms in a fatty acid, the longer it is. The more hydrogen atoms attached to those carbons, the more saturated the fatty acid is.

Saturated   Monounsaturated   Polyunsaturated

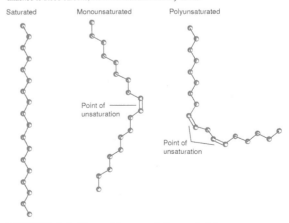

Point of unsaturation

Point of unsaturation

FIGURE 4.8 Three Types of Fatty Acids

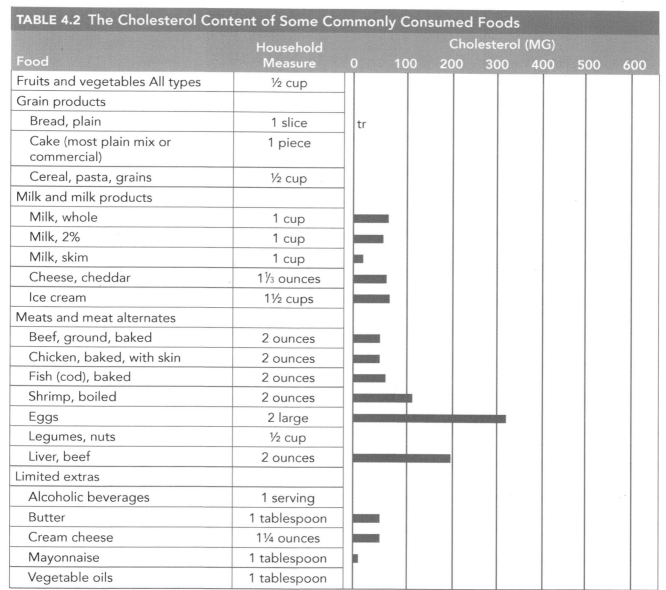

TABLE 4.2 The Cholesterol Content of Some Commonly Consumed Foods

Food	Household Measure	Cholesterol (MG)
Fruits and vegetables All types	½ cup	
Grain products		
Bread, plain	1 slice	tr
Cake (most plain mix or commercial)	1 piece	
Cereal, pasta, grains	½ cup	
Milk and milk products		
Milk, whole	1 cup	
Milk, 2%	1 cup	
Milk, skim	1 cup	
Cheese, cheddar	1⅓ ounces	
Ice cream	1½ cups	
Meats and meat alternates		
Beef, ground, baked	2 ounces	
Chicken, baked, with skin	2 ounces	
Fish (cod), baked	2 ounces	
Shrimp, boiled	2 ounces	
Eggs	2 large	
Legumes, nuts	½ cup	
Liver, beef	2 ounces	
Limited extras		
Alcoholic beverages	1 serving	
Butter	1 tablespoon	
Cream cheese	1¼ ounces	
Mayonnaise	1 tablespoon	
Vegetable oils	1 tablespoon	

Data Sources: 1) United States Department of Agriculture. 1976–1990. *Revised agricultural handbook no. 8 series.* Washington, DC: USDA. 2) Human Nutrition Information Service. 1989. *Agricultural handbook, no. 8, 1989 supplement.* Washington DC: USDA. 3) Pennington, J.A.T. 1989. *Food values of portions commonly used.* New York Harper & Row.

as the origin of vitamin D and is also used to synthesize bile. **Bile** is necessary in fat digestion. Cholesterol also synthesizes **steroid hormones** such as testosterone and estrogen. It is a part of every cell membrane and is needed by the body to function and to survive.

Lipid Requirements

Table 4.3 presents recommendations for total fat, saturated fat, trans fat, and cholesterol. Over the years many individuals have made an attempt to decrease their fat intake. Data from part one of the National Health and Nutrition Examination Survey (NHANES) III, conducted from 1988 to 1991, concluded that 34% of calories in the American diet were from fat, as compared to the 40%–42% estimated in the 1950s.[4] Vegetable oils have also gained in importance in diets and their availability has increased consistently over the past 30 years.[5]

TABLE 4.3 The Recommendations for Total Fat, Saturated Fat, Trans Fat and Cholesterol

Total Fat

Dietary Guidelines 2015[a]

Age Group	Total Fat Limits
Children ages 1 to 3	30%–40% of total calories
Children and adolescents ages 4 to 18	25%–35% of total calories
Adults, ages 19 and older	20%–35% of total calories

American Heart Association[b]

- Limit fat to 25%–35% of total calorie intake

Saturated Fat

Dietary Guidelines 2015

- Consume less than 10% of calories from saturated fatty acids by replacing them with monounsaturated and polyunsaturated fatty acids

American Heart Association

- Limit saturated fat to less than 7% of total energy

Trans Fat

Dietary Guidelines 2015

- Keep trans-fatty acid consumption as low as possible, especially by limiting foods that contain synthetic sources of *trans* fats, such as partially hydrogenated oils, and by limiting other solid fats

American Heart Association

- Limit trans fat intake to less than 1% of total daily calories

Cholesterol

American Heart Association

- Limit cholesterol to less than 300 milligrams per day

[a]*Source*: Dietary Guidelines for Americans, 2015. United States department of Agriculture, Center for Nutrition and Policy Promotion. http://health.gov/dietaryguidelines/2015/guidelines/executive-summary/

[b]*Source*: AHA Dietary Guidelines: Revision © 2000, 2003, 2011 Copyright American Heart Association. http://www.americanheart.org/

Lipid Functions

Lipids have important functions both in food systems and in the body. In moderation, fat is not bad; a little is good but more is not better. To look at the functions of fat, it is important to first separate fats in foods from fats in the body. Below is a list of functions of fat in food and in the body.

Fats in foods:

- Provide the essential fatty acids linoleic and linolenic
- Provide a concentrated energy source (9 kcal/gram)
- Serve as a medium to transport the fat-soluble vitamins A, D, E, and K and to assist in their absorption
- Provide sensory characteristics
- Stimulate the appetite
- Contribute to a feeling of fullness

Fats in the body:

- Are the principal form of stored and reserve energy during times of illness
- Provide the bulk of energy for muscular work
- Protect the internal organs (fat in the abdominal cavity)
- Provide insulation against temperature extremes (fat under the skin)
- Are a major material found in cell membranes
- Serve as starting material for other useful compounds such as bile and hormones
- Brain development in the fetus and child

Lipid Digestion and Absorption

Fats, unlike proteins and carbohydrates, face a unique problem in digestion because they are hydrophobic (not water-soluble), while the enzymes needed to break them down are hydrophilic (water-soluble). Fats separate as they travel through the digestive tract while fat-digesting enzymes remain in solution. A step-by-step description of the digestive process of fats follows. The objective of fat digestion is to take large fats, namely triglycerides, and to break them down to their component parts: monoglycerides, fatty acids, and glycerol. (Figure 4.9)

The Mouth

There is minimal activity in the mouth concerning fat digestion. As fats enter the mouth, the hard fats begin to melt when they mix with saliva. The salivary glands in the tongue produce a fat-digesting enzyme known as a lipase (lip = lipid, ase = enzyme). This lipase enzyme is responsible for digesting fatty acids and is very active in young infants but only slightly active in adults.

The Stomach

Little fat digestion also occurs in the stomach. In the stomach, the mixture is churned and mixed and the fat separates by floating to the top of the mixture while the digestive enzymes are in the bottom of the solution. The contact between fat and the enzymes is limited, but a minimal amount of digestion of fatty acids occurs, due to gastric lipase.

The Intestines

The presence of fat in the upper portion of the small intestine triggers the release of a hormone known as cholecystokinin (CCK). CCK sends a message to the gall bladder to release bile into the small intestine. Bile is used to emulsify the fat and then make it available to the fat-digesting enzymes that are secreted from the pancreas. (Figure 4.10)

Lipase breaks off the fatty-acid chains leaving monoglycerides and a glycerol molecule. These smaller units of fat digestion can simply diffuse into the intestinal cells and become absorbed directly into the blood stream. Monoglycerides and longer chain fatty acids enter into micelles where they are reassembled into triglycerides in the intestinal cells. These triglycerides, as well as phospholipids and cholesterol, are then picked up by chylomicrons and are transported via the lymphatic system into the bloodstream. If fatty-acid chains are attached to sterols, they are not absorbed and move to the large intestine. A small amount of fatty material may pass through the digestive tract without being digested. This fat is removed from the body along with other waste products.

Lipid Transportation

The transportation of lipids through the bloodstream cannot occur without the help of a carrier. Fat-soluble monoglycerides and glycerol molecules need the assistance of lipoprotein (a transport molecule containing

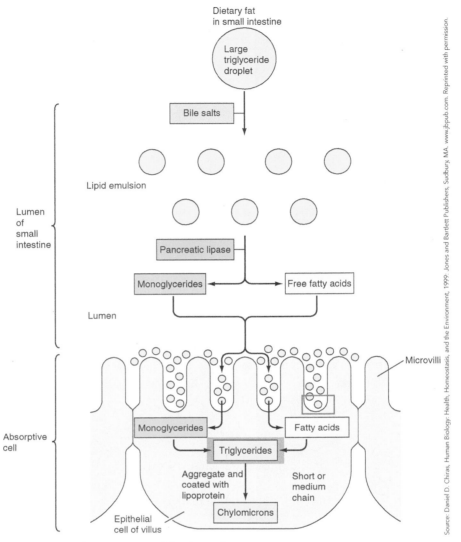

Source: Daniel D. Chiras, Human Biology: Health, Homeostasis, and the Environment, 1999. Jones and Bartlett Publishers, Sudbury, MA. www.jbpub.com. Reprinted with permission.

FIGURE 4.9 The Digestion of Triglycerides

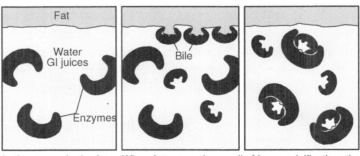

In the stomach, the fat and watery GI juices tend to separate. The enzymes are in the water and can't get at the fat.

When fat enters the small intestine, the gallbladder secretes bile. Bile has an affinity for both fat and water, so it can bring the fat into solution in the water.

After emulsification, the fat is mixed in the water solution, so the enzymes have access to it.

FIGURE 4.10 Bile is used to emulsify fat and to make it available to the fat-digesting enzymes.

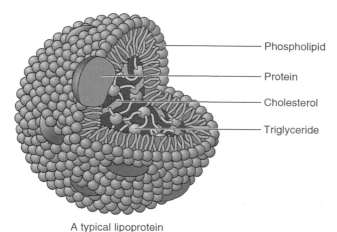

A typical lipoprotein

— Phospholipid
— Protein
— Cholesterol
— Triglyceride

FIGURE 4.11 Lipoproteins help transport dietary lipids through the body.

lipids and proteins) to help transport dietary lipids from the small intestine throughout the body. Four types of lipoproteins assist in transporting fat in the blood: Chylomicrons, VLDL (very low-density lipoproteins), LDL (low-density lipoproteins), and HDL (high-density lipoproteins). (Figure 4.11)

Chylomicrons

Once a triglyceride is broken down to monoglycerides and glycerol it can pass through the intestinal wall. During this passage, long-chain fatty acids and monoglycerides are reassembled by mucosal cells back into triglycerides. These triglycerides then combine with cholesterol, phospholipids, and a small amount of protein to form the lipoprotein known as a chylomicron. Chylomicrons are then absorbed into the lymphatic system and eventually into the bloodstream, bypassing the liver. Chylomicrons are responsible for the delivery of triglycerides to body cells. Lipoprotein lipase exists on the cell surface and dismantles the triglyceride into fatty acids and glycerol that can then be used by the cell for fuel. It may also be resynthesized, in the cell, to a triglyceride and stored. The remains of the chylomicron return to the liver where they are disassembled.

Very Low-Density Lipoproteins (VLDL)

The liver is able to make triglycerides from both short- and medium-chain fatty acids, and glycerol. It is also the major site of cholesterol synthesis. Newly synthesized particles are carried through the blood via VLDLs. VLDLs, made in the liver, transport lipids from the liver, and deliver triglycerides to the body cells. As the VLDLs lose triglycerides to the cells, they are replaced with cholesterol found in circulating lipoproteins in the blood, which then become low-density lipoprotein or LDL. The VLDLs contain less triglycerides and more cholesterol than chylomicrons. Although most of the cholesterol is returned to the liver, about one-third is transformed in the blood to LDLs.

Low-Density Lipoproteins (LDL)

LDLs contain a high level of cholesterol and are the primary cholesterol delivery system in the blood. At the cell site, an LDL receptor on the cell membrane allows the LDL to enter the cell. Once inside the cell, the cell utilizes the cholesterol.

High-Density Lipoproteins (HDL)

The cell uses cholesterol that is broken down, while cholesterol that cannot be used by the cell is returned, intact, to the liver to be eliminated by the body. This removal process is accomplished by HDLs. HDLs are a transport system that circulate and remove cholesterol from tissue, returning it to the liver for disposal, or to other cells that have a higher cholesterol requirement.

Lipid Metabolism

Fatty acids have two possible fates; they can be used for fuel for the body or they can be reassembled into triglycerides and stored for later use. In muscle cells, fatty acids and glycerol are used primarily to produce ATP (adenosine triphosphate) for energy. The remaining fatty acids and glycerol are sent to the adipose tissue (fat cells), where the reassembled triglycerides are stored. During the day, triglycerides may be removed from storage if needed for energy by the body. Feasting and fasting will determine whether triglycerides are put into storage or are removed for energy use.

Feasting

Excess energy intake results in the storage of triglycerides in adipose tissue. Adipose tissue contains cells that have an enzyme known as lipoprotein lipase on their surface. This enzyme gathers the triglycerides from the circulating lipoproteins, hydrolyzes them into fatty acids and monoglycerides, and then takes them into the adipose cell. Once inside, these components are reassembled into triglycerides and tightly packed for storage. When excess energy comes from fat in the diet, the triglycerides are transported directly to the adipose tissues in chylomicrons. Excess energy from protein and carbohydrates must first stop at the liver where it is synthesized to fatty acids, assembled into triglycerides, and eventually transported to the adipose tissue via VLDLs. More energy is then needed to store excess calories derived from protein and carbohydrates. The food source that is most easily stored is actually fat itself. The ability to store fat is great because fat cells can greatly increase in size.

Fasting

If energy intake is lower than the body's demand, the adipose tissue is called upon to release some of its stored fat (the body's energy reserves). Within the fat cells lies a hormone-sensitive enzyme known as lipase. This enzyme receives a chemical message to break down stored triglycerides to fatty acids and to glycerol. These fatty acids and glycerol can then be released directly into the bloodstream and taken up by the body cells to eventually produce ATP. When carbohydrates are lacking in the diet, fatty acids are not completely broken down and ketones are formed. Although ketones can be used for some energy, certain areas of the body also require glucose from carbohydrates for their energy production. For a more detailed understanding of fat metabolism refer to Chapter 8.

Health Issues

Heart Disease

Heart disease is the number one cause of death in the United States, in particular atherosclerosis, which is a disease that affects both the heart and blood vessels. This disease is caused by plaque deposits on the artery wall that narrow the artery opening and restrict the blood flow, consequently causing the arteries to lose their elasticity. There are many risk factors involved with atherosclerosis that are controllable and others that are not. Risk factors include high blood cholesterol levels (especially high LDL cholesterol and low HDL cholesterol), cigarette smoking, hypertension, a high fat/saturated fat diet, family history, diabetes, obesity, physical inactivity, and gender (males are at a higher risk). Dietary factors that can be altered to lower the risk of developing atherosclerosis are important and attainable. Dietary intervention studies support the concept that the restricted intake of saturated fat and cholesterol, and the increased consumption of essential fatty acids, especially omega-3 fatty acids, reduces coronary heart disease.[6] An increase in fiber intake can also contribute positively.

Cholesterol

Hypercholesterolemia (a high blood cholesterol level) represents a significant risk for cardiovascular disease. The majority of cholesterol in the body is actually produced by the body in the liver. In most individuals, the amount the body synthesizes decreases as dietary intake increases. When one consumes a cholesterol-rich diet, the liver decreases cholesterol production so that the blood cholesterol levels stay within normal limits. (Table 4.4) Unfortunately, in some individuals this does not occur, and the liver continues to produce cholesterol at its normal rate even when the cholesterol intake is high, resulting in elevated blood cholesterol levels. Choosing foods that are lower in cholesterol may help to keep blood cholesterol in check. However, it should be noted that saturated fats and trans fats play a much more significant role in elevating blood cholesterol. Dietary cholesterol does not impact blood cholesterol as much and some sources of dietary cholesterol, such as egg yolks contain important nutrients. Other dietary interventions such as >25 g soy protein and soluble fibers, such as pectin and oat bran, are also recommended.[7]

TABLE 4.4 Desirable Blood Lipid Values (Milligrams per Deciliter)
▪ Total Cholesterol <200 mg/dl
▪ LDL <100 mg/dl (Less healthy cholesterol)
▪ HDL >40 mg/dl (Healthy cholesterol)
▪ Triglycerides <150 mg/dl

Saturated Fats and Trans-Fatty Acids

The saturated fat content of a diet is of great concern. Saturated fats raise LDL cholesterol (the "bad" cholesterol) and increase the risk of heart disease. Trans-fatty acids (TFA) form when unsaturated fats pass through the hydrogenation process. These fats have been implicated in the alteration of blood cholesterol levels, similar to the way in which saturated fats affect cholesterol levels. Trans-fatty acids raise the LDL cholesterol, lower the HDL cholesterol (the "good" cholesterol), and increase the risk of heart disease.[8] The link between TFA and coronary heart disease (CHD) is strong. A 2% replacement of calories from TFA with unsaturated fats resulted in a 53% reduction in CHD risk in one recent study.[9]

The intake of trans-fatty acids by Americans in the United States ranges from 1.3 g to 12.8 g/day. Data on the actual intake is difficult to assess because of limited data on the content of trans-fatty acids in foods. In 1999 the TFA average intake was 5.3 g/day, which was derived from products containing partially hydrogenated oils, such as margarines, baked goods, crackers, cookies, and snack foods.[10] Table 4.5 outlines the TFA content of some common food items.[11]

As a result of the potential health concerns regarding the consumption of TFA, new food labeling requirements became effective as of January 1, 2006. Trans fats must now be included on the Nutrition Facts label if there are 0.5 g or more per serving. A lesser amount can be labeled as 0 g per serving. The recommendations for TFA intake according to the 2015 Dietary Guidelines are to keep them as low as possible in the diet.[12] The food industry is now developing new products with a lower TFA content. Products are being created by:

- Modifying the hydrogenation process. The production of TFA during hydrogenation can be controlled by temperature, pressure and catalyst concentration.
- Producing oilseeds with modified fatty acid composition through plant breeding and genetic engineering techniques.
- Using tropical oils.
- Employing the interesterification of mixed fats.

TABLE 4.5 TFA Content of Common Foods				
Food	Common Serving Size	Total Fat (G)	Sat Fat (G)	TFA Content (G)
French Fried Potatoes (Fast Food)	Medium (147 g)	27	7	8
Butter	1 tbsp	11	7	0
Whole Milk	1 cup	7	4.5	0
Shortening	1 tbsp	13	3.5	4
Margarine (stick)	1 tbsp	7	1	3
Potato chips	Small bag (42.5 g)	11	2	3
Candy	1 (40 g)	10	4	3
Cake, pound	1 slice (80 g)	16	3.5	4.5

Major food manufacturers such as Frito-Lay, Kraft, and Pepperidge Farms have introduced retail products that employ some of the techniques mentioned above to produce lower or no trans-fat chips, crackers and margarines.[13]

Exceptions to The Rule: Stearic Acid

There are some exceptions to the rule for saturated fats. Stearic acid is saturated fatty acid found in animal products that does not seem to behave as other saturated fats do in relation to heart health. Compared to other saturated fatty acids and trans fatty acids, stearic acid displays a favorable impact on plasma LDL-cholesterol and also on the ratio of total cholesterol/HDL cholesterol. As a result, stearic acid fats would make an acceptable substitution for trans fats and other saturated fats in foods such as baked goods, shortenings, spreads, and margarines[14].

Polyunsaturated and Monounsaturated Fats

Polyunsaturated fats have been found to lower LDL levels, but have little or no effect on HDL levels. It has been determined that monounsaturated fats lower LDL levels and have the added benefit of increasing HDL levels.

A monounsaturated fat of particular importance is olive oil. Olive oil is classified as a monounsaturated fat because it is composed mainly of this type of fatty acid. In the Mediterranean diet, olive oil is one of the main components, along with fruits, vegetables, and legumes. It has been suggested that olive oil has promising health benefits such as reducing the risk of heart disease, preventing several types of cancers, and improving immune responses.[15, 16, 17] Olive oil contains a high level of monounsaturated fats and is a good source of phytochemicals, particularly phenolic compounds.[18]

Phytochemicals in the body prevent disease and help combat the development of reactive oxygen species (ROS). ROS damage biological macromolecules such as DNA, carbohydrates, and proteins. Unsaturated fatty acids, in particular polyunsaturated fatty acids, are most vulnerable to ROS. Antioxidants derived from the diet, help to reduce the activity of ROS. Diets rich in monounsaturated fatty acids increase the fluidity of the cells and decrease the potential hazards of lipid peroxidation of polyunsaturated fatty acids in the cell membrane. The antioxidants in olive oil scavenge the ROS (also known as free radicals) and prevent damage from occurring. Olive oil also decreases LDL cholesterol and increases HDL levels in the blood to reduce the chance of heart disease. Its consumption is also said to lower the risk of breast and colorectal cancer by reducing the number of circulating free radicals, which if left alone,

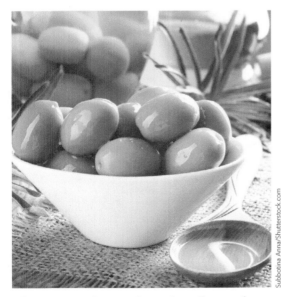

Olives are used to produce olive oil, one of natures only "fruit" oils.

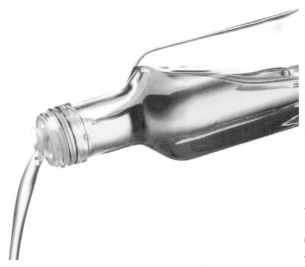

Olive oil is a good choice for chefs to use.

can cause damage to the cell integrity. Olive oil also shows promise in the treatment of autoimmune diseases such as rheumatoid arthritis.[19] A diet high in antioxidants can help prevent or delay the occurrence of pathological changes associated with oxidative stress.[20]

Olive oil can be found in a variety of forms: extra virgin olive oil, virgin olive oil, olive oil, and olive pomace oil. Extra virgin olive oil, derived from the first cold press of olives without the use of chemicals, is said to have the best nutritional value as well as the best sensory components. Table 4.6 provides examples of the culinary uses of olive oil and the types that might be used in these processes. Table 4.7 shows the amount of olive oil needed to replace hard fat in a recipe.

TABLE 4.6 Culinary Uses of Olive Oil

- Sautéing
- Extra virgin olive oil, virgin olive oil, olive oil
- Deep frying
- Olive oil, light olive oil, or olive pomace oil
- Roasting
- Extra virgin olive oil
- Baking
- Extra virgin olive oil, virgin olive oil, olive oil, extra light olive oil
- Marinade, sealant, baste, salad dressings
- Extra virgin olive oil, virgin olive oil, flavor-infused olive oils

TABLE 4.7 Olive Oil Substitutions for Hard Fat

Instead of Butter or Solid Fat in this Amount	Use Olive Oil in this Amount
1 teaspoon	¾ teaspoon
1 tablespoon	2¼ teaspoons
2 tablespoons	1½ tablespoons
¼ cup	3 tablespoons
⅓ cup	¼ cup
½ cup	⅓ cup
¾ cup	½ cup + 1 tablespoon
1 cup	¾ cup

Avocado Oil

Another oil that exhibits healthful properties is avocado oil. Oleic acid is the primary fatty acid in mature avocado fruit. Oleic acid is also the predominate monounsaturated fatty acid (MUFA) in olive oil (between 55-83%).[21] The heart-health benefits of this monounsaturated fatty acid have been well documented. They include a lowering of blood cholesterol as well as a lower potential for lipid oxidation which can lead to atherogenic effects.[22] A diet high in monounsaturated fats has shown a positive impact on lowering blood cholesterol levels as well as improving lipid profiles, hence reducing cardiovascular disease risk. Oleic acid lowers total cholesterol and low-density lipoproteins (LDL) level when it replaces saturated fatty acids in the diet.[23] Women may benefit more than men from a high monounsaturated fat diet because it may reduce total cholesterol and LDL levels without reducing HDL cholesterol. Low HDL cholesterol levels is a greater determinate for cardiovascular risk in women than in men.[24] Tissue membranes that are rich in MUFA are less susceptible to oxidation by free radicals than membranes rich in polyunsaturated fatty acids.[25] This has a protective effect on tissue membrane stability. Oleic acid also has been shown to help decrease inflammation in endothelial cells.[26]

In addition to fatty acids, avocado oil contains several known phytochemicals. Pigments including chlorophylls and carotenoids produce the distinctive color of the avocado. The presence of tocopherols, especially α-tocopherol, is another phytochemical of importance and the plant sterol of sitosterol.

The chlorophyll and carotenoid pigments act as antioxidants and may help in disease prevention. One of the predominate carotenoid pigments found in avocado oil is lutein. Lutein is particularly important in eye health. Lutein and a second carotenoid pigment, zeazanthin, are found in abundance in both the lens and the retina, and specifically in the cone-rich area of the macula. This is the area that helps see fine details.[27] Age-related macular degeneration (AMD) is the leading cause of loss of vision in the older population and lutein is believed to protect the cells of the macula from light-induced damage.[28] Consumption of food-based antioxidants like α-carotene lutein and zeaxanthin seem to be useful for the treatment of macular degeneration and cataracts.[29] These pigments must be obtained by the diet, though, as the body is unable to synthesize them on its own. Avocado oil contains about two times as much lutein as olive oil.[30]

Alphatocopherol is a form of vitamin E that is readily absorbed by humans. Vitamin E is essential to life and acts as a powerful antioxidant in the body. Its job is to prevent the formation of free radicals in the body as it undergoes normal oxidative processes. These powerful antioxidants are associated with the reduction of cardiovascular disease.[31] The level of vitamin E in New Zealand cold pressed avocado oil is comparable to that of olive oil, 70-190 μg/g of oil and 100-140 μg/g of oil, respectively.[32] Betasitosterol is the main plant sterol in avocado oil. Naturally present dietary plant sterols may contribute to reduction of cholesterol absorption especially when combined with other cholesterol-lowering plant foods. The mechanism of action in the body is such that, chemically, sterols look a lot like cholesterol so when they travel through the digestive tract, they can prevent cholesterol from being absorbed into your bloodstream and, hence, lower blood cholesterol levels. β-sitosterol levels in New Zealand cold pressed avocado oil are significantly higher than that found in olive oil (220-450 mg/100 g oil vs. 162-193 mg/100 g oil).[33] Plant sterols have such a positive impact on the reduction of coronary heart disease that the Food and Drug Administration has given it the status of an approved health claim.[34]

Omega-3 and Omega-6 Fatty Acids

Research shows a connection between the consumption of fish that is rich in omega-3 fatty acids and the reduced frequency of coronary heart disease (CHD).[35] A higher consumption of fish and omega-3 fatty acids has been associated with a lower risk of CHD in both men and women.[36] Fish and fish oils are the primary sources of omega-3 fatty acids in the human diet. Table 4.8 lists the omega-3 fatty acid content in foods. Excessive consumption of omega-6 fatty acids, along with an inadequate intake of omega-3 fatty acids, can lead to the increased likelihood of heart attacks, strokes, tumor formation, and various inflammatory conditions.[37] Plant oils are high in omega-6 fatty acids. The U.S. Department of Health (1994) recommends an increase in the consumption of omega-3 fatty acids to overcome the imbalance in the ratio of omega-3 to omega-6 polyunsaturated fatty acids in the diet.[38] The current ratio of omega 6 to omega 3 is 10:1 (in contrast to the 1:1 ratio of primitive man).[39] Another source high in omega-3 fatty acids is flaxseed. Flaxseed contains 73% polyunsaturated fatty acids made up of 57% omega-3 and 16% omega-6 fatty acids.[40] Flaxseed is a rich source of omega-3 fatty acids, and also contains beneficial fiber, lignin (acting as phytoestrogens), and powerful antioxidants. Milled flaxseed or oil is more beneficial because the seeds must be crushed to release potent health components.[41] Flaxseed oil is a long chain fatty acid (18-carbon chain).

Powerful health benefits for heart disease come from the very long, highly unsaturated fatty acid chains, eicosapentaenoic acid (EPA-20 carbon chain) and docosahexaenoic acid (DHA-22 carbon chain). EPA is associated with a decrease in platelet aggregation, the promotion of vasodilation, the inhibition of the inflammatory response, and a decreased risk of a heart attack. DHA is found in high quantities in the brain and is important in the development of the brain in the fetus. DHA also contributes to the health of the retina. The body is able to convert a small percentage

TABLE 4.8 The Omega-3 Fatty-acid Content in Foods

Food Item	MG of Certain Omega-3 Fatty Acids[a] Per 2 OZ. of Fish
Finfish	
Anchovy, European	0.8
Bass, striped	0.5
Bluefish	0.7
Catfish	0.2
Dogfish, Spiny	1.1
Halibul, Greenland	0.5
Herring (sardines)	1.0
Mackerel, Atlantic	1.5
Pike, walleye	0.2
Pompano, Florida	0.4
Salmon, different varieties	0.5–0.8
Trout, lake	1.0
Tuna	0.3
Whitefish, lake	0.8
Crustaceans and mollusks	
Clams, softshell	0.2
Shrimp, different varieties	0.2–0.3
Oysters	0.2–0.4
Squid	0.2

aOmega-3 fatty acids are considered here to be equal to the content of eicosapentaenoic acid (EPA) and docosahexaenoic acid (DHA).

Source: Reprinted from Journal of the Academy of Nutrition and Dietetics (AND), Volume 86, Hepburn R.N., J. Exler, and J.L. Weihrauch,

Provisional tables on the content of omega-3 fatty acids and other fat components of selected foods.

(less than 5%) of the 18-carbon fatty acid found in flaxseed to the longer chain EPA and to a lesser extent DHA.[42] Flaxseed should not be considered an important source of EPA or DHA. Fatty fish are the primary sources of EPA and DHA in the diet, as is demonstrated in Table 4.8.

Fiber

The addition of soluble fibers, in the form of pectin and oat bran, has also shown a positive correlation in the reduction of heart disease. These diets are effective at lowering LDL cholesterol but do not decrease HDL cholesterol. A study evaluating the effect of oat bran and wheat bran shows that oat bran lowers LDL cholesterol a full 12% more than wheat bran without any significant change in HDL cholesterol levels.[43]

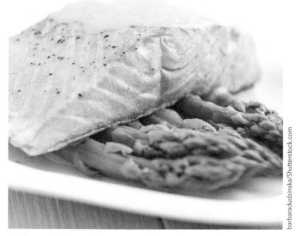

Fish and fish oils such as those found in salmon provide valuable sources of Omega-3 fatty acids.

Culinary Considerations

Healthy eating was at one time associated with food that lacked taste and variety. Today's chefs face the challenge of creating recipes that are both healthy and tasty, to answer the growing demands of health-conscious consumers. A knowledge and understanding of the connection between health and diet is necessary to accomplish this goal. Modifications such as trimming the visible fat on meat prior to cooking it, or removing the skin from chicken can greatly reduce fat calories. Pasta and grains can be cooked in broth and accented with herbs, pepper, nutmeg, or hard, flavorful cheese. Fruit or vegetable purées/juices, and monounsaturated fats such as olive oil may be used in lieu of salad dressing. They can lower unhealthy fats and are also higher in nutrient-dense carbohydrates. Desserts pose the greatest challenge of all and creativity in product selection is needed. Artificial sweeteners, non-dairy products, and egg substitutes are helpful in replacing higher caloric items. Others believe that consumption of smaller portions of flavorful, less processed foods that may also be nutrient dense, lead to optimal nutritional health.

In the category of fats and oils, a careful evaluation of saturated vs. unsaturated fats is necessary. The use of beef fat, chicken fat or sunflower oil is an important consideration. Beef fat is the firmest (due to its high level of saturated fats), and chicken fat the more pliable (due to its lower saturated fat and higher unsaturated fat composition). Sunflower oil is primarily unsaturated and therefore liquid at room temperature. The harder or firmer a fat is, the more saturated the fatty acids of the fat are. To determine whether the oil you use contains saturated fats, place the oil in a clear container in the refrigerator and watch for cloudiness. The least-saturated oils remain the clearest. An understanding of the connection between food and nutrition, and the ability of chefs to accommodate customer needs is critical in today's food service industry.

Fat Alternatives

Fat Replacers

The U.S. recommendations for total fat and saturated fat are 20%–35% and less than 10% respectively for the general population. To achieve this goal it is recommended that consumers eat more fruits, vegetables, nuts, seeds and whole grains, and decrease saturated fat and total fat consumption. Americans are obviously responding to these recommendations because the proportions of calories consumed that are derived from fat are decreasing in the United States.[44, 45] The introduction of fat substitutes or fat replacers has had an impact on lowering fat in the diet. Fat substitutes are compounds that are incorporated into food products to supply the good taste, texture, and cooking properties of fat. The most popular reduced-fat foods are fat-free or low-fat milk products, salad dressings, sauces, mayonnaise, and cheese/dairy products.[46]

Fat substitutes are typically categorized by their macronutrient source (protein, carbohydrate, or fat), and their caloric value can range anywhere from 0 to 9 calories per gram. The functional properties of food determine the type of fat substitute used. Federal regulations govern the fat substitutes that can be used in each type of food product. Olestra may be included in savory snack foods such as chips, but it cannot be used to replace fat in most other food products.[47] Protein-based and microparticulated protein-based fat substitutes are used to provide a smoother texture. Carbohydrate-based fat substitutes use plant polysaccharides to retain moisture and to provide textural qualities. Fat-based fat substitutes are chemically modified to decrease absorption of the fat or to enlist a smaller quantity of fat in the product, and to maintain similar quality characteristics. (Table 4.9)

Negative health-related issues from the use of carbohydrate-based or protein-based fat substitutes have not yet been identified. These do not seem to impact digestion, absorption, or metabolism of other nutrients. Fat-based substitutes, on the other hand, may affect nutritional status by altering the absorption of fat-soluble nutrients.[48]

The use of fat substitutes has a definite place in the marketplace but should not be expected to result in immediate and long-term improvements in weight control. Lifelong behavior changes that include dietary modification and an increase in physical activity are key elements to successful weight management and improved health.

TABLE 4.9 Examples of Fat Replacers

Protein-Based Fat Replacers

Microparticulated Protein (Simplesse®)

This reduced-calorie (1-2 calorie/gram) ingredient is made from whey protein or milk and egg protein. It is digested as a protein and has many applications, including: dairy products (e.g., ice cream, butter, sour cream, cheese, and yogurt), salad dressing, margarine- and mayonnaise-type products, as well as baked goods, coffee creamer, soups and sauces.

Modified Whey Protein Concentrate (Dairy-Lo®)

Controlled thermal denaturation results in a functional protein with fat-like properties. Its possible applications include: milk/dairy products (cheese, yogurt, sour cream, and ice cream), baked goods, frostings, as well as salad dressing and mayonnaise-type products.

Other (K-Blazer®, ULTRA-BAKE™, ULTRA-FREEZE™, Lita®)

One example of this type of reduced-calorie fat substitute is based on egg white and milk proteins. It is similar to microparticulated protein but made by a different process. Another example is a reduced-calorie fat replacer derived from a corn protein. Some blends of protein and carbohydrate can be used in frozen desserts and baked goods.

Carbohydrate-Based Fat Replacers

Cellulose (Avicel® cellulose gel, Methocel™, Solka-Floc®)

Various forms of these fat replacers are available. One is a non-caloric purified form of cellulose ground to microparticles, which when dispersed, form a network of particles with mouthfeel and flow properties similar to fat. Cellulose can replace some or all of the fat in dairy-type products, sauces, frozen desserts and salad dressings.

Dextrins (Amylum, N-Oil®)

Four calorie/gram fat replacers, dextrins, can replace all or some of the fat in a variety of products. Food sources for dextrins include tapioca. Applications include salad dressings, puddings, spreads, dairy-type products and frozen desserts.

Fiber (Opta™, Oat Fiber, Snowite, Ultracel™, Z-Trim)

Fiber can provide structural integrity, volume, moisture-holding capacity, adhesiveness and shelf stability in reduced-fat products. Applications include baked goods, meats, spreads and extruded products.

Gums (KELCOGEL®, KELTROL®, Slendid™)

Gums are also called hydrophilic colloids or hydrocolloids.

Examples of these include guar gum, gum arabic, locust bean gum, xanthan gum, carrageenan and pectin. Virtually non-caloric, they provide a thickening or sometimes a gelling effect and they can also be used to promote a creamy texture. Used in reduced-calorie, fat-free salad dressings and to reduce the fat content in other formulated foods, including desserts and processed meats.

Inulin (Raftiline®, Fruitafit®, Fibruline®)

This reduced-calorie (1–1.2 calorie/gram) fat and sugar replacer is a fiber and bulking agent extracted from chicory root. It may be used in yogurt, cheese, frozen desserts, baked goods, icings, fillings, whipped cream, dairy products, fiber supplements and processed meats.

Maltodextrins (CrystaLean®, Lorelite, Lycadex®, MALTRIN®, Paselli®D-LITE, Paselli®EXCEL, Paselli®SA2, STAR-DRI®)

Maltodextrins consist of 4 calorie/grams of gel or powder that are derived from carbohydrate sources such as corn, potato, wheat and tapioca.

(Continued)

TABLE 4.9 Examples of Fat Replacers (*Continued*)

Carbohydrate-Based Fat Replacers

They are used as fat replacers, texture modifiers or bulking agents. Their applications include baked goods, dairy products, salad dressings, spreads, sauces, frostings, fillings, processed meat, frozen desserts, extruded products and beverages.

Nu-Trim

This beta-glucan rich fat replacer is made from oat and barley by using an extraction process that removes coarse fiber components. The resulting product can be used in foods and beverages such as baked goods, milk, cheese, and ice cream.

Oatrim [Hydrolyzed oat flour] (Beta-Trim™, TrimChoice)

A water-soluble form of enzyme treated oat flour; Oatrim contains beta-glucan soluble fiber and is used as a fat replacer, or bodying and texturizing ingredient. It has reduced calories (1–4 calories/gram) and is used in baked goods, fillings and frostings, frozen desserts, dairy beverages, cheese, salad dressings, processed meats, and confections.

Polydextrose (Litesse®, Sta-Lite™)

This reduced-calorie (1 calorie/gram) fat replacer also serves as a bulking agent. It is a water-soluble polymer of dextrose containing minor amounts of sorbitol and citric acid and is approved for use in a variety of products including baked goods, chewing gums, confections, salad dressings, frozen dairy desserts, gelatins and puddings.

Polyols (many brands are available)

A group of sweeteners that provides the bulk of sugar, polyols have fewer calories than sugar (1.6–3.0 calories per gram, depending on the polyol). Due to their plasticizing and humectant properties, polyols may also be used to replace the bulk of fat in reduced-fat and fat-free products.

Starch and Modified Food Starch (Amalean® I & II, Fairnex™ VA15, & VA20, Instant Stellar™, N-Lite, OptaGrade®, Perfectamyl™ AC, AX-1, & AX-2, PURE-GEL®, STA-SLIM™)

These reduced-calorie (1–4 calories/gram as used) fat replacers are bodying agents and texture modifiers that may be derived from potato, corn, oat, rice, and wheat or tapioca starches. They can be used with emulsifiers, proteins, gums and other modified food starches. Applications include processed meats, salad dressings, baked goods, fillings and frostings, sauces, condiments, frozen desserts, and dairy products.

Z-Trim

Z-Trim is a calorie-free fat replacer made from insoluble fiber from oat, soybean, pea and rice hulls or corn or wheat bran. It is heat stable and may be used in baked goods (where it can also replace part of the flour), as well as in burgers, hot dogs, cheese, ice cream and yogurt.

Fat-Based Fat Replacers

Emulsifiers (Dur-Lo®, EC™ -25)

Examples of these fat replacers include vegetable oil mono- and diglyceride emulsifiers. Used with water, they can replace all or part of the shortening content in cake mixes, cookies, icings, and numerous vegetable dairy products. They have the same caloric value as fat (9 calories/gram), but a smaller amount is used, resulting in a fat and calorie reduction. Sucrose fatty acid esters may also be used for emulsification in products such as those listed above. Additionally, emulsion systems using soybean oil or milk fat can significantly reduce fat and calories by replacing fat on a one-to-one basis.

Salatrim (Benefat™)

Salatrims consist of short and long-chain acid triglyceride molecules. They are a five calorie-per-gram family of fats that may be adapted for use in confections, baked goods, dairy, and other such applications.

Lipid (Fat/Oil) Analogs
Esterified Propoxylated Glycerol (EPG) **
This reduced-calorie fat replacer may be used to partially or fully replace fats and oils in all typical consumer and commercial applications, including the preparation of formulated products, and in baking and frying.
Olestra (Olean®)
A calorie-free ingredient, Olestra is made from sucrose and edible fats and oils. It is not metabolized or absorbed by the body. It is approved by the FDA for use in replacing the fat needed to make salty snacks and crackers, and is stable under high heat food applications such as frying. Olestra is also used in other food applications.
Sorbestrin**
Sorbestrin is a low-calorie, heat stable, liquid fat substitute composed of fatty acid esters of sorbitol and sorbitol anhydrides. It has approximately 1.5 calories per gram and is suitable for use in all vegetable oil applications including fried foods, salad dressings, mayonnaise and baked goods.

Source: Copyright © 2000 Calorie Control Council.

* brand names are shown in parentheses as examples.

**may require FDA approval.

Modified Fats

Modification of lipids changes the role that fats and oils play in food, nutrition, and health applications. Structured lipids (SL) are designed to improve nutritional and/or physical properties by incorporating new fatty acids or adjusting the position of existing fatty acids on the glycerol backbone chain. Lipid modification can be achieved by chemically, enzymatically or by genetically engineering oilseed crops. SLs can be useful in total parenteral nutrition (TPN) and in the food industry to adapt the functionality of the fat to the food. The most common oils used in these modifications for total parenteral nutrition (TPN) are soybean and safflower oils. SLs may provide the most effective means of delivering desired fatty acids for nutritive or therapeutic purposes, and for targeting specific diseases and metabolic conditions.[49] The food industry uses a process of interesterification to produce trans-free margarines, cocoa butter substitutes, and reduced calorie foods. Consequently, SLs are designed to incorporate various fatty acids based on their potential benefits for improvements in nutrition or functionality in food products.[50]

Culinary Corner
What Is Aquaculture?

An increased awareness of the importance of Omega 3 Fatty Acids in the diet has put a spotlight on foods that best serve as sources of this nutrient. Among these offerings, it is widely believed that fatty type fish are excellent sources of Omega 3 Fatty Acids. The growing demand for this type of fish has generated a growing interest in Aquaculture.

Aquaculture refers to the breeding, rearing, and harvesting of plants and animals in all types of water environments, including ponds, rivers, lakes, and the ocean. Similar to agriculture, aquaculture can take place in the natural environment or in a manmade environment. Using aquaculture techniques and technologies, researchers and the aquaculture industry are growing, producing, culturing, and farming all types of freshwater and marine species. Species used in aquaculture include: fish such as catfish, salmon, cod, and tilapia; crustaceans, including shrimp, lobster and crayfish; and mollusks such as mussels, oysters, scallops and clams.[51]

In 1999, farm salmon production worldwide surpassed salmon fishery production for the first time. In the years between 1985 and 2000, farm salmon sales grew from 6%–58% worldwide, while fishery salmon saw a market decline of 94%–42%. Aquaculture industries are responding to this increased demand by expanding the production of farm raised fish. Fish produced from farming activities currently accounts for over one-quarter of all fish directly consumed by humans.[52] By the year 2010, the aquaculture production will reach 50% of the fish consumed by humans.[53]

In general, salmon farmers can produce salmon more cheaply than fishermen. They are able to control the genetic makeup and the diet of the fish they raise to create a product that is in line with market preferences. Salmon farmers can also offer different hues of flesh in salmon by adding varying amounts of synthetic carotenoid to the feed.[54] The health benefits of salmon are derived from their omega-3-fatty acids, ecosopentanoic acid (EPA) and docoshexinoic acid (DHA).

Sensory characteristics have been extensively compared between farm-raised and wild aquaculture species of salmon. A panel of tasters found that farmed salmon were at least as acceptable as wild salmon in terms of appearance, odor, flavor, texture, aftertaste and overall acceptability.[55] Consumers are demanding equal and consistent product quality at an affordable price, and aquaculture is helping to meet this demand.

References

1   C. A. Drevon, "Marine Oils and Their Effects," *Nutrition Reviews* 50 (1992): 38–45.
2   J. E. Brown, Nutrition Now, 3rd ed. Belmont, CA: Wadsworth/Thomson Learning, 2002.
3   J. P. Higgins and L. Flicker, "Lecithin for Dementia and Cognitive Impairment," Cochrane Database of Systematic Reviews 4 (2002): CD0010115.
4   M. A. McDowell, R. R. Briefel, K. Alaimo, et al., Energy and Macronutrient Intake of Persons Age 2 Months and Over in the United States: Third National Health and Nutrition Examination Survey—Phase 1988–1991. Hyattsville, MD: National Center for Health Statistics, 1994, Vital and Health Statistics Publication 255.
5   A. Trichopoulou and P. Lagiou, "Worldwide Patterns of Dietary Lipids Intake and Health Implications," *American Journal of Clinical Nutrition* 66 (1997): 961S–964S.
6   E. J. Schaefer, "Lipoproteins, Nutrition, and Heart Disease," *American Journal of Clinical Nutrition* 75 (2002): 191–212.
7   R. J. Nicolosi, T. A. Wilson, C. Lawton, and G. J. Handelman, "Dietary Effects of Cardiovascular Disease Risk Factors: Beyond Saturated Fatty Acids and Cholesterol," *Journal of the American College of Nutrition* 20 (2001): 421S–427S.
8   D. Kromhout, "Diet and Cardiovascular Disease," *Journal of Nutrition, Health, and Aging*, 5 (2001): 144–149.
9   F.B. Hu et al., "Dietary Fat Intake and the Risk of Coronary Heart Disease in Women," *New England Journal of Medicine* 337 (1997): 1491–1499.
10   Federal Register 68(133): 7/11/03 pg. 41446.
11   Revealing Trans Fats, FDA Consumer Magazine, September-October 2003 issue Pub No. FDA05-1329C.
12   Questions and Answers about Trans Fat Nutrition Labeling, CFSAN Office of Nutritional Products, Labeling and Dietary Supplements July 9, 2003; Updated March 3, 2004, June 25, 2004, August 1, 2005, September 6, 2005, and January 1, 2006, accessed June 15, 2007, http://www.cfsan.fda.gov/~dms/qatrans2.html#s2q1.
13   M. T. Tarrago-Trani et al., "New and Existing Oils and Fats Used in Products with Reduced Trans-Fatty Acid Content," *Journal of The Academy of Nutrition and Dietetics (AND)* 106 (2006): 867–880.
14   Hunter, JE, Zhang, J., Kris-Etherton, PM. 2010. Cardiovascular disease risk of dietary stearic acid compared with trans, other saturated, and unsaturated fatty acids: a systematic review. *American Journal of Clinical Nutrition* 91: 46–63.
15   A. H. Stark and Z. Madar, "Olive Oil as a Functional Food: Epidemiology and Nutritional Approaches," *Nutrition Reviews* 60 (2002): 170–176.

16 A. Trichopoulou and P. Lagiou, "Worldwide Patterns of Dietary Lipids Intake and Health Implications," *American Journal of Clinical Nutrition* 66 (1997): 961S–964S.

17 R. W. Owen, A. Giacosa, W. E. Hull, R. Haubner, G. Wurtele, B. Spiegelhalder, and H. Bartsch, "Olive Oil Consumption and Health: The Possible Role of Antioxidants," *Lancet Oncology* 1 (2000): 107–112.

18 R. W. Owen, A. Giacosa, W. E. Hull, R. Haubner, B. Spiegelhalder, and H. Bartsch, "The Antioxidant/Anticancer Potential of Phenolic Compounds Isolated from Olive Oil," *European Journal of Cancer* 36 (2000): 1235–1247.

19 L. Alarcon de la, M. D. Barranco, V. Motilva, and J. M. Herrerias, "Mediterranean Diet and Health: Biological Importance of Olive Oil," *Current Pharmaceutical Design* 7 (2001) 933–950.

20 D. Giogliano, "Dietary Antioxidants for Cardiovascular Prevention," *Nutrition, Metabolism, and Cardiovascular Disease* 10 (2000): 38–44.

21 D. N. Carroll and M. T. Roth, "Evidence for the Cardioprotective Effect of Omega-3 Fatty Acids," *Annals of Pharmacotherapy* 36 (2002): 1950–1956.

22 http://www.oliveoilsource.com/page/chemical-characteristics

23 S.M. Grundy, "Comparison of Monounsaturated Fatty Acids and Carbohydrates for Lowering Plasma Cholesterol in Man," New England Journal of Medicine 314 (1986): 745–748.

24 NCEP: Expert Panel on Detection, "Third Report of the National Cholesterol Education Program Expert Panel on Detection, Evaluation, and Treatment fo High Blood Cholesterol in Adults," (Adult Treatment Panel III) Final Report 2002, www.ncbi.nlm.nih.gov/pubmed/12485966.

25 P.M. Kris-Etherton, "Monounsaturated Fatty acids and Risk of Cardiovascular Disease," American Heart Association, Nutrition Committee, AHA Science Advisory, Circulation 1999, 100 (11), 1253–1258.

26 E. Gimeno, et. al. "Effect of Ingestion of Virgin Olive Oil on Human Low-Density Lipoprotein Composition," *European Journal of Clinical Nutrition* 56 (2002): 114–120.

27 M. Toborek, et.al., "Unsaturated Fatty Acids Selectively Induce an Inflammatory Environment in Human Endothelial Cells," *American Journal of Clinical Nutrition* 75 (2002): 119–125.

28 J. Mares, "Eat Smart: Which Foods are Food for What," Nutrition Action Health Letter 38 (2011): 1–7.

29 H.H., Koh, et.al., "Plasma and Macular Response to Lutein Supplement in Subjects With and Without Age-Related Maculopathy: A Pilot Study," *Experimental Eye Research* 79 (2004): 21–27.

30 V. Agte and K. Tarwadi. "The Importance of Nutrition in the Prevention of Ocular Disease with Special Reference to Cataract," *Ophthalmic Research* 44 (2010): 166–172.

31 M.N Criado, et.al, "Comparative Study of the Effect of the Maturation Process of the Olive Fruit on the Chlorophyll and Carotenoid Fractions of Drupes and Virgin Oils from Arbequina and Farga Cultivars," *Food Chemistry* 100 (2007): 748–755.

32 W.A. Pryor, "Vitamin E and Heart Disease: Basis Science to Clinical Intervention Trials," *Free Radical Biology and Medicine* 28 (2000): 141–164.

33 R. Turner, et.al., Are the Health Benefits of Fish Oils Limited by Products of Oxidation?," *Nutrition Research Reviews* 19 (2006): 53–62.

34 K.M., Phillips, et.al., "Free and Esterified Eterol Composition of Edible Oils and Fats," *Journal of Food Composition and Analysis* 15 (2002): 123–142.

35 http://www.fda.gov/Food/GuidanceComplianceRegulatoryInformation/GuidanceDocuments/FoodLabelingNutrition/FoodLabelingGuide/ucm064919.htm

36 F. B. Hu, L. Bronner, W. C. Willett, M. J. Stampfer, K. M. Rexrode, C. M. Albert, D. Hunter, and J. E. Manson, "Fish and Omega-3 Fatty Acid Intake and Risk of Coronary Heart Disease in Women," *Journal of the American Medical Association* 287 (2002): 1815–1821.

37 W. E. M. Lands, "Fish and Human Health: A Story Unfolding," *World Aquaculture* 20 (1989): 59–62.

38 Department of Health, Report on Health and Social Subjects. No 46. Nutritional Aspects of Cardiovascular Disease, London: HMSO, 1994.

39 S. B. Eaton, S. B. Eaton III, M. J. Konner, and M. Shostak, "An Evolutionary Perspective Enhances Understanding of Human Nutritional Requirements," *Journal of Nutrition* 126 (1996): 1732–1740.

40 D. H. Morris, "Essential Nutrients and Other Functional Compounds in Flaxseed," *Nutrition Today* 36 (2001): 159–162.

41 K. Fitzpatrick, Flaxseed Oil: Health Benefits and Uses. AOCS 98th Annual Meeting, Quebec City, May 2007.

42 E. Hernandez, Current Status of The Use of Omega-3 fats in Foods. AOCS 98th Annual Meeting, Quebec City, May 2007.

43   J. W. Anderson, D. B. Spencer, C. C. Hamilton, S. F. Smith, J. Tietyen, C. A. Bryant, and D. Oeltgen, "Oat Bran Cereal Lowers Serum Total and LDL Cholesterol in Hypercholesterolemic Men," *American Journal of Clinical Nutrition* 52 (1990): 495–499.

44   M. A. McDowell, R. R. Briefel, K. Alaimo, et al., Energy and Macronutrient Intake of Persons Age 2 Months and Over in the United States: Third National Health and Nutrition Examination Survey 1988–1991. Hyattsville, MD: National Center for Health Statistics, 1994, Vital and Health Statistics Publication 255.

45   E. T. Kennedy, S. A. Bowman, and R. Powell, "Dietary Fat Intake in the U.S. Population," *Journal of the American College of Nutrition* 18 (1999): 207–212.

46   Calorie Control Council. Fat Replacers: Food Ingredients for Health Eating, accessed June 27, 2000, http://www.caloriecontrol.org/fatreprint.html

47   J. Wylie-Rosett, "Fat Substitutes and Health: An Advisory from the Nutrition Committee of The American Heart Association, Circulation 105 (2002): 2800.

48   "Position of Academy of Nutrition and Dietetics (AND): Fat Replacers," *Journal of the Academy of Nutrition and Dietetics (AND)* 98 (1998): 463–468

49   K. T. Lee, and C. C. Akhoh, "Structured Lipids: Synthesis and Applications," *Food Reviews International* 14 (1998): 17–34.

50   H. T. Osborn, and C. C. Akhoh, "Structured Lipids-Novel Fats with Medical, Nutraceutical, and Food Applications," *Comprehensive Reviews in Food Science and Food Safety* 13 (2002): 93–103.

51   http://www.fao.org/docrep/w2333e/w2333e00.HTM

52   R. L. Naylor, R. J. Goldberg, J. H. Primavera, N. Kautsky, M. C. M. Beveridge, MCM. J. Clay, C. Folke, J. Lubshenco, H. Mooney, and M. Troell, "Effect of Aquaculture on World Fish Supplies," *Nature* 405 (2000): 1017–1024.

53   A. M. Rora, B. C. Regost, and J. Lampe, "Liquid Holding Capacity, Texture and Fatty Acid Profile of Smoked Fillets of Atlantic Salmon Fed Diets Containing Fish Oil or Soybean Oil," *Food Research International* 36 (2003): 231–239.

54   J. Eagle, R. Naylor, and R. Smith, "Why Farm Salmon Out Compete Fishery Salmon." http://pangea.stanford.edu/research/Oceans/GES205/fish.pdf

55   L. J. Farmer, J. M. McConnell, and D. J. Kilpatrick, "Sensory Characteristic of Farmed and Wild Atlantic Salmon," *Aquaculture* 187 (2000): 105–125.

Put It into Practice

Define the Term

Review the definitions of atherosclerosis and cardiovascular disease (CVD). List the major risk factors for atherosclerosis and indicate which factors are controllable.

Myth vs. Fact

Determine if the following statement is a myth or fact and support your position with evidence from three research articles on the topic. *Statement: "Eggs are very high in cholesterol, so you should avoid eating them."*

For each research article, summarize each component below.

A. Abstract
B. Methods
C. Results
D. Discussion
E. Conclusion

The Menu

Make list of foods that you might consume in a typical dinner including an appetizer, an entrée, a starch, a vegetable, and a dessert. Identify which of the foods contain saturated fat, Trans fat, monounsaturated fat, and polyunsaturated fat. Create a nutrient dense dinner meal consisting of an appetizer, an entrée, a starch, a vegetable, and a dessert that is moderately low in saturated fat and high in monounsaturated and polyunsaturated fat, yet tasty and appealing in sensory components. How does this meal compare with your typical meal?

Website Review

Navigate the North American Olive Oil Association website: http://www.naooa.org. State the Association's Mission and click on "Learn All About Olive Oil" to review the facts, health, and recipe information. See the Banana Bread Recipe below; how would a chef use olive oil in this recipe? How would it improve the nutritional content, flavor, texture, and sensory appeal?

Banana Bread Recipe

Ingredients	Amount
Bananas	3 each
Flour	1 ¼ cup
Butter	1/2 cup
Sugar	1 cup
Baking Soda	1 tsp
Vanilla	1 tsp
Salt	1/2 tsp
Egg	1 each

Build Your Career Toolbox

Review the Culinary Corner in the chapter entitled "What is Aquaculture"? Develop a job description for a chef or a dietitian in the field of aquaculture, which is the agriculture of the oceans. Include salary range, education, and experience requirements. This person must provide education, information, and resources to key food and nutrition associations as well as to the consumer. How can you meet the consumer demand for quality and affordability of popular aquaculture species, such as salmon, swordfish, cod, tilapia, sturgeon, mollusks, and crustaceans?

Linda's Lipid Profile

Growing up on the U.S.-Mexico border, Linda never thought twice about the cholesterol—laden fried beef and pork tacos that were a staple in her family. According to Linda, "Mom's tacos and other traditional Mexican dishes are just a delicious part of life in Brownsville, Texas." Linda's hobbies are watching movies at home and playing video games; she does not regularly participate in any form of regular physical activity. Poor heart health is also a part of life for Linda's family. "Heart disease is something we were pretty much resigned to," said Linda, whose grandmothers both died of heart attacks when they were in their 30s. Her father also has high cholesterol and high blood pressure. Linda has always believed that "this is just what happens to people over time."

A few months before Linda left home for college, she saw her doctor to have a physical exam and to have clinical blood work done for cardiac risk factors. Here are her results:

Total Cholesterol, 266 mg/dl, LDL: 146 mg/dl, HDL: 63 mg/dl, Triglycerides: 283 mg/dl

After her lab results came back, Linda's doctor sent her and her mom to meet with a dietitian. She has also met with an exercise specialist and will begin an exercise program that includes walking at least 5 days a week with a group of people her age. The dietitian reviewed heart healthy diet guidelines and some healthy cooking techniques with mom, but Linda is unsure about what kind of foods she may be able to eat at home and once she goes away to college. They have contacted you for ideas on foods that Linda could eat at home to get her on the road to good health before she goes away to college in a few weeks.

Wt: 165 lbs   Ht: 5'3"   BMI: 29.3 kg/m² (overweight)
No recent weight change

Dietitian Recommendations

Calorie Needs: 1600–1800 (for weight loss)
Protein Needs: 70–80 g/day
Fat: Goal of 28%–32% calories from fat, <10% calories from saturated fat
Fiber: 20–30 g/day
Sodium: <3 g/day (<3000 mg/day)

Other recommendations: Avoid sweets as much as possible; eliminate soda and juice; add fruits and veggies to every meal (at least 5 servings per day); add monounsaturated fats and omega 3 fatty acids

24-hr Recall

Breakfast: 3 slices of bacon, 2 fried eggs with 2 tbsp cheddar cheese, 1 cup fried potatoes (cooked in 1 tbsp of bacon fat), 1 slice of white bread with 1 tbsp butter + a dash of salt and pepper, and 12-oz orange juice

Lunch: 3 corn tortillas (prepared with lard), 5-ozs carnitas, 2 tbsp sour cream, 1/2 cup refried beans, 1/2 cup seasoned rice, 2 tbsp chopped cilantro, 1 radish, 2 tbsp chopped tomato mixed with onion; 20-oz cola

Snack: 1 individual bag of Hot Cheetos, 10 oz apple juice

Dinner: 3 slices pepperoni pizza, 2 garlic bread sticks (2 oz bread sticks with 1 tbsp butter, 1 tsp garlic), 1 cup romaine lettuce (with 1 tbsp cheddar cheese, 1 tbsp black olives, ¼ cup ranch dressing); 20 oz Sprite

Preferences: Dislikes fish and peanuts; has never eaten many fruits or veggies; likes traditional Mexican foods

Study Guide

Student Name _____   **Date** _____

Course Section _____   **Chapter** _____

TERMINOLOGY

Phospholipid_____	A. A fatty acid chain with only one point of unsaturation
Hydrophilic_____	B. The process that adds hydrogen into unsaturated fats to make them more saturated
Cholecystokinin (CCK)_____	C. The property of having a strong affinity for water. To dissolve or mix with water
Monounsaturated_____	D. Fatty acids that must be supplied by the diet. Linolenic and linoleic fatty acids
Sterols_____	E. A compound that has a phosphorus molecule attached to the glycerol chain
Atherosclerosis_____	F. A fatty acid chain with more than one point of saturation
Hydrogenation_____	G. A hormone produced in the upper small intestine that sends a message to the gall bladder to release bile into the small intestine
Triglycerides_____	H. A disease where there is clogging or hardening of the arteries and blood vessels
Essential fatty acids_____	I. Fatty acids produced through the hydrogenation process that has a negative health impact
Polyunsaturated_____	J. Three fatty acids attached to a glycerol molecule
Trans fatty acids_____	K. A lipid with multiple ring structures that functions in bile, vitamin D and hormone production

Student Name _____   Date _____

Course Section _____   Chapter _____

FAMILY HISTORY RISK ASSESSMENT

1. Develop a family medical tree with as many relatives you can investigate.

2. Fill in the information on each member of your family as listed in the table below.

Determine any medical conditions your family member may have/ had that you are aware of or able to investigate. (List as many medical conditions as you can, using the table below for some ideas.)

Anemia			
Arthritis		Heart Attack	
Asthma		High Blood Pressure	
Cancer		Kidney Disease	
Type 1 Diabetes		Stroke	
Type 2 Diabetes		Thyroid Disorder	

Student Name _____ Date _____

Course Section _____ Chapter _____

Family Members	Age	Living/ Deceased	Medical History
Maternal Grandmother (MOTHER SIDE)			
Maternal Grandfather			
Paternal Grandmother (FATHER SIDE)			
Paternal Grandfather			
Mother			
Father			
Sibling			
Sibling			
Sibling			

After filling in your family medical history tree, answer the following questions

a. What diseases are seen most frequently in your family?

b. What lifestyles choices (diet, exercise, smoking, alcohol consumption, etc.) can you make to reduce your risk of these diseases?

Student Name _____   **Date** _____

Course Section _____   **Chapter** _____

CASE STUDY DISCUSSION

Linda's Lipid Profile: Hyperlipidemia
Review the section on Health Issues of heart disease and review the case study to answer the following questions.

1. Use the information in Table 4.4 "Desirable Blood Lipid Values" and compare them to Linda's clinical blood work results in the case study. What does this mean for Linda's cardiac profile?

2. Explain three dietary or lifestyle changes that Linda could make to reduce her risk factors for heart disease.

Student Name _____   **Date** _____

Course Section _____   **Chapter** _____

PRACTICE TEST

Select the best answer.

1. An example of a hidden fat is
   a. margarine
   b. mayonnaise
   c. whole milk
   d. vegetable oil

2. The two essential fatty acids are
   a. arachadonic and linolenic
   b. linoleic and linolenic
   c. arachadonic and stearic
   d. stearic and linolenic

3. Monounsaturated fats include
   a. corn oil
   b. olive oil
   c. sunflower oil
   d. soybean oil

4. The type of fat that may contribute to a high risk for cardiovascular disease is
   a. monounsaturated fat
   b. polyunsaturated fat
   c. cis fatty acids
   d. trans fatty acids

5. Cholecystokinin (CCK) is a hormone that
   a. removes fat from the stomach
   b. digests polyunsaturated fats so they can be absorbed
   c. digests sterols so they can be absorbed
   d. signals the gall bladder to release bile for fat digestion

Student Name _____   Date _____

Course Section _____   Chapter _____

TRUE OR FALSE

_____ Flaxseed is high in omega-3 fatty acids.

_____ Lecithin is a phospholipid found in egg yolks.

_____ Soybean oil is a polyunsaturated fat.

_____ When determining whether a fat is solid or liquid at room temperature it is important to remember that the shorter the chain length, the more liquid the fat.

_____ Lipids are hydrophobic compounds.

Calculate the calories <u>from fat only</u> in this meal: _____

3 oz tuna steak (6 grams)

1 cup rice (2 grams)

Steamed green beans (0 grams)

Tossed green salad (0 grams)

2 tablespoons salad dressing (28 grams)

1 cup whole milk (8 grams)

State the type of fat found in the following food sources.

- Fatty fish_____
- Olive oil_____
- Corn oil_____
- Butter_____
- Shortening_____

Protein

5

KEY TERMS

Amino acid	Genistein	Marasmus
Antibody	Homeostasis	Mutual supplementation
Complementary protein	Hormone	Neurotransmitter
Complete protein	Incomplete protein	Nitrogen balance
Denature	Isoflavone	Nonessential amino acid
Edema	Ketone	Osteoporosis
Enzyme	Kwashiorkor	Phenylketonuria
Essential amino acid	Limiting amino acid	

Introduction

Proteins are the most diverse and complex of all the molecules in the body. Proteins can be found in a wide variety of sources, both in plant and animal foods. People in the United States derive most of their protein from animal products, while individuals in many other countries derive theirs from plant sources. It is somewhat apparent that animal protein consumption rises with affluence.

Proteins vary chemically from both lipids and carbohydrates. Although they contain carbon, hydrogen, and oxygen, as do lipids and carbohydrates, they also contain the element nitrogen. (Figure 5.1) It is the presence of nitrogen in proteins that contributes to the many important roles of protein. Protein is needed for almost all body functions. Protein contributes to the structure of cells, organs, and tissues, the regulation of processes involving other nutrients, the transportation of molecules, and the production of energy.

Proteins are structurally similar to lipids and carbohydrates. Lipids are made up of chains of fatty acids, complex carbohydrates are made up of chains of glucose, and proteins are made up of chains of **amino acids**. A list of amino acids is found in Table 5.1. These twenty amino acids are considered the "building blocks" of proteins. Protein molecules all have the same backbone structure but differ in the number, sequence, and specific amino acids involved in making the individual protein. (Figure 5.2)

Amino acids can be classified as either **essential** or **nonessential**. Nine of the twenty amino acids are categorized as essential amino acids. Essential amino acids are those that the body needs, but can only create in insufficient quantities or not at all. These nine amino acids are obtained through the diet. Nonessential amino acids (the remaining eleven), on the other hand, can be made or synthesized in the body as long as nitrogen is available. This process is made possible by a reaction known as transamination, which occurs when the amino group from an essential amino acid is transferred to a different acid group and side chain. The synthesis of a nonessential amino acid can also be generated from

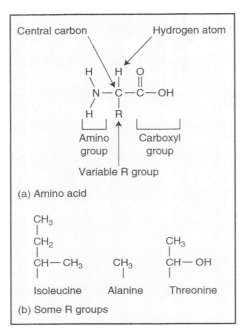

FIGURE 5.1 Proteins contain the elements carbon, hydrogen, oxygen, and nitrogen

| TABLE 5.1 Essential and Nonessential Amino Acids ||
Essential	Nonessential
■ Histidine	■ Alanine
■ Isoleucine	■ Arginine
■ Leucine	■ Asparagine
■ Lysine	■ Aspartic acid
■ Methionine	■ Cysteine
■ Phenylalanine	■ Glutamic acid
■ Threonine	■ Glutamine
■ Tryptophan	■ Glycine
■ Valine	■ Proline
	■ Serine
	■ Tyrosine

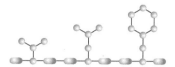

valine   leucine   tyrosine

Single amino acids with different
side chains...

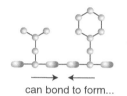

can bond to form...

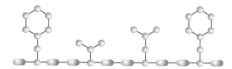

a strand of amino acids, part of a protein.

FIGURE 5.2 Amino acids join
together to make proteins

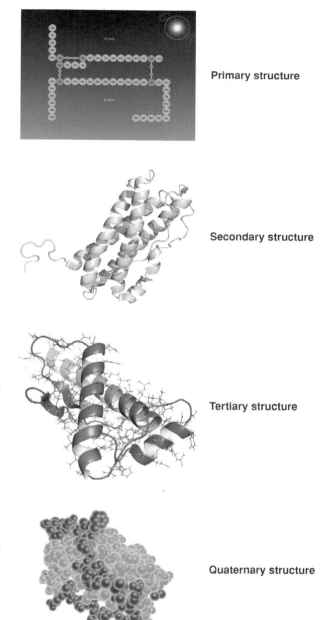

Primary structure

Secondary structure

Tertiary structure

Quaternary structure

FIGURE 5.3 Formations of Proteins (Images ©
Shutterstock.com)

both carbohydrate and lipid sources that contain carbon,
hydrogen, and oxygen in their structures.

A third group, known as conditionally essential
amino acids, consists of nonessential amino acids that
become essential under particular circumstances.
Individuals who suffer from the inherited disease
Phenylketonuria (or PKU) cannot convert the essential
amino acid phenylalanine into the nonessential amino
acid tyrosine, and must therefore obtain tyrosine in their
diet from protein sources. Tyrosine is a conditionally
essential amino acid.

From Amino Acids to Proteins

To form a protein, amino acids must be strung together
like beads on a necklace. The amino group of one amino
acid forms a peptide bond with the acid group of a second amino acid, to form a dipeptide. This reaction is
known as a condensation reaction because a molecule
of water is lost. A polypeptide (protein) is eventually formed as more amino acids are bonded together. The formation of proteins involves very complex structures of twisting and turning amino acid chains. The four levels
of structures are seen in Figure 5.3. The primary structure consists of the sequence of amino acids, while the
secondary structure is the consequent folding of the amino acid chain. The tertiary structure is a more advanced
folding of the chain whereby a three dimensional shape defines the protein. The last structure is the quaternary
structure, which occurs when two or more polypeptides join together. The final configuration allows each protein
to have its own unique function.

Protein Functions in the Body

Protein contributes substantially to almost every function that occurs in the body. It serves either a structural or a regulatory function for cells.

Structural Proteins

Protein is a primary component in the structure of the body because it forms a part of every living cell. It is found in the cell membrane of hair and nails, and in the bones and teeth. An individual's inherited DNA coding determines the way in which these proteins are put together. Deficiencies in protein can result in symptoms such as muscle wasting, hair loss, and loss of skin integrity.

Regulatory Proteins

Most, if not all metabolic functions occur or are influenced by the presence of protein. Protein containing enzymes help to regulate **homeostasis**. **Enzymes** speed up chemical reactions but are not altered during the reaction. Each enzyme is specific for a given reaction and will catalyze only that type of chemical reaction. (Figure 5.4) An enzyme can be used more than once without being destroyed in the process. Enzymes are involved in energy production reactions as well as in joining substances together, as seen in muscle building. They can also break down substances as seen in the digestion process of energy-yielding nutrients. There are thousands of types of enzymes in the body that accomplish a multitude of essential processes.

Proteins also assist in the transport of needed substances in the body. One example of a transport protein is a lipoprotein, which is made up of proteins and lipids. Lipoproteins transport fat-soluble vitamins, cholesterol, triglycerides and other fat-containing molecules through the bloodstream. Another transport protein is hemoglobin which carries oxygen in the blood. A deficiency in protein can prevent the flow of nutrients to their needed destinations. Transport proteins are also involved with the electrolyte balance of sodium and potassium. Under normal circumstances, sodium is in higher concentration outside the cells, whereas potassium is found in larger quantities within the cell. Transport proteins within the cell membrane allow for the proper balance of electrolytes. Body functions such as muscle contraction rely on the balance of these electrolytes and serious problems such as abnormal heart rhythm and muscle weakness can occur if the protein intake is too low.

The formation of **antibodies** also requires protein. Antibodies are a vital part of the body's immune system that helps to destroy or inactivate foreign substances. When an unfamiliar protein (known as an antigen) enters the body, the body produces proteins known as antibodies to destroy the antigen. Deficiencies in protein can compromise the immune system and increase susceptibility to infection. This problem is of a particular concern among the elderly.

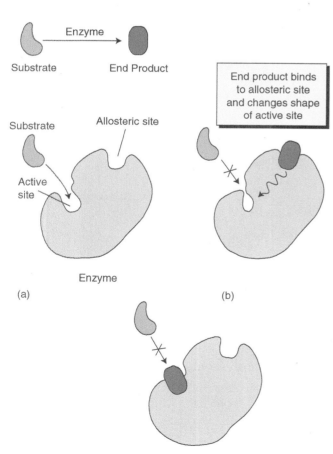

FIGURE 5.4 Enzymes speed up chemical reactions

Hormones also assist in body regulation. Some hormones are protein based and act as chemical messengers. A chemical messenger is a substance that is secreted by one area of the body and travels through the blood to a different destination. At its final destination a "chemical message" is given to this second site to complete a task. The secretion of a hormone is due to a change in the body's environment. The hormone insulin, for example, is secreted by the pancreas in response to elevated blood sugar levels. It then travels through the blood to the cell receptor site where it enables the glucose in the blood to be taken into the cell.

Another regulatory function of proteins is that of muscle contraction. Muscles are actually structural proteins that require regulatory proteins for movement. The two proteins involved with muscle contraction and relaxation are actin and myosin. These muscle filaments align themselves during muscle contraction and separate when the muscle relaxes. Proteins are involved with all body movements.

Fluid balance is yet another regulatory function of protein. Protein helps to regulate the distribution of fluids and particles inside and outside the cell because proteins, themselves, attract fluids. When protein is deficient in the diet, there are no large protein molecules available to keep fluids out of the cell, and fluids collect inside the tissues to cause a medical condition known as **edema** (fluid retention). Edema is often obvious in children in developing countries who exhibit swollen abdomens.

Proteins are responsible for keeping a balance in the amount of acid and base (acid-base balance) in the body. This balance must be present for a chemical reaction to occur. A brief look at fat metabolism will help to explain how this process works. When fat is used as an energy source, a compound known as a **ketone** may be formed. Ketones are acidic in nature and cause acidity levels in the blood to rise. If left unchecked, ketones build up in the blood and cause a condition known as ketosis. As ketosis progresses, the body loses the ability for chemical reactions that are necessary to maintain life. Proteins act as a buffer and neutralize the acidic effect of ketones. Protein side chains (the R groups) have a negative charge that attracts the hydrogen ions (acid) and neutralizes the system.

Proteins also regulate nerve transmission by synthesizing **neurotransmitters** in the body. A neurotransmitter is a chemical messenger that transmits a signal from nerve cells to other parts of the body. The amino acid tryptophan is important in the synthesis of the neurotransmitter serotonin in the brain. Serotonin is a compound that causes a person to feel sleepy.

Energy Production

Although not one of its primary functions, protein contributes to energy production and can provide the body with 4 kcal of energy/gram of protein. The body uses protein as an energy source for survival only when absolutely necessary. When protein is used for energy, the other structural and regulatory processes are denied this source. During a time of famine, protein is taken from body muscle as an energy source. When an individual is well nourished, excess dietary protein is stored as fat. Use of protein for energy production will be discussed in a later chapter.

Protein Requirements

Protein needs fluctuate at various life stages with changes in health conditions. When protein intake matches protein degradation or loss, an individual is said to be in **nitrogen balance**. Nitrogen balance is seen in healthy adults who actively partake in normal daily activity. Individuals who participate in physical activity retain more nitrogen than they excrete due to an increase in muscle growth. This retention of protein results in positive nitrogen balance. During pregnancy and other periods of growth, an individual is usually in positive nitrogen balance. Negative nitrogen balance occurs when the amount of nitrogen lost by the body exceeds the amount retained, possibly during illness or major surgery. In both positive and negative nitrogen balance, protein requirements are greater than usual. Protein is important in the healing of wounds, in the prevention of infection, and in numerous other processes.

Normal protein needs or the Recommended Dietary Allowance (RDA) for protein is set at 0.8 grams per kilogram of body weight for healthy adults. This value is considered by most to be far more accurate than the wide range of protein recommended by the World Health Organization (WHO), which suggests a protein intake of 10%–35% of total calories. Individualized estimates of protein requirements should be based on body weight, age, and health status. The WHO dietary goal is important in determining the overall protein level needs in the diet of the general population and should not be overlooked. As mentioned previously, protein needs increase during growth and pregnancy/lactation; with physical stress such as burns, infections, and surgery; and during periods of exercise. These needs can vary from 1.0 to 1.5 grams per kilogram of body weight, or possibly even higher.

Protein quality is not the same for all protein-containing foods. The presence and quantity of the essential amino acids determine the protein quality of a food. If a food contains a large amount of the essential amino acids it is considered a higher quality protein source. There are a number of methods available to determine protein quality. The method known as protein efficiency ratio (PER) is a measurement of the ability of a protein to support the growth of a weanling rat. It represents the ratio of weight gain to the amount of protein consumed. A potential disadvantage of this method includes the reliability of comparing the requirements of a rat to those of humans for

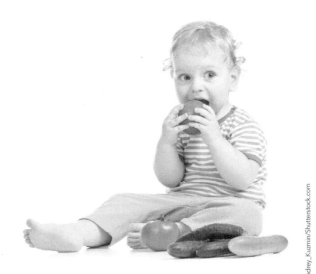

This child is in positive nitrogen balance for his growth needs.

growth and body maintenance. A second method is net protein utilization (NPU), which is the ratio of the nitrogen used for tissue formation as it compares to the amount of nitrogen digested. The third method is called biological value (BV). BV measures the amount of nitrogen retained as it compares to the amount of nitrogen absorbed. The BV and the NPU methods reflect both availability and digestibility, and also provide an accurate appraisal of maintenance needs. In the method known as Protein Digestibility Corrected Amino Acid Score (PDCAAS), the Amino Acid Score includes a digestibility component. The PDCAAS is the measure of protein quality that is currently accepted, based on determinations derived from experiments with animals. Animal products and many soy products are highly digestible and readily absorbed (90%). Grain and vegetable proteins are less digestible and have a lower score of 60%–90%. The Amino Acid Score (AAS) is a chemical rating method that is fast, consistent, and relatively inexpensive. This testing method measures the indispensable amino acids present in a protein and compares these values with a reference protein. The protein is rated based on the absence or the presence of the most limiting indispensable amino acid.

The numerous methods used to measure protein quality are beneficial to determine the protein quality that is available to population groups who may not have good quality protein sources. These methods are not currently used in planning diets for individuals.

Insufficient Protein Intakes

For the most part, protein intake in the United States is adequate to excessive, while in many other countries protein intake is inadequate. When too little protein is consumed a condition known as protein-energy malnutrition (PEM) results. There are two types of PEM: **Kwashiorkor** and **Marasmus**. Kwashiorkor is a deficiency of high-quality protein that occurs even though adequate calories are consumed, and is seen especially in children living in developing countries. A visible characteristic in these children is a swollen belly that is caused by an accumulation of fluids in the abdominal region. Kwashiorkor can result in retarded growth. (Figure 5.5) Marasmus, on the other hand, results from an inadequate intake of both protein and calories. This type of PEM is seen in individuals who live in low-income areas and in the elderly population. The physiological changes caused by aging, poor living conditions, and low income level subsistence are all factors that contribute to PEM in the elderly.[1] Marasmus characteristically causes a wasted skeletal appearance, and if left untreated, also decreases intellectual ability. (Figure 5.6) Table 5.2 outlines the features of Marasmus and Kwashiorkor.

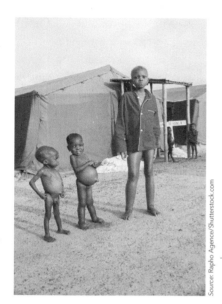

FIGURE 5.5 Kwashiorkor is characterized by a bloated belly

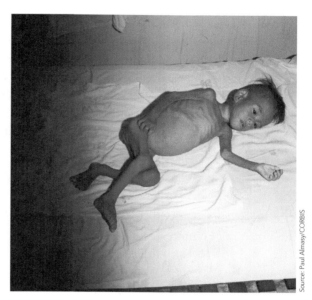

FIGURE 5.6 Marasmus presents as severe wasting

TABLE 5.2 Characteristics of Marasmus and Kwashiorkor	
Marasmus	**Kwashiorkor**
1. The onset is early, usually in the first year of life.	1. Its onset is later, (especially after breast-feeding is stopped), typically from the age of 1–3 years.
2. Growth failure is more pronounced.	2. Growth failure is not very pronounced.
3. There is no edema.	3. Edema is present.
4. Severe muscle wasting and a loss of fat occur.	4. There is some muscle wasting, and lesser amount of fat loss.
5. Skin changes are seen less frequently.	5. Red boils and patches are classic symptoms.
6. The liver is not infiltrated with fat.	6. A fatty liver is seen.
7. Recovery is much longer.	7. The recovery period is shorter with appropriate nutrition therapy.
8. Hair is sparse and dry.	8. Hair is dry and brittle with changes in color.

Excessive Protein Intakes

High protein intakes occur when protein levels reach more than two times the RDA. Several consequences can result from excessive protein intake. The first, and most obvious, is the potential for weight gain due to a higher caloric intake. Since most protein foods come from animal products, saturated fat and cholesterol intake can also be higher than desired. Choosing lower-fat animal proteins may reduce the fat intake but still leave a high level of protein in the diet.

High protein intakes may also have a dehydrating effect on the body. Six to seven times more water is needed to process proteins than to process fats and carbohydrates. The extra nitrogen that is included in protein must also be removed from the body through the kidneys. The kidneys have to excrete more nitrogen so a greater demand is placed on them which, over time, can cause irreparable damage to the kidneys. Another problem associated with higher protein intake involves liver function. One of the liver's many functions is to remove nitrogen from amino acids and to leave the resulting carbon, hydrogen, and oxygen for use as glucose or to be stored as fat (carbohydrates and fats only contain carbon, hydrogen, and oxygen). This additional task places a greater demand on the liver which, over time, may cause liver damage. The last problem related to higher protein intake is the potential for calcium loss from the bones that may lead to the weakening of the body's skeletal structure, resulting in an increased chance of fractures. Post-menopausal women who are already losing calcium in the bones due to changes in hormonal levels should be particularly concerned about osteoporosis. A lower ratio of animal protein to vegetable protein intake appears to be a key factor in the amount of bone loss in post-menopausal women.[2]

Protein Digestion

The process of protein digestion is similar to that of other nutrients: a large component is broken down to an absorbable unit. Large protein molecules must split apart to yield individual amino acids that are then absorbed into the body. Protein digestion is discussed at greater length in the sections that follow.

The Mouth

When food enters the mouth it is chewed, causing the particles to separate. No chemical digestion of protein occurs at this point, but protein foods are broken apart and the surface area for future protein degradation is increased.

The Stomach

The stomach is where protein digestion is initiated by hydrochloric acid. Stomach acid is responsible for denaturing the protein molecule (changing its structure) and for making it more accessible to enzyme attack. Once the protein has undergone the denaturation process, enzymes can begin to break apart the large protein molecule. The enzyme necessary for protein digestion is inactive and must be activated by the presence of acid. Stomach acid prepares the protein for breakdown and activates the enzyme pepsin that is needed to start protein digestion.

The Intestines

Further and more complete digestion of proteins to amino acids takes place in the small intestine. Here, the neutralization of the stomach contents occurs (see Chapter 8), and additional enzymes continue to digest protein by mixing with the liquefied material in the small intestine to complete the digestion process. Once the amino acids are released from the protein molecule, they are ready to be absorbed into the small intestine (Figure 5.7). By the time the ingested material enters the large intestine, there is very little left to digest. Waste material is collected in the large intestine and then excreted.

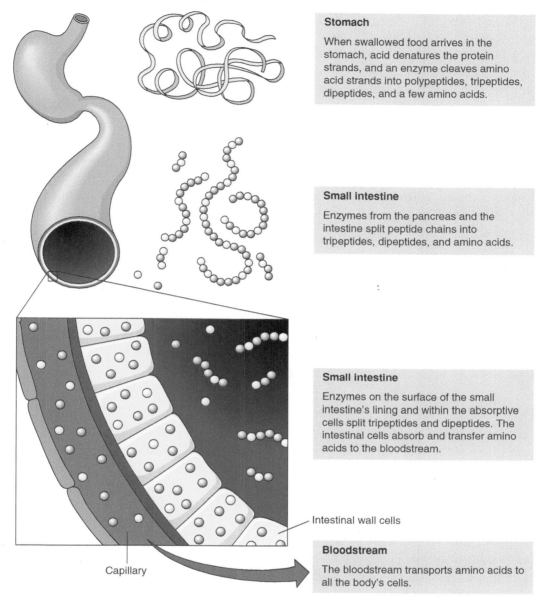

Stomach

When swallowed food arrives in the stomach, acid denatures the protein strands, and an enzyme cleaves amino acid strands into polypeptides, tripeptides, dipeptides, and a few amino acids.

Small intestine

Enzymes from the pancreas and the intestine split peptide chains into tripeptides, dipeptides, and amino acids.

Small intestine

Enzymes on the surface of the small intestine's lining and within the absorptive cells split tripeptides and dipeptides. The intestinal cells absorb and transfer amino acids to the bloodstream.

Intestinal wall cells

Bloodstream

The bloodstream transports amino acids to all the body's cells.

Capillary

FIGURE 5.7 Protein Digestion

Protein Metabolism

Once proteins are broken down into their component parts (amino acids), they are ready to be absorbed in the interior of the body. Amino acids that are absorbed through the intestinal cell wall then travel through the portal system to the liver. The liver determines the fate of the amino acid based on the body's needs. These amino acids may then become hormones or antibodies, or serve to replace certain structures such as skin or hair proteins. Body proteins are continually broken down and resynthesized. The cells lining the gastrointestinal tract are replaced every few days, whereas red blood cells last several months. The rate of synthesis and the breakdown of proteins in the body may be increased or decreased based on the body's needs. For example, the enzyme produced by the liver to break down alcohol speeds up when an individual consumes alcohol, and slows down if a person abstains from consumption.

The synthesis of proteins is similar to an assembly line process. Proteins are made up of long strings derived from twenty amino acids, which are put together in an array of combinations. When it is time for a protein to be assembled, all the necessary amino acids must be present. If an amino acid is missing or is in limited supply, the resultant protein may not be made. Since one transport mechanism is equally shared by all amino acids, the presence of an excess of one particular amino acid will most likely be absorbed at the expense of another amino acid in lesser supply. This absorption leads to the presence of inadequate amounts of a particular amino acid. If the quantity and/or type of amino acid is limited, the synthesis of a protein slows down, or in some cases stops.

A missing amino acid is referred to as a **limiting amino acid**. A limiting amino acid is an essential amino acid that is at its lowest concentration in relation to the body's need. The absence of an amino acid may have serious effects on the body. Hemoglobin, for example, contains the essential amino acid histidine. If histidine (the limiting amino acid) is inadequate in the body, hemoglobin will not be produced. Without adequate hemoglobin the blood cannot carry oxygen to the cells for energy production. Therefore, it is important that a diet contains a healthy blend of all the essential amino acids.

Vegetarianism

Foods that contain all the essential amino acids to make the proteins that the body needs are considered **complete protein sources**. Complete proteins exist in all animal products and in the non-animal product soy. Foods that lack one or more of the essential amino acids are said to be incomplete protein sources. Some individuals do not consume all the essential amino acids due to the consumption of **incomplete protein** source foods. Incomplete protein food products are those of plant origin, with the exception of soy protein.

Vegetarian Diets

The term vegetarian is generally used to describe individuals who do not consume the flesh of animals but who may eat animal by-products. There are three types of vegetarian diets that are generally recognized, and two of these diets include animal sources. The least restrictive vegetarian diet is the lacto-ovo vegetarian diet, which includes all plant products, dairy products, and also egg products. The second type is the lacto vegetarian diet that is similar to the lacto-ovo except it excludes egg products. The third type, and the most restrictive of the three, is the vegan diet. This plant-based diet eliminates all animal sources from the diet and can present a challenge in meeting nutritional requirements. Vegan diets should be carefully designed and monitored.

Vegan diets have increased in popularity over the last few decades. Approximately 1.7 million people in the United States now consider themselves to be vegan.[3] Individuals who follow a vegan diet must carefully evaluate the nutrients they fail to consume when they eliminate particular food groups and the calories that they need to replace. Samples of the Healthy Vegetarian Eating Patterns can be seen in Chapter 2 in Table 2.6.

Mutual Supplementation

Lacto-ovo and lacto vegetarian diets include animal by-products that provide adequate complete proteins. Vegan vegetarian diets often include sufficient quantities of soy protein for complete proteins. Vegan vegetarian diets also provide the necessary essential amino acids by including two incomplete plant sources and combining them to make a full complement of essential amino acids. Individual plant products often do not provide all the essential amino acids, yet when combined with another plant source form a complement of all the essential amino acids. An individual plant protein source is referred to as a **complementary protein** to another plant protein source because what one source lacks the other plant source contains. (Figure 5.8) The method of mixing together two complementary proteins to make a complete protein is known as mutual supplementation. Examples of this process are found in Table 5.3.

AN EXAMPLE OF MUTUAL SUPPLEMENTATION

In general, legumes provide plenty of the amino acids isoleucine (Ile) and lysine (Lys), but fall short in methionine (Met) and tryptophan (Trp). Grains have the opposite strengths and weaknesses, making them a perfect match for legumes.

	Ile	Lys	Met	Trp
Legumes				
Grains				
Together				

FIGURE 5.8 Complementary protein foods complement each other in their amino acid patterns

TABLE 5.3 Examples of Mutual Supplementation

Grains	Legumes And Nuts
Barley	Dried beans
Bulgur	Dried lentils
Cornmeal	Dried peas
Oats	Peanuts
Pasta	Soy products
Rice	Walnuts
Whole-grain breads	

Advantages of Vegan Diets

The vegan diet has many potential health benefits because it includes a high nutrient-dense selection of foods. It is typically lower in fat, particularly saturated fat.

No animal products are consumed and all of the fats are derived from plant products. The vegan diet is also devoid of cholesterol, due to the absence of animal products. It consists of a high content of fiber that is derived from fruits and vegetables, which provide both soluble and insoluble fibers. A higher concentration of phytochemicals and antioxidants is also present in the diet. When planned correctly, vegan diets can offer significant health benefits including a reduced risk of obesity, cardiovascular disease, hypercholesterolemia, hypertension, type 2 diabetes, colon cancer, diverticular disease, and gallstones. Table 5.4 provides an example of a creative vegan menu.

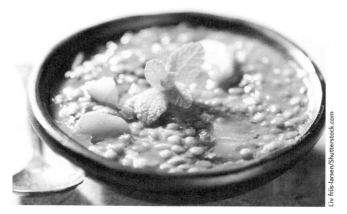

Liv friis-larsen/Shutterstock.com

Lentils and vegetables provide valuable protein, however, they are incomplete proteins as they do not provide all the essential amino acids. The addition of rice to the lentils would make a complete protein.

TABLE 5.4 Sample Vegan Menu

Quinoa Vegetable Miso Soup

Asian and Mushroom Salad

Seitan Steak with Braised Mushrooms

Wild Rice Medley

Stuffed Peppers with Cous Cous

Sweet Potato Biscuit with Strawberries and Glace Topping

Potential Disadvantages of Vegan Diets

The vegan diet frequently fails to provide adequate amounts of vitamin D, vitamin B_{12}, calcium, and iron. Riboflavin and zinc are also nutrients that must be carefully assessed in the vegan diet. The highest source of vitamin D is found in fortified dairy products, which vegans do not consume. Dairy products also contain high amounts of riboflavin. Fortunately, some sources of soy milk are fortified with vitamin D and can be used as a good replacement for cow's milk. Riboflavin intake can be increased by consuming whole grains, legumes, and green leafy vegetables. Vitamin B_{12}, which is found in animal products, is also an essential vitamin that is often lacking. A potential deficiency of vitamin B_{12} can be avoided with the consumption of products such as soy milk and breakfast cereals that are fortified with this vitamin. A diet rich in whole grains, legumes, nuts, and seeds can increase zinc content in the diet as well. Calcium requirements are most easily met with dairy products, plant products, and fortified foods. The best sources of calcium are dark green leafy vegetables, seeds, nuts, beans, fortified soy milk, cereals, and fortified fruit juices. Iron stores are usually also lower in vegans than in meat eaters because the form of iron present in plant products is nonheme iron rather than heme iron, which is more readily absorbed. The best plant sources of iron are legumes, fortified whole grain products, and dried fruits.[4] The health benefits of a vegan diet may outweigh the negatives when the diet is carefully and thoughtfully planned.

Soy Protein

Soybeans contain many beneficial nutrients and are highly adaptable to various recipes. They contain many B vitamins, and minerals such as calcium, phosphorus, and magnesium. Even though they are plant based, they contain complete protein that serves as an excellent substitute for meat. Soybeans also contain valuable phytoestrogens such as **isoflavones**. Phytoestrogens are chemical compounds in plants that act in a similar way to estrogens in the human body. Soy is touted for fiber, protein, and antioxidant contributions. A diet high in soy reduces the risk of heart disease, some forms of cancer, and osteoporosis, and helps in the treatment of menopausal symptoms.

The benefits of soy to heart health are promising. In many parts of the world where soy is an important part of the diet, the incidence of coronary artery disease is lower than in the United States. In 1991, there were approximately 238 deaths from cardiovascular disease for every 100,000 men in Japan, in comparison to a rate of 487 deaths for every 100,000 men in the United States. For women, the total number of deaths is lower, but the percentage of both Japanese and American women is similar to that of men.[4] The Anderson meta-analysis includes 38 studies (with more than 730 volunteers) involving the substitution of soy protein for animal protein in a variety of situations.

Results of these studies show:

- An average reduction in blood cholesterol levels by 9.3%
- An increase in HDL levels of 2.4%
- An average decrease in LDL levels of 12.3%[5]

Replacing animal protein with soy protein helps to lower blood cholesterol levels and improves the ratio of HDLs to LDLs. Soybeans and other similar legumes contain no cholesterol and are high in fiber. The FDA has approved a health claim that the inclusion of soy protein in a diet that is low in saturated fat and cholesterol may reduce the risk of coronary heart disease by lowering blood cholesterol levels.[6]

Soy may also contribute to the prevention of cancer. Reproductive cancers that include breast and prostate cancers make up the greatest percentage. Other cancers in women include uterine and ovarian cancers. In these hormone-related cancers, exposure to estrogen is blamed for increasing the risk of breast cancer, ovarian cancer, and uterine cancer, while exposure to testosterone is thought responsible for increasing the risk of prostate cancer. Soy consumption reduces exposure to estrogen binding sites in reproductive tissue by replacing natural estrogens with weaker phytoestrogens. This replacement leads to a decrease in carcinogenic effects from the natural estrogens or synthetic estrogens found in hormone replacement therapies.[7]

Soy also helps in the prevention and treatment of osteoporosis. Bones, like all body tissue, are constantly restored (older cells are replaced with newer ones). The sex hormones, estrogen and testosterone, and human growth hormone control this cycle. Estrogen preserves bones by preventing the reabsorption of excess amounts of cells. Testosterone stimulates the growth of stronger, denser bone tissue while the human growth hormone directs the pace of new cell production. The ingredient in soy that is credited for producing this activity is the isoflavone **genistein**. Isoflavones serve two purposes: they increase the body's ability to hold onto the calcium derived from the diet, and they supplement and act to preserve (similar to estrogen) and build bone (similar to testosterone). A study done by researchers Messina and Messina at Loma Linda University in California indicates that isoflavones retard bone loss almost as effectively as estrogen in animals whose ovaries had been removed.[8]

The relationship of soy to menopausal symptoms, particularly hot flashes, is also important. A hot flash is a sudden feeling of intense heat over the face and upper body, which is sometimes accompanied by a reddening of the skin and sweating. A decline in estrogen, which occurs during menopause, affects how the body regulates temperature. When estrogen is in short supply, the area in the brain that regulates body temperature by controlling the dilation and constriction of blood vessels does not operate effectively. The result is a hot flash. Soy contains phytoestrogens that are believed to replace the diminishing natural estrogens of the body.

The benefits derived from soy consumption are numerous. Soy protein may be incorporated into food products. Soy comes in a variety of forms including soymilk, which may be consumed by individuals with lactose intolerance to milk. Tofu (soybean curd) is a form of soy that is white in color and shaped into cakes. It is very bland in flavor and works well when combined with foods and seasonings with intense flavor. Tofu comes in a variety of textures and may be incorporated into fruit smoothies; used in a marinade with spices, oils and vinegars; and incorporated into vegetable stir-fries. Tempeh is a form of soy that is made from fermenting soybeans which are then shaped into cakes. It can be barbeque flavored and added to replace meat in meat dishes. Texturized vegetable protein (TVP) is made from the granules of isolated soy protein and then rehydrated before it is used in recipes such as vegetarian "burgers." Additional forms of soy include soy cheeses and soy ice cream.[9] Creativity, appropriate cooking techniques, and flavor enhancers can make the use of soy products a success.

Culinary Corner
Food Allergies

Food allergies are said to affect about 2% of the general population and as many as 6–8% of young children (many of whom outgrow the allergy). Any food may provoke a reaction, however relatively few foods are responsible for the vast majority of food-allergic reactions.[10] A food allergy can be defined as an immune system response to a food that the body mistakenly believes is harmful. A specific antibody called Immunoglobulin (IgE) is created, once the immune system decides that a particular food is harmful. IgE is a type of protein that acts as an antibody and circulates through the blood. It is believed that individuals have an inherited predisposition to form IgE against certain food items. When an individual consumes a particular food for which he/she has an IgE formed, the immune system releases massive amounts of chemicals, including histamine, to protect the body. These chemicals can affect the skin and many systems in the body including the respiratory, digestive, and cardiovascular systems. Although any food can trigger a reaction, eight foods are responsible for approximately 90% of food-allergic reactions:

- Milk
- Eggs
- Peanuts
- Tree nuts (e.g., walnuts, cashews)
- Fish
- Shellfish
- Soy
- Wheat

Food allergens are the food fractions responsible for allergic reactions. They are proteins within the food that are not usually broken down by cooking, stomach acids, or enzymes that digest food.

These proteins cross the gastrointestinal lining and go to target organs where they cause allergic reactions throughout the body. Itching, nausea, vomiting, diarrhea, pain, a drop in blood pressure, hives, swelling, and difficulty breathing may occur. The most severe reaction is called an anaphylactic shock, which is a potentially fatal immune response that may affect any body system.[11, 12]

The presence of food allergies in the US population is increasing. Food allergies can be classified as those that persist indefinitely and those that are transient. Certain foods are more likely than others to be tolerated in late childhood and adulthood.[13] In particular, peanut allergy has become much more common.[14]

Diagnosis of food allergy is best done by a systematic approach including history, laboratory studies, elimination diets, and food challenges. Food allergies are managed by educating the patient to avoid ingesting the responsible allergen, choose substitute foods and to initiate therapy in case of an unintended ingestion.[15] A person who has been diagnosed with a food allergy should consider the following:

- Look for unsuspected ingredients.
- Develop a plan, possibly with the assistance of a registered dietitian, to assure consumption of nutrients provided by the [avoided] food allergens.
- Seek out nutritious, palatable recipes and restaurants that omit the food allergen(s).
- Be prepared to handle an allergic reaction including carrying an EpiPen (a syringe of adrenaline-epinephrine that can be self-administered) at all times, if prescribed.
- Recognize early symptoms of a reaction.
- Teach others how they may help. Wear a medical alert bracelet.
- Get to an emergency room at the earliest signs of a reaction.

Chefs, restaurant staff, manufacturers, school staff, and the general public should be educated about food allergies and anaphylaxis. The importance of proper labeling and ingredient information is crucial.[16] Elimination of certain foods can lead to nutritional deficiencies. People living with a food allergy may need to make substitutions for foods that must be eliminated from the diet. Chefs can prepare creative, flavorful recipes using alternative foods as well. Some examples of allergenic foods and nutritionally similar substitutes are listed in Table 5.5.

In 2012 the Food Allergy and Anaphylaxis Network (FAAN) merged with the Food Allergy Initiative to form the Food Allergy Research and Education organization (FARE). FARE is a valuable source of information concerning food allergies. Professionals who have contributed information to this website are: Doctors, Registered Dietitians, Nurses and Chefs. The FARE website has information for consumers and chefs, including recipes, information on dining out and creating "allergy friendly" restaurant and school environments.[17]

Restaurants should have a food allergy management plan as well as training for employees. Guidelines for restaurants include:

- The ability to supply, upon request, a list of ingredients for the menu items
- Have an employee available who is able to answer questions and deal with special requests from guests with food allergies
- A thorough understanding of cross-contamination
- If an error in a special order occurs, the only acceptable way to address this is to discard the order and remake the menu item
- If a guest has an allergic reaction, call 911 and seek medical attention

For additional information, FARE offers a brochure entitled "Welcoming Guests with Food Allergies, which includes links to helpful videos for restaurant staff and management."[18]

The National Institute of Allergy and Infectious Diseases (NIAID), part of the National Institutes of Health, worked with 34 professional organizations, patient advocacy groups and federal agencies to develop new national guidelines for the diagnosis and management of food allergy, published in December 2010. *The Guidelines for the Diagnosis and Management of Food Allergy in the United States: Report of the NIAID-Sponsored Expert Panel*, reflects long-awaited agreement across medical specialties about what food allergy is and how to diagnose and treat it.[19]

TABLE 5.5 Allergenic Foods and Nutritionally Similar Substitutes	
Eggs in a recipe	– 1 t. baking powder, 1 T. liquid and 1 T. vinegar
	– 1 t. yeast dissolved in ¼ cup warm water
	– 1 ½ T. water, 1 ½ T. oil and 1 t. baking powder
	– 1 packet unflavored gelatin w/2 T. warm water
	– Commercial Product: Ener-G Egg Replacer
	– ¼ cup blended silken tofu
Peanut butter	Sunflower butter or soy butter
Milk	Soy milk
	High Protein Almond Milk
Wheat	Quinoa, amaranth, rice, millet

References

1   B. Blaylock, "Factors Contributing to Protein-Calorie Malnutrition in Older Adults," *Medsurg Nursing* 2 (1993): 397–401.

2   D. E. Sellmeyer, K. L. Stone, A. Sebastian, and S. R. Cummings, "A High Ratio of Dietary Animal to Vegetable Protein Increases the Rate of Bone Loss and the Risk of Fracture in Postmenopausal Women," *American Journal of Clinical Nutrition* 73 (2001): 118–122.

3   D. Aronson. "The Virtues of Vegan Nutrition and the Risks," *Today's Dietitian* 8 (2001): 46–51.

4   C. L. Larsson and G. K. Johansson, "Dietary Intake and Nutritional Status of Young Vegans and Omnivores in Sweden," *American Journal of Clinical Nutrition* 76 (2002): 100–106.

5   J. W. Anderson, et al., "Meta-Analysis of the Effects of Soy Protein on Serum Cholesterol," *New England Journal of Medicine* 333 (1995): 276–282.

6   Food and Drug Administration, "Food Labeling: Health Claims, Soy Protein and Coronary Heart Disease," HHS, Final Rule. *Fed Register* 64 (1999): 57700–57733.

7   C. A. Rinzler, *The Healing Power of Soy: The Enlightened Person's Guide to Nature's Wonder Food*, Rocklin, CA: Prima Publishing, 1998.

8   M. Messina and V. Messina, "Soyfoods, Soybean Isoflavones, and Bone Health: A Brief Overview," *Journal of Renal Nutrition* 10 (2000): 63–68.

9   S. Kapoor, *Professional Healthy Cooking*, New York, NY: John Wiley & Sons Inc., 1995.

10   H. A. Sampson, "Food Allergy," *Journal of Allergy Clinical Immunology* 111 (2003): 540S–547S.

11   Common Food Allergen Fact Sheet, 2003. http://www.foodallergy.org/allergens.html

12   *Food Allergy and Intolerances, NIAID Fact Sheet*, Office of Communications and Public Liaison National Institutes of Health, Bethesda, Maryland, June 2001.

13   S. Kagan, "Food Allergy: An Overview," *Environmental Health Perspective* 11 (2003): 223–226.

14   G. Lack, D. Fox, K. Northstone, and J. Golding, "Avon Longitudinal Study of Parents and Children Study Team," *New England Journal of Medicine* 348 (2003): 977–985.

15   H. A. Sampson, "Food Allergy," *Journal of Allergy Clinical Immunology* 111 (2003): 540S–547S.

16   Food Allergy Research Archives, 2003. http:www.foodallergy.org/research_archive/researcharchive.html

17   www.Foodallergy.org

18   http://www.foodallergy.org/resources/restaurants

19   Guidelines for the Diagnosis and Management of Food Allergy in the United States: Report of the NIAID-Sponsored Expert Panel, *Journal of Allergy and Clinical Immunology* 26 (2010): S1–58.

Put It into Practice

Define the Term

Provide the definition of homeostasis. Using the information in the "Protein Functions in the Body" section, list the ten functions of protein and determine if each function is structural or regulatory.

Myth vs. Fact

Determine if the following statement is a myth or fact and support your position with evidence from three research articles on the topic. *Statement: "It is impossible to get enough protein on a vegetarian diet."*

For each research article, summarize each component below.

    A. Abstract
    B. Methods
    C. Results
    D. Discussion
    E. Conclusions

The Menu

Develop four dinner meals for an upscale restaurant that would meet the needs of each of the following vegetarian diets: Vegan, Lacto, and Lacto Ovo. Each meal must include an appetizer, an entrée, a starch, a vegetable, and a dessert. List the sources of complete and incomplete protein, as well as any forms of mutual supplementation.

Website Review

Review the "Culinary Corner: Food Allergies" section in the textbook and then navigate the Food Allergy and Anaphylaxis Network website: www.foodallergy.org. List a few of the network's goals and accomplishments. List the eight foods that account for 90% of all food-allergic reactions and explain four unexpected or hidden food sources for each.

Build Your Career Toolbox

Review the textbook section entitled "Vegetarianism" and Table 5.4 Sample Vegan Menu. Develop a job description for a "Vegan Chef." Include salary range, education, and experience requirements. This person must provide vegan menu choices for an upscale hotel foodservice establishment serving breakfast, lunch, dinner, buffet catering, and room service.

Denzel's Case Study

Denzel is a 35-year-old man who has just been diagnosed with cancer. He has had one cycle of high-dose chemotherapy, and he will continue on this high dose treatment every other month for the next 6–8 months. Since getting diagnosed with cancer, Denzel has stopped eating meat and has become a vegetarian. He has said that there are a lot of foods that make him nauseous, and he has had some mouth pain that makes eating difficult. He said that most of the foods he's been eating are room temperature or cool, and he has found it easier to eat soft foods with the pain he's been having.

You are a personal chef, and Denzel's dietitian is hoping you can help him come up with a sample menu to help him better meet his energy and protein needs to prevent further weight loss. Denzel is excited about working with you so that you can come up with ways to help maintain his weight and keep his immune system strong during his treatment. His wife often cooks and bakes at home so she'll be helping him as well.

Wt: 220 lbs   Ht: 6'1"   BMI: 29 kg/m² (overweight)
Weight loss of 20 lbs over the past 2 months because of poor appetite

Dietitian Recommendations
   Calorie Needs: 2400–2600 (for weight maintenance)
   Protein Needs: 130–140 g/day
   Fat: 30%–35% of calories, <10% calories from saturated fat
   Fiber: 30–35 g/day

Other Recommendations: Spread protein foods throughout the day (a bit of protein in each meal/snack); try vegetarian protein sources (though he reports that he and his wife don't know how to cook them); include "healthy" fats; prevent further weight loss; avoid "high risk" foods like sushi, runny eggs, and other foods that may cause foodborne illness

24-hr Recall

Breakfast: 1 cup Rice Krispies cereal well soaked in 3/4 cup 2% milk, 1 banana, 12-ozs black coffee with 2 tbsp nonfat vanilla creamer, and 2 tsp sugar

Snack: 2 slices of soft wheat bread (untoasted), 2 tbsp apricot jam

Lunch: 1/2 cup cottage cheese, 1 cup canned peaches, 1/2 cup unsweetened applesauce; 1 slice of soft wheat bread with 1/4 avocado (sliced) with a pinch of salt

Dinner: 5-ozs boiled spaghetti (made with salt) mixed with 1 diced Roma tomato (raw), 2 tbsp olive oil, 1/2 cup soft steamed green beans, 1/4 cup steamed spinach, 2 tbsp cooked chickpeas, a pinch of salt and pepper; 1 navel orange

Snack: 1 dairy-free mango popsicle or 1/2 cup sorbet

Preferences: Vegetarian, doesn't like eggs but will eat them in baked goods; Nothing strong smelling (garlic, onions, strong herbs/spices, etc.); nothing crunchy or hard to chew; wants to limit dairy products to no more than 1–2 cups per day; interested in making smoothies that he can bring to the treatment center to have during his treatments; no reported food allergies

Study Guide

Student Name _____   **Date** _____

Course Section _____   **Chapter** _____

TERMINOLOGY

Edema_____	A. The measure of protein intake in the diet contrasted with that which is used and excreted by the body
Marasmus_____	B. A deficiency of high-quality protein which can result in retarded growth
Nitrogen balance_____	C. An amino acid that must be supplied by the diet because the body cannot make them in sufficient quantities
Essential amino acid_____	D. To change the structural configuration of a protein
Complementary protein_____	E. The retention of fluid in the body
Homeostasis_____	F. The building blocks of protein
Complete protein_____	G. A severe deficiency of protein and calories in the diet, often characterized by a wasted skeletal appearance
Kwashiorkor_____	H. Two food sources providing an amino acid profile so that all essential amino acids are present
Amino acid_____	I. A balance of bodily functions
Denature_____	J. A food that contains all the essential amino acids

Student Name _____   **Date** _____

Course Section _____   **Chapter** _____

NITROGEN BALANCE AND PROTEIN REQUIREMENTS

Define:

Nitrogen Balance-

Positive Nitrogen Balance-

Negative Nitrogen Balance-

Determine whether the following conditions are examples of positive, negative, or nitrogen balance and explain your reason for each. Using the formula reviewed in the chapter, calculate the grams of protein needed per day for each individual according to their RDA:

1. A pregnant woman, weighs 140 pounds. RDA: 1.5gm/kg

2. A 2-year-old child, weighs 36 pounds. RDA: 1.3gm/kg

3. A marathon runner, weighs 150 pounds. RDA: 1.4gm/kg

4. A cancer patient, weighs 130 pounds. RDA: 1.2gm/kg

5. A healthy adult, weighs 145 pounds. RDA: .8gm/kg

Student Name _____   **Date** _____

Course Section _____   **Chapter** _____

"FOOD CHOICE" MENU PLANNING

Individual menu plan_____

Develop a one day meal plan including breakfast, lunch, one snack and dinner for one of the individuals listed on the previous page. Using Appendix B "Choose Your Foods Lists for Meal Planning" in your text book, calculate the grams of protein in the entire menu. You must meet the protein needs of this individual.

Meal	Grams of Protein

TOTAL PROTEIN_____ gm

Student Name _____   Date _____

Course Section _____   Chapter _____

CASE STUDY DISCUSSION

Denzel's Case Study: Staying Strong When Health Is Compromised

Review the sections in Chapter 5 on "Protein Requirements" and "Vegetarianism". After reading the case study, use the information to answer the following questions:

1. Is Denzel in nitrogen balance? Why or why not?

2. What general dietary recommendations would you provide Denzel to help him meet his protein needs while following a vegetarian diet and keep his immune system strong during his illness?

3. Using Table 5.3 "Examples of Mutual Supplementation" describe 5 vegan meals for Denzel and his wife to prepare which combine Grains + Legumes and Nuts to create a complete protein source.

Student Name _____ Date _____

Course Section _____ Chapter _____

PRACTICE TEST

Select the best answer.

1. The element contained in protein and not in carbohydrates or fats is
   a. carbon
   b. hydrogen
   c. oxygen
   d. nitrogen

2. Proteins are made up of
   a. amino acids
   b. fatty acids
   c. monosaccharides
   d. triglycerides

3. An essential amino acid
   a. is found in all foods
   b. must be obtained in the diet
   c. can be manufactured by the body
   d. is needed in large quantities

4. Which of the following is known as a chemical messenger?
   a. enzyme
   b. hormone
   c. antibody
   d. ketone

5. The condition where fluids collect in the tissues and is retained there is called
   a. edema
   b. fluid overload
   c. hypertension
   d. bloating

Student Name _____   Date _____

Course Section _____   Chapter _____

TRUE OR FALSE

_____ A deficiency of protein but not calories can lead to kwashiorkor.

_____ All plant proteins are incomplete proteins.

_____ Eggs and dairy products are part of a lacto-ovo vegetarian diet.

_____ Regulatory proteins maintain homeostasis.

_____ An antibody is produced by the body in response to an antigen.

List the 8 most common food allergens.

- _____
- _____
- _____
- _____
- _____
- _____
- _____
- _____

Calculate the recommended amount of protein per day for a college student who weighs 180 pounds and the RDA is .8gm/kg.

Calculate the recommended amount of protein per day for an athlete who weighs 210 pounds and the RDA is 1.5gm/kg.

Calculate the calories, from protein only, in the following meal:

3 oz fish (21 grams)

1 medium baked potato (4 grams)

1 cup green beans (4 grams)

1 cup skim milk (8 grams)

Vitamins

6

KEY TERMS

Anticoagulant
Bioavailability
Carcinogenesis
Carotenoids
Cholecalciferol
Coenzymes
Cofactor
Deficiency
Epidemiology

Epithelial
Ergocalciferol
Fat-soluble vitamin
Hyperkeratosis
Malabsorption
Menaquinone
Micronutrient
Neuromuscular
Osteomalacia

Phylloquinone
Prothrombin
Rickets
Thrombin
Tocopherol
Toxicity
Vitamins
Water-soluble vitamin
Xerophthalmia

Introduction

Vitamins are essential nutrients. They are required by the body and are obtained primarily through the diet. The daily dosage of vitamins needed is very small. Vitamins are measured in milligrams and micrograms, rather than in grams. Vitamins are considered **micronutrients**. Vitamins provide no caloric value. Many are present in the body to assist with protein, carbohydrate, and lipid breakdown, although they contribute no energy value in and of themselves. Vitamins are important for most body processes and they help to promote and regulate chemical reactions in the body. Vitamins also play a role in building body structures such as bones and teeth. They are organic compounds, in contrast to water and minerals, which are inorganic.

Vitamins were often discovered by accident. The classic tale of British sailors who developed bleeding gums, and who lost their teeth during long sea voyages, is well known. Not familiar with the effects of vitamins and vitamin deficiencies at that time, sailors tried a variety of foods to alleviate the problem, and eventually discovered that if they drank lime juice every day the symptoms ceased. Hence, the term "limey" is often used to describe British sailors.

As early as Roman times, the effects of vitamin D deficiency were seen in children who suffered from skeletal deformities (bowed legs). This vitamin D deficiency disease came to be known as rickets. In the 1800s, it was discovered that consuming cod liver oil could prevent the development of rickets, yet it took another 100 years before scientists identified that vitamin D was the component responsible for curing rickets.

Vitamins can be broken down into two categories: **fat-soluble** and **water-soluble** vitamins. The fat-soluble vitamins include vitamins A, D, E, and K, and the water-soluble vitamins consist of vitamin B complex and vitamin C. Each category of vitamins has its own unique absorption and transportation properties, and is stored and excreted differently. The body's need for a particular vitamin in the diet is dependent upon its use and storage in the body. Table 6.1 provides a summary of the two vitamin categories.

TABLE 6.1 Overall Summary Tables of Water-soluble and Fat-soluble Vitamins		
	Water-Soluble	Fat-Soluble
Absorption	Directly into blood	First in lymph, then blood
Transport carriers	Travel freely	May require protein
Storage	Circulate in water-filled parts of the body	Trapped in cells associated with fat
Excretion	Kidneys remove excess in the urine	Remain in fat-storage sites
Toxicity	Possible if supplements are consumed	Likely if supplements are consumed
Requirements	Frequent doses (daily or every other day)	Periodic doses (several times per week)

Body Regulation

It is important to know how vitamins are absorbed into the body and then used. The term bioavailability refers to how well a nutrient can be absorbed and used by the body. For most nutrients the degree of bioavailability increases when nutrients are consumed in foods rather than in their simple form. The presence of other nutrients in foods usually helps to enhance the absorption of vitamins. Milk, for example, is a good source of calcium. Manufacturers have added vitamin D to milk because vitamin D and calcium work together in absorption and function. A simple supplement of calcium may not result in as high a bioavailability of calcium as when calcium is consumed in vitamin D fortified milk.

The bioavailability of vitamins may vary from 40%–90%. Determining the bioavailability of a vitamin is not an easy process because of the many factors that influence the absorption and utilization of vitamins. Such factors include:

- The efficiency of digestion of energy yielding nutrients and the time of transit through the GI tract
- The previous nutrient intake and nutrition status
- The other foods simultaneously consumed

- The method of food preparation (raw, cooked, processed)
- The source of the nutrient (synthetic, fortified, naturally occurring)

There is tremendous interaction between vitamins and other dietary components. Although vitamins do not work in isolation, it is easiest to discuss them individually and to clearly delineate their functions, sources, and intakes, and the effects of their deficiencies and toxicities.

Fat-Soluble Vitamins

There are four fat-soluble vitamins: vitamin A, vitamin D, vitamin E, and vitamin K. Although each vitamin has its own distinct set of functions, some generalities can be made about the group as a whole. Vitamins are present in the fatty portions of foods and in the oils that an individual consumes. Fat-soluble vitamins can only be absorbed if bile is present in the small intestinal tract. After their absorption, they are transported by chylomicrons in the lymphatic system and stored in the liver and in the adipose tissue (fatty tissues). They are not excreted in the urine. A daily intake of fat-soluble vitamins is not as essential as the intake of water-soluble vitamins. Deficiencies of fat-soluble vitamins are rare in healthy individuals, due to the body's storage capacity of these vitamins. Deficiencies can be seen in diets that are very low in fat or in a person who has a malabsorption problem in the intestinal tract. Another factor that may precipitate a deficiency in fat-soluble vitamins is a protein deficiency known as Kwashiorkor (the nutritional disease seen in infants and children characterized by fluid retention in the abdominal region). Liver disease can also influence or precipitate a deficiency when there is no bile produced. Toxicity issues are of even greater concern. When fat-soluble vitamins are stored, and continue to build up in the liver and adipose tissue, toxicity problems may arise. This problem is uncommon unless excessive vitamin supplements are included in a diet. The fat-soluble vitamins will now be discussed individually. (See Table 6.2 for the functions, deficiencies, and toxicities, and sources of fat-soluble vitamins.)

TABLE 6.2 The Functions, Deficiencies, and Toxicities and Sources of Fat-soluble Vitamins

Fat-Soluble				
Name	Function	Deficiency	Toxicity	Sources
Vitamin A (retinol, retinal, retinoic acid)	vision, epithelial cells, mucous membranes, bone/tooth growth, reproduction, immunity	night blindness, hyperkeratosis, anemia, diarrhea, cessation of bone growth, impaired enamel formation, tooth decay, depression, infections	red blood cell breakage, bone pain, growth retardation, headaches, nausea, vomiting, diarrhea, blurred vision, muscle weakness, fatigue, dry skin, hair loss, liver damage, birth defects	fortified dairy foods, eggs, liver, beta-carotene in dark, green leafy vegetables and deep orange fruits and vegetables
Vitamin D (calciferol, cholecalciferol, dihydroxy vitamin D, cholesterol is precursor)	bone mineralization	abnormal growth, bowed legs, joint pain, malformed teeth, muscle spasms	elevated blood calcium, soft tissue calcification, excessive thirst, headaches, nausea, loss of appetite, kidney stones	self-synthesis with sunlight, fortified milk products, eggs, liver, sardines, fortified milk alternatives such as soy milk, almond milk.

(Continued)

TABLE 6.2 The Functions, Deficiencies, and Toxicities and Sources of Fat-soluble Vitamins (*Continued*)

Fat-Soluble				
Name	Function	Deficiency	Toxicity	Sources
Vitamin E (tocoperol, a-tocopherol)	antioxidant, cell membrane stability, oxidation reactions, protects vitamin A and PUFAs	anemia, breakage of red blood cells, leg cramps, weakness	mental/physical retardation, nausea, blurred vision, fatigue, enhances anti-clotting medication	polyunsaturated plant oils, green and leafy vegetables, wheat germ, whole grains, nuts, seeds
Vitamin K (phylloquinone, naphthoquinone)	synthesis of blood-clotting proteins, proteins involved in bone mineralization	hemorrhage, poor mineralization of bones	interferes with anti-clotting medication	synthesized by intestinal bacteria, green leafy vegetables, soybeans, vegetable oils

Vitamin A

Vitamin A was the first fat-soluble vitamin to be discovered. This vitamin takes on three active forms in the body: retinol, retinal, and retinoic acid. Together these compounds form the group known as retinoids. Retinoids are found in animal products as retinyl esters, and are converted to retinol in the intestine. Vitamin A is also found in plant sources in the form of carotenoids (a plant pigment referred to as provitamin A). This pigment can then be converted by the liver into active vitamin A. The most important carotenoid is beta-carotene. Beta-carotene is found in deep orange and yellow fruits and vegetables. Once absorbed, vitamin A is sent to the liver. It can be stored in the liver, or when needed, it can be picked up and transported into the blood by a special retinol building protein. Each cell then has its own protein receptor, which enables the vitamin to enter the cell.

Vitamin A has many functions, but it is most well-known for its contribution to vision. Light entering the eye must be changed into nerve impulses that are further converted by the brain into visual images. The transforming

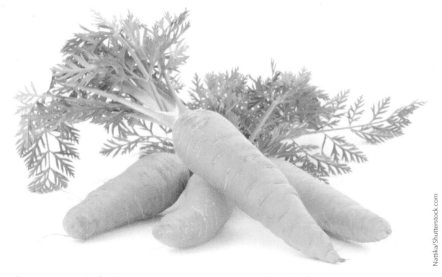

Nattika/Shutterstock.com

Carrots contain beta-carotene, a precursor to vitamin A.

molecule responsible for this is a pigment known as rhodopsin, which is found inside the cells of the retina. Rhodopsin contains retinal that separates itself from rhodopsin after it absorbs light. The remaining part of rhodopsin, known as opsin, then changes and sends a nerve impulse to the brain to identify the image. Retinal can then rejoin with opsin to form the pigment rhodopsin. Some of the retinal does become oxidized and is then no longer useful. When vitamin A is deficient, vision is impaired and a condition known as night blindness occurs. Night blindness is an early sign of vitamin A deficiency and is characterized by an inability to see in dim light, or a slow recovery of vision after observing a flash of bright light at night (similar to the effect produced on the eyes by the high beams of an approaching car).

Other functions of vitamin A are also of great importance. These contributions include the maintenance of healthy skin and epithelial tissue, immunity, the support of reproduction, and the growth of the body. Retinoic acid acts much like a hormone in the process of cell differentiation and contributes to the health and maintenance of the epithelial tissue. The epithelial tissue covers all body surfaces, both inside and out. Inside, it protects the mucous membranes found in areas such as the mouth, stomach, intestine, and lungs. On the outer surface, the epithelial tissue is what is known as the skin. Advances in medicine incorporating vitamin A derivatives have brought about treatments for skin ailments such as acne. Vitamin A aids in immunity by maintaining healthy epithelial tissue that fights infection from bacterial and viral attacks. The vitamin A form known as retinol is primarily involved in reproductive functions such as sperm production and fetal development. Vitamin A has a definitive role in bone development as it assists in breaking down old bone so that newer, stronger bones can develop.

A list of the functions of vitamin A would not be complete without the mention of beta-carotene. Beta-carotene is a naturally occurring orange pigment in the carotinoid family that is found in plants, and which the body is able to convert to vitamin A (referred to as a precursor to vitamin A or provitamin A). Beta-carotene that is left intact (not used to make vitamin A), functions as an antioxidant to protect the body against disease such as certain forms of cancers. They function at the cellular level to protect cell membranes from oxidation and to inhibit the growth of cancer cells.

A deficiency of vitamin A is a well-known problem in developing countries. Approximately 250,000 million preschool children suffer from vitamin A deficiency. Many of these children become permanently blind and many die within one year of losing their vision. Death is generally due to infectious diseases that might easily be treated in developed countries.[1]

Up to a year's supply of vitamin A can be stored in the body (90% of which is found in the liver). Deficiency symptoms will appear when this supply is depleted. In addition to night blindness, diseases such as xerophthalmia and hyperkeratosis may occur. Xerophthalmia is caused when vitamin A is not sufficiently present to allow the epithelial cells to produce mucus. The eye becomes very dry and leaves the cornea susceptible to infection and hardening, resulting in a permanent loss of vision. Hyperkeratosis is characterized by rough and bumpy skin resulting from a buildup of the protein keratin in hair follicles. This disease can also interfere with the normal function of sweat glands and make the skin very dry. In hyperkeratosis, mucus production may be decreased in the epithelial cells of the mouth, the eyes and other tissues as well, which can then lead to increased chances of infections in the respiratory and urinary tracts. Vitamin A deficiency may take one to two years to appear, but once the deficiency is apparent, the effects are pronounced and severe. Individuals at risk for vitamin A deficiency include the elderly with low nutrient intakes, newborn or premature infants with lower liver stores of the vitamin, and young children with low intakes of fruits and vegetables. Individuals with Crohn's disease, celiac disease or diseases of the liver, pancreas, or gall bladder may be at risk due to a malabsorption of fat.

Toxicity is rare if a balanced diet is consumed and no supplements are added. Children are most susceptible to deficiency and more prone to toxicities due to their more limited vitamin A requirements. Vitamin A toxicity in a developing fetus can cause birth defects. Beta-carotene, when converted to vitamin A, although not toxic, can build up in fat deposits under the skin to give the skin a yellowish tint.

The best sources of vitamin A are foods of animal origin such as liver, dairy products, and eggs. Plants do not contain vitamin A, but do contain carotene. Plant products that are dark green and deep orange in color are sources of beta-carotene. The RDA for vitamin A varies based on age and gender. Vitamin A and beta-carotene requirements are expressed in retinol activity equivalents (RAE: 1 RAE = 1 microgram retinol = 12 micrograms of beta-carotene).

Vitamin D

Vitamin D is a vitamin unlike the others because it can be produced in the body. Vitamin D occurs in two forms: cholecalciferol and ergocalciferol. The former is found in animal products and the latter in plant products. Vitamin D is frequently referred to as the "sunshine" vitamin because the liver produces a vitamin D precursor that can be converted to vitamin D with the assistance of the ultraviolet rays of the sun and the kidneys. Vitamin D is referred to as a vitamin but actually works as a hormone in the body. Vitamin D receptors are found on every tissue in the body and are the primary regulator for at least 1,000 genes in the body.[2]

The major association of vitamin D with bone growth and development is also well documented. Vitamin D plays an active part in a team of nutrients and compounds that work together to support bone growth and maintenance. These vitamins include A, C, and K, the hormones parathormone and calcitonin, the protein collagen, and the minerals calcium, phosphorus, magnesium, and fluoride. The key role of vitamin D is to make calcium and phosphorus available in the blood that surrounds the bones, and allow the bones to absorb and deposit the necessary minerals to form a denser bone structure. Vitamin D works to maintain calcium levels in the blood and bones. Acting as a hormone, vitamin D can mobilize calcium from the bones into the blood and increase the absorption of calcium from the digestive tract. It can also influence the kidneys in recycling calcium back to the blood rather than excreting it in the urine. The functions of vitamin D are numerous and have great health implications, including contributions in the brain and the nervous system, the pancreas, the skin, the muscles and cartilage, and in the reproductive organs.[3] There has been much research on some of the lesser known health benefits of vitamin D. Two of these benefits include vitamin D's relationship to cancer prevention and the prevention/treatment of cardiovascular disease. Although the results of studies related to cancer are inconsistent, most conclude that when vitamin D levels are low in the blood, supplementation to bring the levels back to normal do, in fact, reduce the incidence of some forms of cancer (breast and colorectal). On the other hand, if blood levels are normal, supplementation with a vitamin D supplement has no apparent effect and these high levels seem to increase the risk.[4, 5] Bringing blood levels of vitamin D back to normal has also shown some benefit in the treatment of hypertension and cardiovascular disease.[6]

A deficiency in vitamin D may also result in calcium deficiency because vitamin D is necessary for calcium absorption. A low blood calcium level and abnormal bone development in children may result in the disease known as rickets. When bones do not calcify as they should, growth retardation and abnormalities of the skeletal system occur. Weakened bones bend in an attempt to support the body's weight and cause a bowed-leg appearance. In adults this disease is known as osteomalacia, or adult rickets. When calcium is released from the bones to keep blood levels normal, the bones become weak and may fracture in the weight-bearing bones such as the hips and spine. Fifty percent of women over age 50 will have a bone fracture resulting in approximately $131 billion dollars in health care costs alone.[7] Vitamin D, in conjunction with calcium, can improve bone mass density although there is no complete agreement as to the actual requirements needed to do so. To better understand the deficiency problems associated with vitamin D, it is suggested that vitamin levels in the blood should be assessed. According to NHANES III, there is an increase in mortality with both low and high levels of serum vitamin D.[8]

Toxicities in vitamin D show their effects in the soft tissues of the body. Calcium absorption from the GI tract is increased and calcium from the bone is released into the surrounding blood. High blood calcium levels can deposit in the soft tissue to form stones. The kidneys are particularly susceptible to these calcium deposits. There may also be cardiovascular damage from high blood calcium levels. Although the intake of vitamin D from food sources is not known to cause toxicity, vitamin D is recognized as one of the most toxic of all the vitamins. Consuming four to five times the RDA of vitamin D can result in toxicity-related problems.

The recommendation for vitamin D is set for food sources only. The DRI is set to establish the recommended levels of the vitamin in the blood. Exposure to sunlight may meet the body's needs for vitamin D, although this source is not considered when the DRI is set because it cannot be quantified and shows high variations. An individual's ability to obtain vitamin D through sunlight depends on a number of factors such as skin color, climate and season, clothing, use of sun-blocking lotions (SPF of 8 or above), the amount of pollution (smog), and the presence of tall buildings. Most individuals should not rely on sun exposure for adequate vitamin D levels because of the accompanying increased risk of skin cancers. Overexposure to the sun cannot cause vitamin D toxicity because the skin's mechanism for converting the precursor to an active vitamin D form is prevented. Vitamin D is also found naturally in food sources such as egg yolks, liver, fatty fish, and butter.

Vitamin E

In the early part of the twentieth century, vitamin E was identified as a fat-soluble component of grains that was necessary for reproduction in rats. Many years later it was also determined that it was needed for human reproduction. The biologically active form of vitamin E has the chemical name tocopherol (which means to bring forth birth). There are four tocopherol compounds: alpha, beta, gamma, and delta. Of these compounds, alpha tocopherol is the most abundant and biologically active in nature.

The primary function of vitamin E is that of an antioxidant. In many chemical reactions that occur in the body, harmful compounds known as free radicals are created. Free radicals have been shown to cause cell damage in the body and to lead to the development of chronic diseases. It is the job of vitamin E, along with other antioxidant nutrients, to neutralize these free radicals before cell damage can occur. Vitamin E will donate an electron to a free radical, hence stabilizing it so no damage can be caused to other molecules in the body. Vitamin E is particularly important in preventing the oxidation of polyunsaturated fatty acids (PUFA) and in helping to maintain the integrity of the cell membrane in nerve cells, red blood cells, immune system cells, or any other cell in the body. Vitamin E also protects LDLs from oxidative damage and thus can lower the risk for developing heart disease.[9] It also helps to protect cells from damage that may be caused by pollutants such as smog or cigarette smoke. Vitamin E works with the mineral selenium to protect cells from oxidative damage, and interacts with vitamin C to rebuild itself.

Deficiencies of vitamin E are very rare because this vitamin is contained in most food supplies and is stored in many of the body's tissues. If a deficiency arose, changes in red blood cells and nerve tissues would result. Red blood cells would rupture, because of the weakening of the cell membrane from PUFA oxidation, and this would lead to anemia. Prolonged vitamin E deficiency can cause neuromuscular problems of the spinal cord and of the eye's retina. Symptoms of vitamin E deficiency include loss of muscle coordination and reflexes, and impaired vision and speech. Deficiencies may occur in individuals who consume low-fat diets for extended periods of time, in those with fat malabsorption due to cystic fibrosis, and in premature infants. Vitamin E toxicity is uncommon and its effects are not as serious as those of vitamin A and D. Doses exceeding 320 times the RDA have shown only few side effects.[10] Extremely large doses of this vitamin may interfere with the blood clotting action of vitamin K, and individuals who take blood-thinning medications should avoid vitamin E supplements.

The RDA for vitamin E is given in tocopherol equivalents (TE). In food, one TE equals 1 mg of active vitamin E. In vitamin E supplements, the term international unit (IU) may be used on the labels. For this situation, 1 IU of natural vitamin E is equivalent to 0.67 mg TE. In the synthetic form, 1 IU is equal to 0.45 TE. An individual who consumes larger amounts of PUFA needs a higher intake of vitamin E in the diet. Vitamin E and PUFA are typically found in food sources such as vegetable oils and products made from vegetable oils (margarine and salad dressings). Animal fats contain little vitamin E, but many fruits, nuts, seeds and vegetables serve as good sources of this vitamin. Vitamin E is absorbed with fat in the diet and then incorporated into the chylomicrons. Most of the vitamin E is transported to the liver, transferred to VLDLs and LDLs and sent into the blood to the tissues. Excess vitamin E is stored primarily in the adipose tissue, unlike vitamins A and D, which are mainly stored in the liver.

Vitamin K

The last fat-soluble vitamin, vitamin K, was also discovered inadvertently when chicks that were fed a vitamin K-deficient diet developed a bleeding disorder that only disappeared when an extract from green plants was introduced into the diet. The name vitamin K is derived from the Danish word koagulation (coagulation or blood clotting). The primary function of vitamin K in the body is blood clotting. Vitamin K activates several proteins that are involved in the formation of a blood clot. The most well-known of these proteins is **prothrombin**, which is manufactured by the liver as a precursor to **thrombin**. Whether from injuries, or from normal wear and tear, blood vessels break and blood loss ensues. Blood clotting is necessary to repair such injuries.

Another function of vitamin K is the production of bone proteins. Vitamin K helps minerals bind to proteins in the bone and to protect against **osteoporosis**. Diets high in vitamin K may be associated with a reduction in bone fractures and a vitamin K supplementation may increase bone density in individuals with osteoporosis.[11]

Vitamin K is found both in animal and plant sources. The plant form of vitamin K is called **phylloquinone**, while the form of vitamin K that is synthesized by bacteria in the large intestine, and found in animal products, is known as **menaquinone**.

A secondary vitamin K deficiency may occur when there is a fat malabsorption problem in the body because of the connection between fat and bile production. Inadequate fat absorption reduces bile production and limits the absorption of vitamin K. The use of antibiotics also destroys vitamin K-producing bacteria that are naturally present in the intestinal tract. **Anticoagulant** medication, used in the treatment of strokes and heart attacks, can interfere with vitamin K metabolism and activity as well. If a deficiency does arise, it can prove to be fatal if the blood fails to clot. Vitamin K supplements are given to newborns orally, or by injection, because of their sterile digestive tract (devoid of vitamin K-producing bacteria). This supplement provides the infant with an adequate supply of vitamin K until intestinal bacteria is sufficiently produced. Toxicity is not a common problem that is connected to vitamin K unless supplements are ingested. High levels of vitamin K can decrease the effectiveness of anticoagulant medications that are taken to prevent blood clotting. Symptoms of toxicity include red blood cell breakage (hemolytic anemia), the release of the yellow pigment bilirubin (jaundice), and brain damage. It is for these reasons that vitamin K supplements are available only by prescription.

An RDA has been established for vitamin K because the amount produced by intestinal bacteria is inadequate. Foods such as liver, green leafy vegetables and cruciferous vegetables help to provide adequate amounts of vitamin K. Significant levels can also be obtained from milk, meats, eggs, cereals, fruits, and vegetables. Absorption of vitamin K is dependent on bile and increased with the presence of dietary fat. Most absorption occurs in the jejunum and ileum of the small intestine. Like vitamin E, vitamin K is transported by the chylomicrons through the lymphatic system and eventually to the liver. Vitamin K can be found in the liver. Smaller amounts of this vitamin are stored in the bone and adipose tissue.[12]

Water-Soluble Vitamins

Water-soluble vitamins have different characteristics than fat-soluble vitamins. Water-soluble vitamins include the eight B vitamins and vitamin C. These vitamins are found in the watery compartments of foods and in the water-filled areas of our bodies. When blood levels of the water-soluble vitamins get too high, the excess is excreted in the urine. Although toxicity of water-soluble vitamins is rare, deficiency problems are more common, and these vitamins should be supplied in the diet daily. (See Table 6.3 for a description of the functions, deficiencies, toxicities, and sources of water-soluble vitamins.)

TABLE 6.3 The Functions, Deficiencies, Toxicities, and Sources of Water Soluble Vitamins

Water-Soluble				
Name	Function	Deficiency	Toxicity	Sources
Thiamin (vitamin B_1)	part of coenzyme involved in energy metabolism, nervous system function, normal appetite	edema, abnormal heart rhythms, wasting, apathy, irritability, loss of reflexes, mental confusion, anorexia	none reported	pork products, liver, whole and enriched grains, legumes, nuts
Riboflavin (vitamin B_2)	part of coenzyme involved in energy metabolism, normal vision, skin health	cheilosis (cracks at mouth corners) magenta tongue, sore throat, skin rash, sensitivity to light	none reported	dairy products, meat, liver, leafy green vegetables, whole and enriched grains
Niacin (vitamin B_3, nicotinic acid, nicotinamide, niacinamide, tryptophan is precursor)	part of coenzyme involved in energy metabolism	diarrhea, glossitis (bright red, swollen, smooth tongue), loss of appetite, mental confusion, flaky skin rash, irritability, weakness	nausea, vomiting, painful flushing, liver damage, impaired glucose tolerance	all protein-containing food
Folate (folic acid, folicin, pteroglutamic acid)	part of coenzyme involved in new cell synthesis	anemia, glossitis, gastrointestinal discomfort, frequent infections, mental confusion, neural tube defects	masks vitamin B_{12} deficiency	leafy greens, vegetables, asparagus, orange juice, legumes, seeds, liver, enriched grains
Vitamin B_{12} (cyanocobalamin)	part of coenzyme involved in new cell synthesis, helps to maintain nerve cells	anemia, glossitis, hypersensitivity of skin, fatigue, degeneration leading to paralysis	none reported	animal products
Vitamin B_6 (pyridoxine, pyridoxal, pyridoxamine)	part of coenzyme involved in amino acid and fatty acid metabolism, helps convert tryptophan to niacin, helps make red blood cells	anemia, rashes, greasy, scaly dermititis, depression, confusion, convulsions, abnormal brain wave patterns	bloating, fatigue, impaired memory, irritability, nerve damage, loss of reflexes, skin lesions, depression	meat, fish, poultry, liver, legumes, fruits, potatoes, whole grains, soy products
Pantothenic Acid	part of coenzyme involved in energy metabolism	ntestinal upset, insomnia, fatigue, hypoglycemia	occasional edema	widespread

(Continued)

TABLE 6.3 The Functions, Deficiencies, Toxicities, and Sources of Water Soluble Vitamins (*Continued*)

Water-Soluble				
Name	Function	Deficiency	Toxicity	Sources
Biotin	cofactor for several enzymes involved in energy metabolism, fat synthesis, amino acid metabolism, and glycogen synthesis	abnormal heart function, nausea, depression, muscle pain, fatigue, numbness of extremities, dry around nose, eyes, and mouth	none reported	widespread
Vitamin C (ascorbic acid)	collagen synthesis (scar tissue, blood vessel walls, bone growth), antioxidant, thyroxine synthesis, amino acid metabolism, increased infection resistance, assists iron absorption	anemia, pinpoint hemorrhages, frequent infections, loose teeth, bleeding gums, muscle degeneration and pain, depression, hysteria, joint pain, rough skin, poor wound healing	intestinal distress, excessive urination, headache, fatigue, insomnia, skin rash, aggravation of gout, interferes with medical tests	citrus products, cabbage-type vegetables, dark green vegetables, cantaloupe, peppers, strawberries, lettuce, tomatoes, potatoes, mangoes, papayas

Functions of B Complex Vitamins

The eight B complex vitamins include thiamin (B_1), riboflavin (B_2), niacin (B_3), folate, vitamin B_6, vitamin B_{12}, pantothenic acid, and biotin. For the most part, B complex vitamins act as coenzymes in the body. A coenzyme is a molecule that binds to an enzyme so that the enzyme can do its metabolic work in the body. The B vitamins help the body to obtain energy from the energy-yielding nutrients; carbohydrates, proteins, and lipids. (Figure 6.1) Even though B vitamins do not provide energy to the body, the body can feel tired when there is a deficiency of these vitamins.

The B vitamins thiamin, riboflavin, niacin, pantothenic acid, and biotin assist in the release of energy from the energy-yielding nutrients. Vitamin B_6 acts as a coenzyme in the metabolism of amino acids that are derived from the energy-yielding nutrient protein. Folate and vitamin B_{12} help cells to multiply and deliver nutrients for the body's energy-yielding reactions. The B vitamins work closely with one another, and it is at times difficult to distinguish which vitamin is responsible for a given effect. Nutrients are inter-dependent, and the presence or absence of one impacts the absorption, metabolism, and excretion of another.

Thiamin (B_1)

Thiamin or vitamin B_1 was the first vitamin identified as necessary for human health and well-being. Thiamin plays a role in the metabolism of energy because it forms a part of the coenzyme thiamin pyrophosphate (TPP), the coenzyme that converts pyruvate to acetyl CoA in the glycolytic pathway for energy production (see chapter 8 for more information). Other specific functions of thiamin include its role as a coenzyme in the metabolism of branched-chain amino acids (leucine, isoleucine, and valine) that are used for energy in muscle. Thiamin also aids in the production of DNA and RNA for protein synthesis, and it helps in the production of neurotransmitters by working at the nerve cell membrane.

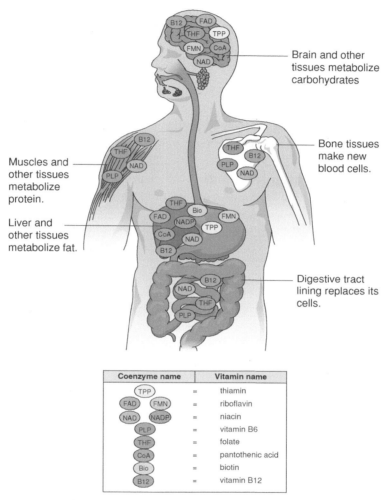

FIGURE 6.1 The B Vitamins Play an Important Part in Metabolism.

Thiamin requirements are based on caloric intake because thiamin is needed for energy metabolism. Typically, persons who consume adequate calories to meet their energy needs have sufficient thiamin to maintain a healthy lifestyle. Individuals at risk for deficiencies of thiamin include people with eating disorders, the elderly, and long-term dialysis patients. Thiamin deficiency may also be apparent in the homeless population because of inadequate dietary intake. The deficiency disease associated with thiamin is known as beriberi. The disease results in muscle wasting due to the body's inability to metabolize energy. If left untreated, nerve damage may occur and result in paralysis. If the heart muscle is affected, an individual may die of heart failure. Individuals suffering from alcoholism may develop Wernicke-Korsakoff's syndrome, a thiamin deficiency resulting in memory impairment, confusion, and muscle tremors. Heavy use of alcohol interferes with the absorption of thiamin and the liver's ability to utilize thiamin to make TPP.[13]

The best food sources of thiamin are pork products, whole grains and enriched grain products, and legumes. Under normal circumstances, thiamin toxicity is not a problem as the excess intake is excreted by the kidneys.

Riboflavin (B$_2$)

Riboflavin (B$_2$) was the second B vitamin to be discovered. It is also important in the production of energy and is a component of two coenzymes; flavin mononucleotide (FMN) and flavin adenine dinucleotide (FAD). These coenzymes are involved in the Kreb's Cycle or the electron transport chain (see chapter 8). They are also involved with the metabolism of all 3 energy-yielding nutrients; protein, carbohydrates and lipids. Riboflavin supports normal vision and skin health.

Riboflavin requirements in the United States are easily met, and like thiamin, they are based on energy intake. Deficiencies in riboflavin may occur under the same circumstances seen in thiamin deficiency, where total energy intake is at risk. The deficiency disease associated with riboflavin is known as ariboflavinosis. Symptoms include cheilosis (dry, scaly lips with cracking at the mouth corners), a magenta-colored tongue, sore throat, a skin rash and sensitivity to light.

A high quantity of riboflavin is present in dairy products. About one-third of the RDA for this vitamin is supplied by milk in the diet of Americans. A decline in the consumption of milk and milk products in Western countries may contribute to the poor riboflavin status reported in segments of the population, particularly among young people.[14] Riboflavin is light-sensitive and is therefore easily destroyed by light. It is for this reason that milk is stored in opaque or light-blocking containers.

Niacin (B$_3$)

Niacin (B$_3$) is comprised of two different vitamin entities, nicotinic acid and nicotinamide. Nicotinamide is the major form found in the blood and nicotinic acid can be easily converted to nicotinamide in the body. The functions of niacins are closely associated with those of thiamin and riboflavin in energy production. There are two coenzymes, nicotinamide adenine dinucleotide (NAD) and nicotinamide adenine dinucleotide phosphate (NADP), that are needed to breakdown carbohydrates, proteins, and lipids to energy in the metabolic pathways (see chapter 8).

Niacin requirements are closely tied to protein intake because this vitamin can be synthesized from the amino acid tryptophan. To make 1 mg of niacin the body needs 60 mg of tryptophan from the diet. Because of this relationship, niacin is measured in niacin equivalents (NE). One NE equals 60 mg of tryptophan. A food containing 1 mg of niacin and 60 mg of tryptophan would have the equivalent of 2 NE.

A deficiency of niacin is rare, except in some parts of India, China, and Africa where protein intake is limited. The disease associated with niacin deficiency is known as pellagra. Pellagra was also common in the southern United States during the early 1900s where income was low and corn products were the major dietary staple.[15] In the United States, deficiencies can also be observed in those who chronically abuse alcohol. Pellagra is sometimes referred to as the 4 Ds due to the progression of its symptoms: diarrhea, dermatitis, dementia, and ultimately death if left untreated.

High doses of niacin can affect the nervous system and result in a flushing of the skin that is caused by dilation of the blood vessels. Physicians have prescribed pharmacological doses of niacin in the treatment of cardiovascular disease. Pharmacologic doses of nicotinic acid, (but not nicotinamide), have been used to reduce serum cholesterol since 1955.[16] An increase in niacin intake of 6.2 mg has also been associated with a 40% decrease in cases of cancers of the mouth and throat. An increase of 5.2 mg increase in niacin intake has also been associated with a similar decrease in cases of esophageal cancer.[17, 18] It should be mentioned that high doses of niacin do come with some potential hazardous side effects including liver damage.

Sources of niacin consist of protein-containing foods such as meat, fish and poultry, as well as enriched grain products. Toxicity from food sources does not occur but an UL has been established for niacin because of its potential harmful impact on the body when supplements are taken in large doses.

Folate

Folate is a broad term for a part of the B-complex family of water-soluble vitamins. Other names for folate include folic acid, folacin, and pteroylglutamic acid (PGA). The primary functions of folate occur in the enzymes involved with DNA synthesis, cell differentiation and amino acid metabolism. Folate also has a critical role in embryonic development in a woman during her first few weeks of pregnancy. Folate is needed for the synthesis of new cells, as well as for the repair of damaged cells.

The requirement for folate is set at a higher value because folate has a low bioavailability. An amount less than 50% of folate is absorbed through food sources.[19] The synthetic form (folic acid) is highly bioavailable at between 85%–100%, which includes the folic acid that is found in fortified grain products.[20] Since there is a discrepancy in the bioavailability between synthetic folic acid and the folate naturally occurring in food, the requirement for folate is measured in dietary folate equivalents (DFE).

A deficiency in folate can have several negative outcomes. Since the functions of folate involve new cell synthesis and cell differentiation, the results from a deficiency are numerous, including a form of anemia known as macrocytic anemia. Macrocytic anemia is characterized by large, immature red blood cells that contain less hemoglobin and thus diminishes the ability of the red blood cells to carry oxygen. Folate deficiency can be compounded with vitamin B_{12} deficiencies and can lead to elevated levels of homocysteine in the blood. High levels of homocysteine in the blood have been associated with an increase in heart disease.[21] One of the more frequently published consequences of folate deficiency is the development of neural tube deficits (NTD) in the developing fetus of a pregnant woman. Since the neural tube is what eventually develops into the infant's central nervous system, malformations of the brain and spinal cord may occur with a folate deficiency.

The only known toxicity noted with folate is its ability to mask a vitamin B_{12} deficiency. Folate itself has no toxic symptoms. The sources for folate, as already mentioned, can be either naturally occurring in food in the form of folate, or synthetically produced for use in food fortification and supplements (folic acid). The word folate means foliage. Leafy green vegetables such as spinach are rich sources of folate, as are other leafy greens. Legumes can also add folate in the diet. Protein-containing foods, on the other hand, are poor sources of folate. Because the need for this vitamin is so critical in the diet of pregnant women, the U.S. Food and Drug Administration authorized the addition of folic acid to enriched grain products in March of 1996, with a mandatory compliance by January 1998. A 19% reduction in NTD birth prevalence has occurred following folic acid fortification of the U.S. food supply.[22]

Vitamin B_{12}

Vitamin B_{12} is also known as cyanocobalaminn because of the presence of cobalt in its structure. As with the previously mentioned water-soluble vitamins, vitamin B_{12} is part of a coenzyme. This coenzyme functions in DNA synthesis, particularly in relation to the formation of red blood cells. It is also responsible for the maintenance of the myelin sheath that covers nerve fibers. Vitamin B_{12} is known to function jointly with folate to lower homocysteine levels and to lower the risk of cardiovascular disease.

The absorption of vitamin B_{12} is quite different from that of any other vitamin. This vitamin is attached to the protein in food and needs to be released for absorption to occur. It is released from the protein, in the stomach, by the presence of stomach acid and then subsequently binds to another protein known as R-binder protein. Another protein known as intrinsic factor is also produced in the stomach. The vitamin B_{12}-R-binder protein complex and the intrinsic factor then travel to the small intestine. In the small intestine, the R-binder protein is enzymatically removed from the B_{12} molecule. Intrinsic factor and vitamin B_{12} then join together to allow vitamin B_{12} to be absorbed. The receptor site for vitamin B_{12} absorption only recognizes this complex of vitamin B_{12}-intrinsic factor and not that of vitamin B_{12} itself. Once absorbed, the vitamin B_{12} is transported to the cells and the excess is temporarily stored in the liver.

Individuals who consume animal products do not normally have problems with meeting their vitamin B_{12} requirements because vitamin B_{12} is found in all animal products. Vegans need to consume vitamin B_{12} fortified foods to meet their needs. Since the absorption of vitamin B_{12} is dependent upon a series of steps, including the presence of stomach acid, anything that reduces acid production in the stomach may result in a decline in vitamin B_{12} absorption, and hence a deficiency even though sufficient quantities of the vitamin are consumed in the diet. One research study has shown that fifteen percent of adults older than 65 had laboratory evidence of vitamin B_{12} deficiency.[23] Up to 30% of adults over the age of 50 experience a thinning of the stomach lining, which results in decreased production of intrinsic factor. The use of gastric acid-blocking agents can lead to decreased vitamin B_{12} levels and may have a role in the development of vitamin B_{12} deficiency.[24]

A deficiency in vitamin B_{12} typically results in macrocytic anemia. Other signs that indicate a vitamin B_{12} deficiency include gastrointestinal problems, **peripheral neuropathy** (a problem with the nerves that carry information to and from the brain and spinal cord to the rest of the body—can produce pain, a loss of sensation, and an inability to control muscles), depression, irritability, and memory impairment.[25]

No evidence has been reported to demonstrate adverse effects of high levels or toxic levels of vitamin B_{12}.

Because all animal products have vitamin B_{12}, a diet that includes these foods will usually contain an adequate supply for most individuals. The consumption of a combination of low-fat, protein-rich foods such as beef, fish, poultry, and dairy also contributes to healthy vitamin B_{12} levels.

Vitamin B_6

Vitamin B_6 is a family of compounds that includes pyridoxine, pyridoxal, and pyridoxamine, as well as their phosphate forms. Like many of the previously mentioned vitamins, vitamin B_6 has a key coenzyme role in energy metabolism, particularly in amino acid metabolism. It contributes to a process called transamination, where the nonessential amino acids are synthesized. Without adequate vitamin B_6, all amino acids would become essential. Vitamin B_6 is also involved in the production of the enzyme glycogen phosphorylase, which allows the release of glucose from glycogen stores in the liver when blood sugar levels start to dip. Vitamin B_6 works in conjunction with vitamin B_{12} and folate in the metabolism of homocysteine. It also works in the synthesis of hemoglobin, which is required for oxygen transport through the blood.

A deficiency of vitamin B_6 results in skin, blood, and central nervous system disorders. Symptoms include irritated, dry patches on the skin, anemia, depression, and confusion. Homocysteine levels increase with low levels of vitamin B_6, vitamin B_{12}, and folate, which also increase the risk for cardiovascular disease.

Toxic vitamin B_6 levels from food sources alone are not known to cause problems, but very high doses (200 mg or more per day) of vitamin B_6 can cause neurological disorders, such as loss of sensation in the legs and imbalance. Supplemental doses to treat premenstrual syndrome and carpel tunnel syndrome have been studied but results are controversial.[26] Adequate amounts of vitamin B_6 can be found in animal products and in enriched grain products and starchy vegetables.

Pantothenic Acid

Pantothenic acid is a water-soluble vitamin in the B complex family that is also involved in energy production. Pantothenic acid is utilized in the body to make coenzyme A (CoA), which is needed for the production of energy from all energy-yielding nutrients (see chapter 8 on digestion), as well as for the synthesis of fatty acids. A second compound made from pantothenic acid is called acyl carrier protein (ACP). This protein is involved with the synthesis of fatty acids, steroids and cholesterol.[27]

Cases of pantothenic acid deficiencies are extremely rare and there are no apparent adverse effects from the intake of high levels of this vitamin. Pantothenic acid is common in a large array of foods such as animal proteins and whole grain products.

Biotin

Biotin also functions as a coenzyme in the body. This B-complex vitamin is involved in fatty acid synthesis, gluconeogenesis, and the metabolism of energy-yielding nutrients. A deficiency in biotin is rare, except if a person consumes raw egg whites for an extended period of time. A protein found in raw egg whites can bind to biotin and make it unavailable for absorption. Biotin in excess of requirements appears to have no health implications. The biotin content of food is rarely reported and may not be available in food composition tables.

Deficiencies of B Complex Vitamins

The deficiency of a single B vitamin is rare and is usually accompanied by the deficiency of other B vitamins. B vitamin deficiencies typically affect many areas of the body because of their involvement with the energy-yielding pathways. When energy is unavailable, the functioning of all body processes is impaired. The need for B complex vitamins is great, and an inadequate level of their presence may cause the impairment of many bodily functions.

Toxicities of B Complex Vitamins

Toxicity from water-soluble vitamins is rarely caused solely by food sources, but toxicity from supplements is known to occur. Supplements provide a concentrated source of the nutrient, which can quickly overwhelm the cells. A 2-milligram capsule of vitamin B_6 contains the same amount of vitamin B_6 as is found in 3,000 bananas, 6,600 cups of rice, or 3,600 chicken breasts. The cells usually try to excrete the excess amounts, but if they are not able to keep up with the high levels, toxic levels may occur.

Food Sources of B Complex Vitamins

Appropriate selections from each food group in ChooseMyPlate help to ensure an adequate supply of necessary B vitamins. The grain group provides thiamin, niacin, riboflavin, and folate. Fruits and vegetables also contribute to folate. The meat, poultry, and dry bean groups supply significant amounts of thiamin, niacin, vitamin B_6, and vitamin B_{12}. The dairy group is well known for its riboflavin and vitamin B_{12} content. A well-balanced diet, that includes foods from all of the groups, helps to ensure adequate B complex vitamin intakes.

B Vitamins and Cardiovascular Disease

Epidemiological studies have implicated high homocysteine levels in the blood as a risk factor for the development of cardiovascular disease. Homocysteine is a sulfur-containing amino acid that is found primarily in animal proteins. The B vitamins are key components in regulating homocysteine metabolism. There are ongoing studies on the use of B vitamin supplementation for the prevention of cardiovascular disease in select population groups.[28] Studies are also being conducted on the efficacy of using folic acid with other B vitamins to treat and prevent cardiovascular disease to determine the potential benefit of these supplementations.[29] It is believed that a multivitamin/mineral supplementation can improve plasma homocysteine levels in older adults who are concurrently consuming a folate-fortified diet.[30] Although epidemiological studies indicate relationships between homocysteine levels and cardiovascular disease, and connections between folic acid, B_6, B_{12}, and homocysteine metabolism, a direct connection that links supplementation and a decrease in cardiovascular disease remains speculative and needs further testing.[31]

Vitamin C

The value of vitamin C (also known as ascorbic acid or ascorbate) was discovered more than two hundred years ago when two-thirds of British sailors who were at sea for long voyages developed the disease scurvy. Those who traveled for shorter periods of time showed no signs of the disease. A physician, at the time, theorized about the cause of this phenomenon based on the availability of particular foods when a voyage was lengthy. Fresh fruit and vegetable supplies were depleted early on during the voyage and only grains and animal products remained for consumption. Based on this observation, sailors were divided into groups and provided with diets consisting of cider, vinegar, sulfuric acid, seawater, oranges, or lemons. Those who consumed citrus products were able to alleviate the symptoms of scurvy. Today we know that citrus products contain high levels of Vitamin C. The amount of vitamin C needed to prevent scurvy is only 10 mg daily.

Even though vitamin C is a water-soluble vitamin, similar to the B complex vitamins, it functions very differently. Vitamin C helps enzymes in numerous reactions and also acts as an antioxidant. Vitamin C is involved with the reactions that make the structural protein collagen, which is the most important protein in connective tissues and in the formation of bones and teeth. Collagen is responsible for forming scar tissue and is essential in the arteries and in the capillary walls where expansion and contraction take place for the flow of blood.

As an antioxidant, vitamin C protects substances found in foods and in the body from oxidation. Most of the oxidized vitamin C is readily recycled to an active form to be reused.[32] Population studies show that high intakes of vitamin C have a protective effect against chronic diseases such as heart disease, cancer, and eye diseases. Vitamin C is thought to reduce the oxidative damage caused by oxidation. A lower rate of chronic diseases in these studies may also reflect a more healthful lifestyle and diet.[33] Whenever the immune system becomes more active, vitamin C is used as an antioxidant. Recent research has studied the effects of vitamin C consumption on the common cold because vitamin C is said to reduce histamine levels. Nasal congestion develops in response to elevated histamine levels and people often take antihistamines for relief. Vitamin C also deactivates histamine.[34]

The RDA for vitamin C is 75 mg per day for women and 90 mg for men. Consumption of these amounts allows tissues to reach saturation levels. After the tissues are saturated, the remaining vitamin C is excreted. Under stressful conditions such as infections and burns, exposure to extremes in temperature (both high and low), intakes of toxic heavy metals such as lead and mercury, or the continued use of medications such as aspirin, barbiturates, and oral contraceptives, the need for vitamin C increases. Exposure to cigarette smoke, especially when accompanied by low intakes of vitamin C, depletes the body's supply in both active and passive smokers. The RDA increases from 75 to 110 mg for female smokers and from 90 to 125 mg for males.

When vitamin C intake is consistently low for several weeks, the symptoms of scurvy may appear. The first indications are bleeding gums and pinpoint hemorrhages under the skin caused by the weakening, and ultimately the breakage of, capillaries. Scurvy is rarely seen except in the elderly population, in drug or alcohol abusers, or in infants fed only cow's milk.

High intakes of vitamin C have been associated with nausea, abdominal cramps, and diarrhea. Since there has been much published about the health benefits of vitamin C, many consume levels well above the RDA. Doses between 100 and 300 mg do not appear to have any harmful effects. Levels above 2,000 mg, on the other hand, can compromise the results of urine and blood tests that are used as diagnostic procedures for diabetes and can also interfere with the action of anticoagulant medications.

The most widely known sources of vitamin C are fruits and vegetables. Consuming a cup of orange juice at breakfast, a salad for lunch and one-half cup of broccoli and a potato at supper provides more than 300 mg of vitamin C. Raw fruits and vegetables provide higher levels of vitamin C than their cooked counterparts. Grains, meats, cow's milk, and legumes, on the other hand, are poor sources of this vitamin.

Culinary Corner
Functional Foods and Nutritional Supplements

Functional foods include whole foods, fortified foods, and enriched, and/or enhanced foods. They are defined as similar in appearance to conventional foods, with demonstrated physiological benefits that reduce the risk of chronic disease beyond basic nutritional functions. The simplest form of a functional food is a whole food, which is an unmodified food such as a fruit or vegetable. An example of a whole food that would be considered a functional food is broccoli because of its high physiologically active compounds of sulforaphane and beta carotene. Fortified foods include those that have been fortified with nutrients, or enhanced with phytochemicals or botanicals. Examples of fortified foods include eggs with increased omega-3 fatty acids, fortified margarines with stanol esters, and orange juice with calcium. An enriched food is one that has had nutrients added to replace nutrients that were lost during manufacturing and storage. Iron and several types of vitamin B, for example, are added to wheat flour after processing. Additional levels of vitamins and minerals may also be added to foods during the enrichment process. Examples of enriched foods include enriched white flour and white rice. A tremendous growth in the development of functional food products has been actively monitored by Food Technologists, who feel that this growth will continue through the 21st Century.[35]

The consumption of nutritional supplements such as fortified food products is increasing in popularity. A nutritional supplement is taken orally, and usually contains one or more dietary ingredients such as vitamins, minerals, herbs, amino acids, and enzymes. Nutritional supplements are also called dietary supplements. Dietary supplements are readily available on the internet, and at pharmacies, grocery stores, and health food stores. They are used by millions of people in the United States and their sales generate billions of dollars annually. The U.S. Food and Drug Administration (FDA) regulates dietary supplements. They are not considered "drugs" and are therefore not required to show evidence of efficacy or safety prior to marketing. There are no FDA regulations to ensure the identity, purity, quality, composition, or strength of dietary supplements, and the FDA must demonstrate that a product is unsafe before it can take regulatory action. It has been suggested that new legislation is needed for defining and regulating dietary supplements.[36]

Individuals should carefully consider the benefits and potential risks of nutritional supplements. Some supplements contain very concentrated forms of single nutrients and may pose a greater risk than food sources for toxicity, interactions with other nutrients or drugs, and adverse reactions. Nutritional supplements may, on the other hand, prove beneficial for persons following dietary regimens. Vegan vegetarians who lack vitamin B_{12}, individuals who are lactose intolerant and need calcium and vitamin D supplementation, and people on a caloric-restricted diet for weight loss may benefit from a nutritional supplement. Persons at different stages of the lifecycle may also benefit from an increase in certain nutrient supplements that are lacking because of disease or conditions such as iron deficiency.[37]

Herbal nutritional supplements, derived from all parts of the plant including the leaves, stems, roots, bark, seeds, and flowers, are also popular. Traditionally they have been used to season foods, yet over the past several years, interest in using these plant sources to treat certain ailments and to improve athletic performance (ergogenic aids) has grown. This use of herbs in the treatment of diseases is not new. The medicinal properties of plants have been lauded for thousands of years. The pharmaceutical industry actually grew from herbal treatment, and continues to use plant extracts to make drugs. The drug digitalis that is used to treat heart disease comes from the foxglove plant and morphine is derived from the opium poppy. About 25% of today's prescription drugs are at least partially derived from plants.[38] Table 6.4 presents various herbs and their uses.

Herbal supplements are available in many forms. Care should to be taken in self-dosing with herbs because of a lack of standardized formulas and the possibility of their interaction with certain medications as seen in Table 6.5. Individuals who use nutritional supplements should inform their health care providers of their use, especially if they are taking medication. A balanced variety of nutrient-dense foods consumed in moderation should always serve as the primary foundation of a healthy diet.

TABLE 6.4 Various Herbs and Their Effects on the Body

Herbs	Uses	Possible Side Effects
Aloe (Aloe barbadensis)	The gel from the inner leaves work externally to reduce inflammation as a result of minor burns, skin irritations, and infections.	Taken internally, may cause cramps and diarrhea.
Black Cohosh (Cimicifuga racemosa)	The root contains substances that act like the female hormone estrogen. May help with menstrual discomfort, menopause, and PMS.	May cause diarrhea, nausea, and vomiting. Can contribute to abnormal blood clotting and liver problems
Chamomile (Matricaria recutita)	Elements of the oil of the chamomile flower can calm the central nervous system and relax the digestive system.	Rare, unless allergic to other daisy family plants.
Dong Quai (Angelica Sinensis)	The root contains substances that may help with menstrual problems and poor blood circulation.	Rare.
Echinacea (Echinacea spp.)	The root contains substances that have anti-infective properties. Also an immune stimulant.	Rare if taken as directed, unless other daisy family plant allergy is present. Should not be taken continuously for more than a few weeks, or if suffering from any immune system disorder.
Ephedra (Ephedra sinica, also known as Ma Huang)	The root and other parts of the plant contain active substances that are central nervous system stimulants. Opens bronchial passages, activating the heart, increasing blood pressure and speeding up metabolism.	Increased blood pressure, or heart rate, heart palpitations, and death.
Feverfew (Chrysanthemum parthenium)	Feverfew leaves are believed to contain the chemical parthenolide, which blocks the inflammatory substances from the blood to help treat headaches.	From the dairy family, allergic response will be similar. May interfere with the blood's clotting ability.
Garlic (Allium sativium)	Garlic's active ingredient, allicin is believed to have antibiotic, and antifungal properties. It also may lower blood cholesterol.	Rare, but may interfere with the blood's clotting ability.
Ginger (Zingiber officinale)	Substances from the root include gingerols and are believed to help alleviate motion sickness, dizziness, and improve digestion.	Heartburn.
Ginkgo (Ginkgo Biloba)	Extracted from the leaves, ginkgo biloba extract (GBE) dilates blood vessels to improve blood flow. Also used to treat vascular diseases.	Irritability, restlessness, diarrhea, nausea.
Ginseng (American, Panax quinquelfolium)	The root contains panaxosides that are thought to restore energy, calm the stomach and brain, and act as a stimulant to vital organs. American ginseng is said to be milder than Asian ginseng.	Headache, insomnia, anxiety, and skin rash. More serious side effects include asthma attacks, increased blood pressure, and heart palpitations.

TABLE 6.4 Various Herbs and Their Effects on the Body

Herbs	Uses	Possible Side Effects
Ginseng (Asian, Panax gingseng)	The root contains ginsenosides, which are said to boost the immune system and increase the body's ability to handle fatigue and stress. It is more potent than the American version.	Same as American ginseng.
Guarana (Paullinia cupana)	Substances from the seed contain a high amount of caffeine for increased stimulant effect.	Nervousness, insomnia, irregular heartbeats.
Goldenseal (Hydrastis Canadensis)	The substances found in the root are believed to act as a stimulant. They seem to affect the body's mucous membranes by drying up secretions and reducing inflammation.	Irritation of the skin, mouth, and throat.
Licorice (Glycyrrhiza glabra)	Substances in the root are thought to help relieve skin irritations. Internally it is said to help digestive disturbances.	Upset stomach, diarrhea, headache, and edema.
Milk thistle (Silyubum, marianum)	Substances found in the seeds including silymarin, may have antioxidant effects and are thought to help in the regeneration of liver cells.	Diarrhea.
Peppermint (Mentha piperita)	Its principal active ingredient is menthol, which stimulates the stomach lining and relaxes the muscles in the digestive process.	Rare.
Saw Palmetto (Serenoa repens)	The active ingredient found in the berries of the plant may be helpful in benign prostatic hyperplasia, nasal congestion, and coughs due to colds.	Rare.
St. John's Wort (Hypericun perforatum)	The substances found in the leaves and flowers are said to contain psychoactive substances used to treat mild depression and nervous conditions.	High blood pressure, headaches, nausea, vomiting, and sun sensitivity.
Valerian (Valeriana officinalis)	Substances in the root can have mild tranquilizing effects, and are often used for insomnia, anxiety, and nervousness.	Headache, upset stomach, and morning grogginess.

Source: Adapted from Varro, Tyler, *The Honest Herbal,* 3rd ed., The Hawthorne Press, Binghamton, NY, 1993, and Health and Wellness Library, The Southwestern Co. Nashville, TN, 2000. http://www.nccam.nih.gov/health/acai/ataglance.htm

TABLE 6.5 Potential Herb and Drug Interactions

Herb	Drug	Interaction
Feverfew	Aspirin, ibuprofen, and other nonsteroidal anti-inflammatory drugs	Drugs negate the effect of the herb for headaches.
Feverfew, garlic, Ginkgo, ginger, and ginseng	Warfarin, coumadin (anticlotting drugs, "blood thinners")	Prolonged bleeding time; danger of hemorrhage
Ginseng	Estrogens, corticosteroids	Enhanced hormonal response.

(Continued)

TABLE 6.5 Potential Herb and Drug Interactions (*Continued*)

Herb	Drug	Interaction
Kyushin, licorice, plantain, uzara root, hawthorn, ginseng	Digoxin (cardiac antiarrhythmic drug derived from the herb foxglove)	Herbs interfere with drug action and monitoring.
Ginseng, karela	Blood glucose regulators	Herbs affect blood glucose levels.
Kelp (iodine source) St. John's wort, saw palmetto, black tea	Synthroid or other thyroid hormone replacers	Herb may interfere with drug action.
Echinacea (possible immunostimulant)	Iron	Tannins in herbs inhibit iron absorption.
Evening primrose oil, borage	Cyclosporine and corticosteroids (immunosuppressants) Anticonvulsants	May reduce drug effectiveness Seizures.

Source: L. G. Miller, Herbal medicinals. Selected clinical considerations focusing on known or potential herb-drug interactions. Archives of Internal Medicine 158 (1998): 2200–2211. Copyright © 1998. American Medical Association. All rights reserved.

References

1   World Health Organization (WHO) 2009, Micronutrient deficiencies; Vitamin A deficiency. www.wgo.int/nutrition/topics/vad/en/.

2   G. A. Plotnikoff, "Vitamin D and Cardiovascular Disease: What you need to know," Presented at American Oil Chemists Society Annual Meeting, May 3rd, 2011.

3   A. W. Norman, et al., "Differing Shapes of 1 Alpha, 25-Dihydroxyvitamin D3 Function as Ligands for The D-Binding Protein, Nuclear Receptor and Membrane Receptor: A Status Report," *Journal of Steroid Biochemistry and Molecular Biology* 56 (1996): 13–22.

4   M. Chung, E. M. Balk, M. Brendel, et al., Vitamin D and Calcium: A Systematic Review of Health Outcomes, Evidence report number 183 Rockville, MD: Agency for Healthcare Research and Quality, 2009. (AHRQ publication no. 09-E015.)

5   International Agency for Research on Cancer. Vitamin D and Cancer-A Report of The IARC Working Group on Vitamin D, Lyon, France: World Health Organization Press, 2008.

6   G. A. Plotnikoff, "Vitamin D and Cardiovascular Disease: What You Need to Know," Presented at American Oil Chemists Society Annual Meeting, May 3rd, 2011.

7   C.M. Weaver, "Vitamin D, Calcium, and Bone Health: Strength of The Evidence Towards The New DRIs," Presented at The American Oil Chemists Society Annual Meeting, May 3rd, 2011.

8   A. A. Ginde, R. Scragg, R. S. Schwartz, and C. A. Camargo, "Prospective Study of Serum 25-Hydroxyvitamin D Level, Cardiovascular Disease Mortality, and All-Cause Mortality in Older U.S. Adults," *Journal of The American Geriatric Society* 57 (2009): 1595–1603.

9   The HOPE and HOPE-TOO Trial Investigators. 2005, "Effects of Long-Term Vitamin E Supplementation on Cardiovascular Events and Cancer. A Randomized Controlled Trial," *Journal of the American Medical Association* 293 (2009): 1338–1347.

10 A. Bendich and L. J. Machlihn, "Safety of Oral Intake of Vitamin E," *American Journal of Clinical Nutrition* 48 (1988): 612–619.

11 P. Weber, "Vitamin K and Bone Health," *Nutrition* 17 (2001): 880–887.

12 FAO and WHO 2002, Vitamin K: Human Vitamin and Mineral Requirements, Report of A Joint FAO/WHO Expert Consultation. www.micronutrient.org/idpas/pdf/846.10-chapter10.pdf.

13 N. D. Vo, Wernicke-Korsakoff Syndrome Presentation 2003. http://www.med.unc.edu/medicine/web/Wernicke%20Korsakoff%20syndrome.pdf

14 H. J. Powers, "Riboflavin (B$_2$) and Health," *American Journal of Clinical Nutrition* 77 (2003): 1352–1360.

15 Y.K. Park, C.T. Sempos, C.N. Barton, J.E. Vanderveen, and E.A. Yetley, "Effectiveness of Food Fortification in The United States: The Case of Pellagra," *American Journal of Public Health* 90 (2000): 727–738.

16 R.H. Knopp. "Drug Treatment of Lipid Disorders," *New England Journal of Medicine* 341 (1999): 498–511.

17 E. Negri, S. Franceschi, C. Bosetti, et al., "Selected Micronutrients and Oral and Pharyngeal Cancer," International *Journal of Cancer* 86 (2000): 122–127.

18 S. Franceschi, E. Bidoli, E. Negri, et al., "Role of Macronutrients, Vitamins and Minerals in the Etiology of Squamous-cell Carcinoma of the Oesophagus," *International Journal of Cancer* 86 (2000): 626–631.

19 M. H. Stipanuk, Biochemical, Physiological, and Molecular Aspects of Human Nutrition, W. B. Saunders, Philadelphia, 2006, pgs. 693–732.

20 C. M. Pfeiffer, L. M. Rogers, L. B. Bailey, and J. F. Gregory, "Absorption of Folate from Fortified Cereal-grain Products and of Supplemental Folate Consumed With or Without Food Determined Using a Dual-label stable-isotope Protocol," *American Journal of Clinical Nutrition* 66 (1997): 1388–1397.

21 L. J. Riddell, A. Chrisholm, S. Williams, J. I. Mann, "Dietary Strategies for Lowering Homocysteine Concentrations," *American Journal Clinical Nutrition* 71 (2000): 1448–1454.

22 A. Margaret, J. Leonard, T. J. Mathews, J. Erickson, C. Lee-Yang Wong, "Impact of Folic Acid Fortification of the US Food Supply on the Occurrence of Neural Tube Defects." *Journal of the American Medical Association* 85 (2001): 2981–2986.

23 L. C. Pennypacker, R. H. Allen, J. P. Kelly, L. M. Matthews, J. Grigsby, K. Kaye, "High Prevalence of Cobalamin Deficiency in Elderly Outpatients," *Journal of American Geriatric Society* 40 (1992): 1197–204.

24 G. S. Bradford, C. T. Taylor, "Omeprazole and Vitamin B12 Deficiency," Annuals *Pharmacotherapy* 33 (1999): 641–3.

25 R. C. Oh, and D. L. Brown, "Vitamin B12 Deficiency," *American Family Physician* 67 (2003): 979–986.

26 University of Maryland Medical Center website, "Vitamin B6 (Pyridoxine)," (accessed May 5, 2011). http://www.umm.edu/altmed/articles/vitamin-b6-000337.htm

27 Linus Pauling Institute at Oregon State University, Micronutrient Information Center. http://lpi.oregonstate.edu/infocenter/vitamins/pa/

28 S. E. Lenhart and J. M. Nappi, "Vitamins for The Management of Cardiovascular Disease: A Simple Solution to a Complex Problem?" *Pharmacotherapy* 19 (1999): 1400–1414.

29 J. Blacher and M. E. Safar. "Homocysteine, Folic Acid, B Vitamins, and Cardiovascular Risk," *Journal of Nutrition, Health, and Aging* 5 (2001): 196–199.

30 D. L. McKay, G. Perrone, H. Tasmussen, G. Dallal and J. B. Blumberg, "Multivitamin/Mineral Supplementation Improves B-Vitamin Status and Homocysteine Concentration in Healthy Older Adults Consuming a Folate-Fortified Diet," *Journal of Nutrition* 30 (2000): 3090–3096.

31 J. W. Eikelboom, E. Lonn, G. Genest and S. Yueuf, "Homocysteine and Cardiovascular Disease: A Critical Review of The Epidemiologic Evidence," *Annals of Internal Medicine* 131 (1999): 363–375.

32 G. Wolf, "Uptake of Ascorbic Acid by Human Neutrophils," *Nutrition Reviews* 11 (1993) 337–338.

33 R. A. Jacob and G. Sotoudeh. "Vitamin C Function and Status in Chronic Disease," *Nutrition in Clinical Care* 5 (2002): 66–74.

34 S. Mendiratta, Z. C. Qu and J. M. May, "Erythrocyte Ascorbate Recycling: Antioxidant Effects in Blood," *Free Radical Biology and Medicine* 24 (1998): 789–797.

35 Position of the Academy of Nutrition and Dietetics: Functional Foods, *Journal of the Academy of Nutrition and Dietetics*, 104 (2004): 814–826.

36 P. Fontanarosa, et al., "The Need for Regulation of Dietary Supplements-Lessons from Ephedra," The *Journal of the American Medical Association* 289 (2003): 1568–1570.

37 Position of the Academy of Nutrition and Dietetics: Fortification and Nutrition Supplements, *Journal of the Academy of Nutrition and Dietetics* 105 (2005): 1300–1307

38 Time/Life Books, *Health & Wellness Library, Volume 2*. Nashville, TN: The Southwestern Company, 2000, p. 69.

Put It into Practice

Define the Term

Fruits and vegetables contain many vitamins, though they can be destroyed by cooking and improper holding and storage. It is possible to retain and enhance the absorption of vitamins in fruits and vegetables by using specific techniques. Review the definitions of fat-soluble and water-soluble vitamins in the text. Conduct an online search and list specific preparation, holding and storing techniques that can retain or enhance the absorption of vitamins in fruits and vegetables.

Myth vs. Fact

Determine if the following statement is a myth or fact and support your position with evidence from three research articles on the topic. *Statement: "The more vitamin supplements that you consume, the better it is for your health."*

A. Abstract
B. Methods
C. Results
D. Discussion
E. Conclusion

The Menu

Develop four snack recipes that contain at least two of the fat-soluble and water-soluble vitamins outlined in Tables 6.2 and 6.3 in the text. List the two specific vitamins found in each snack recipe. Each recipe must include the number of servings, an ingredient list, and the method of preparation.

Website Review

Navigate the WebMD website's information on Vitamin D through the following link: www.webmd.com/food-recipes/slideshow-vitamin-d-overview. Review the entire slideshow entitled: "Amazing Vitamin D, Nutrition's Newest Star." In your opinion, how does this information impact college age students? List three ways a chef or dietitian could use the information from the slideshow in the workplace.

Build Your Career Toolbox

The consumption of nutritional supplements such as fortified food products is increasing in popularity and food professionals must be aware of their uses and their potential side effects in the diet. Supplements are readily available on the Internet, as well as at pharmacies, grocery stores, and health food stores. Nutritional supplements are especially popular among high school students. Review the textbook section entitled "Culinary Corner: Functional Foods and Nutritional Supplements," and list three examples of each:

a. Functional food
b. Fortified food
c. Enriched food

Develop a job description for a "Nutrition Educator" for a public school system. Include salary range, education, and experience requirements. This individual is responsible for developing the nutrition education curriculum in the school district and must be available to help with student concerns regarding all aspects of nutrition.

Carol's Osteoporosis Case Study

Carol is a 78-year-old woman who loves to play tennis, work in her garden, and walk 3 miles every day. Throughout her lifetime she had poor calcium intake due to lactose intolerance. She sprained her ankle due to a recent fall. She went to see her doctor and had a DEXA bone scan to check her bone mass. She was diagnosed with osteoporosis. She met with a dietitian who suggested getting more calcium, protein, and vitamin D in her diet. Bones are largely made up of a protein. Vitamin D helps your body absorb calcium so it can do its job building strong bones. Most adults should get between 600 and 800 international units (IUs) of vitamin D every day, and between 1000 and 1300 milligrams (mg) of calcium daily. The higher levels are for postmenopausal women, adolescent girls, and women who are pregnant or nursing.

Carol does not have the ability to go food shopping or cook because she needs rehabilitation and physical therapy for her ankle. She seeks the assistance from a personal chef to shop, plan, and prepare meals on a weekly basis. She is slightly overweight but does not want to lose weight at this time. She is afraid of gaining weight because she will not be as active.

Wt: 160 lbs   Ht: 5'7"   BMI: 26 kg/m^2 (overweight)

Dietitian Recommendations
   Calorie Needs: 1600–1800 calories (for weight maintenance)
   Protein Needs: 60–90 g
   Calcium Needs: 1300 mg
   Vitamin D: 800 IU

24-hr Recall

(B) none, usually skips breakfast except for morning coffee: 3–10-oz cups black coffee

(S) 1 banana

(L) 1/2 sandwich ham and mustard on white bread, 2 cups black coffee, 1-oz potato chips

(D) small bowl of chicken noodle soup, 8 saltine crackers, small tossed salad with iceberg lettuce, cucumber, and sliced tomato with 3 tablespoons of balsamic vinaigrette dressing, water to drink

(S) 2–6-oz glasses of red wine, 6 medium size pretzel sticks

Preferences

Likes: deli ham, deli turkey, tuna salad, seafood salad, beans, meat pie, orange juice, spinach, nuts, most soups except cream

Dislikes: breakfast food (eggs, cereal, waffles, pancakes, etc.), fish such as salmon or white fish, potatoes, dairy products—milk, cheese, cream due to lactose intolerance

Study Guide

Student Name _____ **Date** _____

Course Section _____ **Chapter** _____

TERMINOLOGY

Vitamin C_____	A. Food sources include pork products
Vitamin A_____	B. A molecule that binds to an enzyme so that the enzyme can do its metabolic work in the body
Folate_____	C. Functions in collagen systems
	D. Functions in blood clotting
Thiamin_____	E. Toxicity can lead to painful skin flushing
Vitamin D_____	F. Food sources include dairy products
Toxicity_____	
Coenzyme_____	G. Found in leafy green vegetables
Niacin_____	H. The overabundance of a nutrient in the body that can potentially cause adverse health problems
Riboflavin_____	I. Particular importance in a vegan diet
Vitamin B12_____	J. Involved in cell membrane stability
Vitamin K_____	K. An inadequate level of nutrients in the body with potential negative health effects
Vitamin E_____	L. Deficiency may lead to night blindness
Deficiency_____	M. How well a nutrient can be absorbed and used by the body
Bioavailability_____	N. Also called the "Sunshine Vitamin"

Student Name _____   Date _____

Course Section _____   Chapter _____

VITAMIN MENU PLANNING

Featured Vitamin:_____

RDA for college age students (19-30 years) _____ *include unit of measure/day

You are the foodservice director of a large university dining facility and you are in charge of planning menus. Create one breakfast and one dinner meal with specific dietary alternatives that provide a good source of your vitamin (using the food sources from your list below). **Use RDA tables in textbook** and **Chapter 6: Vitamin Tables 6.2 and 6.3** summarize the information about your featured vitamin. **Your menu must follow the "Choose Your Foods Lists for Meal Planning" (Appendix B)**. See back for menu plan.

This vitamin is: fat soluble   water soluble   (circle correct answer)

Functions in the body:

Deficiency symptoms:

Toxicity symptoms:

Most common food sources:

Student Name _____   Date _____

Course Section _____   Chapter _____

Vitamin:_____

circle or underline foods with the featured vitamin

Each meal must have at least one good source of your vitamin.

Food Choice Requirements

Breakfast: 2 starch, 1 dairy, 2 protein, 1 fruit, 2 fat

Dinner: 2 starch, 4 protein, 2 veg, 2 fat

Breakfast	Breakfast	Breakfast	Breakfast	Breakfast
-Regular	-Lacto	-Lacto- ovo	-Vegan	-Gluten Free

Student Name _____   **Date** _____

Course Section _____   **Chapter** _____

Dinner	Dinner	Dinner	Dinner	Dinner
-Regular	-Lacto	-Lacto-ovo	-Vegan	-Gluten Free

Student Name _____ **Date** _____

Course Section _____ **Chapter** _____

CASE STUDY DISCUSSION

Carol's Osteoporosis Case Study: The Relationship between Vitamin D and Calcium
Review the section in Chapter 6 on vitamin D and the role of calcium in the body. After reading the case study, use the information to answer the following questions.

1. Explain the major functions of vitamin D.

2. List the names and differences between the two forms of Vitamin D.

3. List the symptoms of vitamin D deficiency.

4. What is the DRI for Vitamin D for adults?

5. List three dietary recommendations for Carol to help increase her intake of vitamin D.

Student Name _____   Date _____

Course Section _____   Chapter _____

PRACTICE TEST

Select the best answer.

1. Vitamins
   a. provide the body with energy
   b. are inorganic
   c. assist body functioning and structures
   d. are macronutrients

2. The fat-soluble vitamins include
   a. folate, D, A, and E
   b. A, D, E, and K
   c. B12, riboflavin, A, and E
   d. niacin, folate, C, and D

3. Bioavailability
   a. refers to how well a nutrient can be absorbed
   b. refers to how well a nutrient is used by the body
   c. decreases when the nutrient is consumed in food rather than as an individual supplement
   d. both a and b

4. A molecule that binds to an enzyme so that the enzyme can do its metabolic work in the body is called a (an)
   a. coenzyme
   b. helper enzyme
   c. peri-enzyme
   d. add-enzyme

5. A good source of folate would be
   a. pork
   b. spinach
   c. banana
   d. mashed potatoes

Student Name _____   Date _____

Course Section _____   Chapter _____

TRUE OR FALSE

_____ Toxicities are a concern with fat-soluble vitamins.

_____ Cholecalciferol is the form of vitamin D found in plants.

_____ Vitamin B$_{12}$ is found in all plant products.

_____ Overexposure to the sun can cause vitamin D toxicity.

_____ Vitamins contribute 2 kcal/gm to your caloric intake.

List 2 characteristics of fat-soluble vitamins and 2 characteristics of water-soluble vitamins.

List the primary function and major food source of the following vitamins

- **Vitamin D** _____
- **Vitamin K** _____
- **Riboflavin** _____
- **Folate** _____
- **Vitamin C** _____

Minerals

7

KEY TERMS

Cofactor	Diuretics	Fluorosis
Cretinism	Electrolyte	Goiter
DASH	Extracellular	Heme
Dehydration	Fluorohydroxyapatite	Hemochromatosis

Homocysteine
Hyperkalemia
Hypertension
Hypokalemia
Hyponatremia
Hypothyroidism

Intracellular
Iron-deficiency anemia
Major minerals
Minerals
Myoglobin
Nonheme

Osteoporosis
Overhydration
Salt-sensitive
Trace minerals

Introduction

Minerals are essential nutrients that are very important for normal body functions. Like vitamins, very small amounts are needed. Minerals are inorganic chemical substances that occur in nature. Their functions in the body are regulatory and structural. Minerals are required to maintain fluid balance and acid-base balance in the blood. Despite the miniscule amounts needed, a lack of these in the diet can be devastating. Inadequate levels of calcium in the diet (which on average is a measly 1,000 mg, or less than one-quarter of a teaspoon per day) over a period of time can increase the risk of developing a devastating loss of bone density termed osteoporosis. Although only about five pounds of our body weight is comprised of minerals, they are certainly a vital component.

Types of Minerals

Minerals that are required in our diet are classified according to the quantities found in the body. Minerals are termed major minerals or trace minerals. Major minerals are essential nutrients found in the body in amounts greater than 5 grams (Table 7.1), while trace minerals are essential nutrients that are found in the body in quantities of less than 5 grams. (Table 7.2) Although a very small amount of trace minerals are needed daily, a slight deficiency in these can cause serious health concerns. Some of these concerns will be discussed later. There is currently no conclusive evidence concerning the importance of the minerals arsenic, vanadium, boron, silicon, and nickel to humans, although some animals require them.

TABLE 7.1 Major Minerals	
Calcium	Chloride
Phosphorus	Potassium
Magnesium	Sulfur
Sodium	

TABLE 7.2 Trace Minerals	
Iron	Manganese
Zinc	Fluoride
Iodine	Chromium
Selenium	Molybdenum
Copper	

Major Minerals

Calcium

Calcium is the most abundant mineral in the body, contributing to about 2% of our total body weight. The majority of calcium, approximately 99%, is stored in the bones and teeth because it is an integral part of their structure. Although the calcium found in body fluids accounts for the remaining 1% of the body's calcium, its functions are numerous. Calcium in body fluids transports ions across cell membranes, aids in nerve transmission, helps to clot blood, assists in muscle contraction, activates cellular enzymes, and is involved with acid-base balance.

Because blood levels of calcium are critical to the functioning of the body, there must be a mechanism to keep the blood levels stable. There are many hormones involved with regulation of blood calcium levels—of particular interest is parathyroid hormone (PTH). When blood levels of calcium begin to decline, the parathyroid glands produce PTH. This, in turn, activates vitamin D. The last step in the process to stabilize blood calcium levels is for PTH and vitamin D to encourage the kidneys to reabsorb calcium and, at the same time, break down bone to release calcium into the blood. Vitamin D will also enhance calcium absorption from the intestines. With these three processes in place, blood calcium levels are maintained.

Excellent dietary sources of calcium include milk (all forms), yogurt, cheese, calcium-set tofu, fortified soymilk, broccoli, and turnip greens. Spinach and chard contain calcium that the body cannot absorb due to the presence of oxalates in these vegetables which inhibits calcium absorption in the intestines. The bioavailability of calcium changes during the lifespan and is also influenced by dietary composition. As a person ages, the amount of calcium absorbed through the intestinal tract can be as low as 25%. In addition, intake of iron, phosphorus, magnesium, vitamins K and D all can influence the absorption of calcium from the diet.[1] High levels of calcium in the diet appear to pose no threat for toxicities. Excess calcium is excreted through the feces. The use of calcium supplements has the potential to lead to high levels in the body and may cause an interference with absorption of other nutrients such as iron, zinc and magnesium.

Calcium Deficiency and Osteoporosis

Calcium deficiency may lead to a drop in blood calcium levels and a loss of calcium in the bones. Over a long period of time, calcium deficiency leads to a loss in bone mass and bone density, with bones becoming fragile and porous. This condition, known as osteoporosis, greatly increases the likelihood of bone fractures and related complications. One in two women and one in five men in the United Kingdom will have an osteoporotic fracture after the age of 50.[2] Causes of osteoporosis include poor nutrition; inadequate calcium and vitamin D consumption; decreased levels of estrogen in women (particularly after menopause); a lack of physical activity; being underweight; the use of alcohol and tobacco; and excess consumption of protein, sodium, caffeine, vitamin A, and soft drinks. Exercise and the adequate intake and/or supplementation of vitamin D and calcium in the diet can help prevent this condition. Medications are available to help treat osteoporosis. The most common ones are called biphosphonates which are relatively inexpensive and have been investigated over long-term clinical trials.[3] Hormone estrogen replacements, calcitonin, and parathyroid hormone treatment can also be used. There are financial costs and side effects associated with those medical therapies so every effort should be made to prevent osteoporosis through lifestyle behaviors. As a person ages, the chances of osteoporotic fractures increase and household safety becomes extremely important.[4] Osteoporosis is a treatable condition when lifestyle changes are implemented, appropriate vitamin/mineral supplementation is utilized and medications are prescribed.

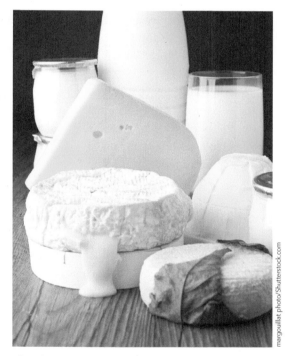

The dairy group is well known for its calcium content.

Phosphorus

Phosphorus is the second most abundant mineral found in the body. It is essential for bone and teeth formation and is combined with calcium in crystals that make up bone and teeth cells. Most of the phosphorus in the body is found in the bone. Phosphorus helps to maintain acid-base balance, forms a part of RNA and DNA makeup, assists in energy metabolism, as it is part of adenosine triphosphate (ATP), and helps to make up phospholipids that are part of cell membranes.

Phosphorus is readily found in many plant and animal sources and is rarely deficient in the diet. Foods particularly high in phosphorus are protein products such as dairy, meat and eggs. Phosphorus can also be found in processed foods and is present in sodas. High intakes of phosphorus, in conjunction with low intakes of calcium, may adversely affect bone mass by disrupting the calcium/phosphorus ratio and leading to a loss of calcium from the bone.[5] The trend of replacing milk with soft drinks, hence reducing calcium intake and increasing phosphorus intake, may negatively affect bone health.[6]

Magnesium

Another mineral needed for numerous metabolic processes is magnesium. This mineral is vital for energy production and use, for adenosine triphosphate (ATP) production, for muscle function, and DNA and protein synthesis. Magnesium is a cofactor for numerous enzymatic systems in the body. Most of the magnesium in the body is found in the bones, with smaller quantities in the muscles, heart, liver, and other soft tissues. The bones supply magnesium when there is a deficiency in the diet, and the kidneys help conserve it. Magnesium deficiency is not common, but can result from inadequate intake, severe vomiting and diarrhea, alcoholism, or protein malnutrition. Magnesium toxicity is rare, but can occur as a result of abusing magnesium containing laxatives, antacids, or other medications. Consequences of toxicity include diarrhea, disturbance in acid-base balance, and dehydration.

Recent studies have investigated the role of magnesium in association with certain forms of cancers. A lower risk of invasive colon cancer was seen in men but not in women when magnesium intake was high.[7] Magnesium is found in a variety of plant and animal foods and is abundant in dark, green leafy vegetables. In some parts of the United States, magnesium levels are high in the water supply, so less magnesium is required from food sources. Fiber will bind with magnesium and prevent its absorption. Protein, on the other hand, will promote magnesium absorption.

Sodium

Sodium is a positive ion that plays a major role in maintaining the body's fluid and **electrolyte** balance system. It helps keep the volume of fluid outside the cell (**extracellular** fluid) and assists in maintaining acid-base balance, muscle contraction, and nerve transmission. Sodium is an electrolyte that makes up the positive ion in sodium chloride (commonly known as table salt). Sodium makes up approximately 40% of the weight of table salt. Sodium is found in naturally low levels in some foods, and naturally higher levels in others such as milk and certain vegetables. Large quantities of sodium chloride are included in processed foods such as luncheon meats, canned vegetables and soups, convenience foods, fast foods, salty snacks, cheeses, and salted and cured foods. Sodium deficiency is rare, as we require only about 500 mg of sodium per day, and this amount is usually consumed in a normal diet without adding table salt. The average American should be concerned about excess sodium consumption rather than its deficiency. The amount recommended by the Dietary Guidelines for Americans 2015 is a maximum of 2,300 mg of sodium per day. Most Americans exceed this level by signicant amounts, consuming 3,500 to 4,000 mg/day, with more than 70% of this derived from sources added by food manufacturers in processed food. Although excess sodium in the diet can be excreted, it creates health risks for certain populations.[8, 9]

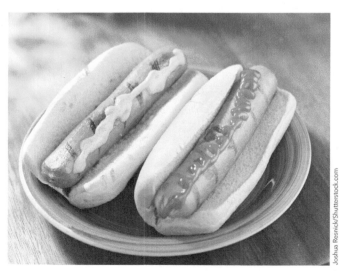

Processed foods such as hot dogs typically contain high amounts of sodium.

Sodium and Hypertension

Excess salt in the diet is linked to **hypertension** (high blood pressure). Although not all people suffering from high blood pressure are affected by sodium intake, some are **salt-sensitive** and experience a rise in blood pressure because of excess salt consumption. Individuals who suffer from kidney disease, are of African American descent, have a family history of hypertension, or are over the age of 50, have a greater risk of salt sensitivity. Too much sodium in the diet can increase calcium secretion that, in turn, can affect bone health. Excess sodium might also be detrimental to a weakened heart or may aggravate kidney problems.

Dash Approach (Dietary Approaches to Stop Hypertension)

Findings on the study of hypertension have focused on the positive effects of lifestyle modification for the prevention and management of this

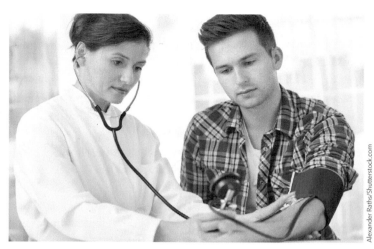

Some individuals who have high blood pressure are salt-sensitive and should lower sodium in the diet.

condition. The DASH approach focuses on a diet rich in fruits, vegetables, nuts, low-fat dairy foods, and reduced saturated and total fats. (Table 7.3)[10] Clinical trials using this approach have found blood pressure levels to be substantially and significantly lower.[11] Studies combining the DASH diet with lowered sodium intake show further benefits to individuals with hypertension.[12]

Chefs can provide menu ideas that incorporate more fruits, juices, and vegetables into the diet to help individuals control blood pressure. Using fruit and vegetable purées in sauces and soups; adding more vegetables to soups, casseroles, and grains; and using fruits in desserts are invaluable suggestions. Ideas for seasoning with less salt by substituting fresh herbs, spices, citrus fruits, vinegars, and wines as flavor enhancers are also helpful.

Chloride

Chloride is an electrolyte that is negatively charged. It is closely associated with sodium in the extracellular fluid and shares the same responsibilities of maintaining fluid and electrolyte balance. It provides the chloride molecule to hydrochloric acid (the acid found in the stomach that aids in digestion) and assists in the transmission of nerve impulses. Chloride sources in the diet are mainly table salt (sodium chloride) and foods made and processed with salt. A deficiency of chloride is rare, but may occur as a result of severe vomiting, resulting in dehydration.

TABLE 7.3 Dash Diet	
Food Groups	**Servings Per Day**
Grains	7–8
Vegetables	4–5
Fruits and Juices	4–5
Milk, nonfat or low-fat	2–3
Meats, Poultry, or Fish	2 or less
Nuts, Legumes, Seeds	1/2–1
Fats and Oils	2–3

(Serving size is listed in Chapter 2 in the USDA Food Guide Pyramid)

Potassium

Potassium, like sodium, is an electrolyte that is a positively charged ion. Potassium, though, is in the intracellular fluid. It is crucial to fluid and electrolyte balance, is necessary for cell integrity, and is crucial to maintaining a normal heartbeat. It also assists in carbohydrate and protein metabolism. Potassium is found in the largest quantities in fresh fruits and vegetables. When food is processed, higher levels of sodium are reached with a consequent reduction in potassium levels. Therefore, consumption of less processed foods and more fruits and vegetables results in a more beneficial potassium intake.

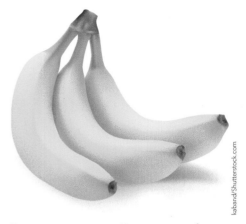

Bananas are an excellent source of potassium.

A deficiency of potassium, known as hypokalemia, is usually caused by health conditions or medications that deplete body potassium, rather than by a deficient intake. Conditions that may deplete body potassium include prolonged diarrhea and vomiting, dehydration, uncontrolled diabetes, kidney disease, and medications such as diuretics that eliminate excess fluids. A prolonged deficiency of potassium may result in muscle weakness, confusion and heart arrhythmias. Potassium toxicity from food is rare, but may occur from supplements that greatly exceed the RDA, or in kidney disease. The kidneys are responsible for the reabsorption of potassium when needed and excretion of potassium when blood levels are elevated. In chronic kidney disease, excess potassium is unable to be excreted and levels may build up in the blood, resulting in hyperkalemia. This can disrupt heart rhythm resulting in a heart attack.

Sulfur

Sulfur is a major mineral that does not function alone in the body, but rather serves to contribute to the makeup of vitamins such as biotin and thiamin. As such, it is involved with metabolism of the energy-yielding nutrients. It is an essential component of several amino acids as well. Sulfur helps to stabilize the shape of amino acids and helps the liver in its role of detoxification. Sulfur may become deficient in the body if an extreme protein deficiency exists in the diet. Aside from protein deficiency, sulfur deficiencies and toxicities symptoms are not seen.

Trace Minerals

Trace minerals are required in the diet in very small amounts, but a lack of these minerals can cause devastating health consequences. Trace minerals assist in chemical reactions, act as cofactors for enzymes, and serve as components of hormones. They are crucial to almost all cell functions including growth and the healthy functioning of the immune system.

Iron

Iron is a crucial trace mineral to the body and is found in every living cell. Despite the fact that it is the earth's most abundant mineral, it is often lacking in the diet. Iron is essential for a number of reactions in the body. The many functions of iron will be explored next.

Functions of Iron

Iron plays a major role in the transport and release of oxygen in the blood. It is a component of hemoglobin, the compound that carries oxygen in the blood. As blood passes through the lungs, it accumulates oxygen and with the help of the iron in hemoglobin, turns blood bright red. Blood that is full of oxygen continues to cells throughout the body, and oxygen is delivered where it is needed. When hemoglobin is depleted of oxygen, it turns a bluish color and must return to the lungs for more oxygen. Iron is also important to the muscle component of myoglobin, the oxygen transporting protein of muscle. Iron is a cofactor for numerous enzymes and is needed for optimal immune functions. It is required for brain and nervous system development in children, and continues to be important in these systems in adults as well. Iron also plays a key role in energy production from carbohydrates, proteins and fats as a component of cytochromes involved with electron transport and its involvement in the enzymes utilized in the Kreb's Cycle.

Sources of Iron

There are two forms of iron in food: **heme** (the ferrous form) and **nonheme** (the ferric form). Heme iron is found in meats, poultry, and fish, while nonheme iron is found in vegetables, fruits, grains, and eggs. Heme iron is in a highly absorbable form of iron that contributes significantly to one's requirement, despite the small percentage that is found in dietary intake. The nonheme form can be changed to the heme form in the presence of stomach acid. Certain dietary factors increase the absorption of both types of iron. Meat, fish and poultry contain a special "meat factor" that enhances absorption of iron in the diet. This meat factor effect comes from the binding of iron with a mixture of peptides from digested proteins and other constituents of meat, such as phospholipids.[13] Foods high in vitamins and sugars (such as wine), and those with a high vitamin C content (such as citrus fruits), enhance the absorption of both heme and nonheme iron sources. Phytates and fibers found in whole grains and nuts, calcium and phosphorus found in milk, and tannic acid present in tea, coffee, and nuts, inhibit absorption.

Deficiency and Toxicity of Iron

Iron deficiency can result from inadequate intake and inadequate absorption. Absorption of iron is very poor. The amount absorbed from the diet can be as low as 14%–18%. However, if iron levels are low in the body, absorption can increase to as high as 40%. It is the most common nutritional deficiency worldwide, particularly in developing countries. Over 30% of the world's population is anemic.[14] In the United States, certain populations such as toddlers and females of childbearing age are particularly at risk.[15] An association between **iron-deficiency anemia** (IDA) and impaired cognitive and psychomotor development in infants and young children has been suggested. However, the results are not definitive because children with IDA usually come from the poorer segments of society where other factors, such as low-birth weight, environmental deprivation, lack of stimulation, poor maternal IQ and education, social stress and other nutritional deficits may be the cause of both the IDA and the developmental deficits.[16] The most severe iron deficiency results through blood loss. Women need more iron than men, due to their regular menstrual losses, and suffer from iron deficiency at a much higher rate. Increased iron needs occur during pregnancy and lactation. During infancy and childhood, a deficiency may occur due to an increased need for iron to support growth.

Iron in hemoglobin helps to carry oxygen to the cells. When the supply of iron is depleted, hemoglobin levels drop and red blood cells become small and pale. People who suffer from this form of anemia often appear uncommonly pale. Symptoms of iron-deficiency anemia include fatigue, weakness, headaches, apathy, pallor, and poor resistance to cold temperatures. Treatment of iron-deficiency anemia first involves identifying the cause of the deficiency (for example, a decreased intake or loss of blood). Once the cause is determined, iron supplementation should be initiated, in the form of ferrous sulfate supplements. Ferrous sulfate is best absorbed on an empty stomach, however, it is not always tolerated. If iron is taken with food, foods that prohibit absorption should be avoided, as well as antacids.[17]

Toxicity of iron, otherwise termed iron overload or **hemochromatosis**, does not occur as frequently as iron deficiency. Causes of iron toxicity include genetics (a gene that enhances iron absorption), repeated blood transfusions, massive doses of dietary iron, metabolic disorders, and alcoholism. Large amounts of iron can be damaging to the liver as well as to other tissues.

Zinc

Zinc is found in almost all cells—but mainly found in the muscles and the bone—and has many important functions. It serves as a **cofactor** (a mineral element that works with an enzyme to assist in chemical reactions) for more than 100 enzymes in the body, and supports numerous proteins in the body. Because of its association with enzymatic functions, zinc is required for metabolism of alcohol, digestion and metabolism of energy-yielding nutrients, bone formation, and the synthesis of hemoglobin. Zinc functions with proteins to maintain the structural characteristics of the protein. A third important function of zinc is in gene regulation. Zinc is involved with turning genes on or off.[18] It is also involved in blood clotting and thyroid hormone function, and influences behavior and learning performance. Zinc is essential in the production of the active form of vitamin A (retinal) found in visual pigment. It is needed for taste perception, to heal wounds, to make sperm, and for proper fetal development. Zinc's role in diabetes has long been established and low levels of this mineral in the pancreas have been linked with diabetes.[19]

Although not common in developed countries, zinc deficiency may occur in pregnant women, young children, the elderly, and the poor. The most common symptom is growth retardation in children. Supplementation of zinc in less developed countries improves growth in underweight or stunted children and should be considered in areas of the world where diets are predominately grain-based.[20] Zinc toxicity is rare, however, intakes exceeding 2 grams can cause vomiting, diarrhea, fever, and exhaustion. High intakes can also interfere with absorption of iron and copper. As with other minerals, toxicity with normal dietary intake poses no health threat. It is the consumption of high doses, in supplemental form, that can lead to toxicity problems. Sources of zinc include protein-rich food such as shellfish (in particular, oysters), red meats, poultry, and liver. Legumes and whole grains are also good sources of zinc. Zinc found in animal-based products is better absorbed than that from plant-based sources. Zinc, like iron, is poorly absorbed, ranging from 10%–35% absorption from the food source.

Iodine

Iodine in a gas form is poisonous to humans. Iodine in foods, however, is converted in the digestive tract to iodide, which is essential for the body. Most of the iodide in the body can be found in the thyroid gland. Iodide is an integral component of two very important hormones in the thyroid gland. These hormones assist in the regulation of body temperature and metabolic rate, reproduction, growth, the production of blood cells, and nerve and muscle function. They essentially control the rate at which cells use oxygen and release energy during metabolism.

A deficiency of iodine in the diet can cause symptoms of lethargy and weight gain. An enlargement of the thyroid gland may also occur when the gland

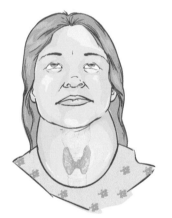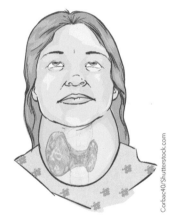

FIGURE 7.1 Iodine deficiency can cause goiter, an enlargement of the thyroid gland

works overtime to retain as much iodine as possible. Ninety percent of all **goiter** (enlargement of the thyroid) cases that occur in about 200 million people, the world over, are caused by iodine deficiency. (Figure 7.1) During pregnancy, an iodine deficiency in the diet may cause irreversible mental and physical retardation of the fetus, known as **cretinism**. Iodine deficiency is one of the world's greatest single causes of preventable brain damage and mental retardation according to the World Health Organization.[21] The condition of hypothyroidism (low levels of thyroid hormone) may also be caused by low iodine levels. Symptoms of **hypothyroidism** include decreased body temperature, sensitivity to cold environments, weight gain and fatigue. Iodine is abundant in the ocean and is, therefore, rich in seafood. Soil concentrations of iodine vary tremendously and cannot be counted on to supply the needed iodine for our bodies. In the early 20th century, goiter was a major health issue in the United States due to the low levels of iodine found in the soil. Individuals living away from the ocean were predominately at risk. As a result, fortification of common table salt with iodine was introduced in the mid-1920's. This supplementation has caused the reduction of total goiter prevalence in the Americas to be less than 5%.[22] Not all salts have been iodized so reading the labels of salt and packaged products is very important. Kosher salt does not contain iodine and sea salt contains very little.

Selenium

Selenium is an essential mineral that is readily absorbed by the body. One function in the body is as an antioxidant. It works closely with the enzyme glutathione peroxidase to prevent free radical formation that damages cells and increases the chances of heart disease and cancer. Selenium works closely with vitamin E in the body to decrease oxidative damage to cell membranes. Selenium also helps to convert thyroid hormones to an active form, making it important in metabolism and maintenance of body temperature.

Selenium is found in a variety of plant and animal sources such as seafood, meat and grains. It is also found in varying amounts in soils where the plants will absorb it. Selenium deficiency is rare but would result in impaired immune response, depression, impaired cognitive function, an enlarged heart, and muscle pain and wasting. Selenium toxicity may occur by ingesting a milligram or more. Symptoms include vomiting, diarrhea, loss of hair and nails, and lesions of the skin and nervous system.

Copper

Copper is found in many body tissues, including muscles, liver, brain, bone, kidneys, and blood. It is an enzyme constituent that is involved in iron metabolism by enabling iron to be transformed from the ferrous form to the ferric form. It serves as an antioxidant, is important in the manufacturing of collagen, and contributes to wound healing. It is involved in reactions that relate to respiration and the release of energy, as well as regulation of neurotransmitters, particularly serotonin.

Copper is widely found in drinking water, meat, legumes, grains, nuts, organ meats, and seeds. Copper deficiency is rare, except in cases of excess zinc consumption, which interferes with copper absorption, and also in extreme cases of malnutrition in children. Copper toxicity is also not common.

Manganese

Manganese is found primarily in the bones, liver, kidney, and pancreas. Like so many of the other trace minerals, it is needed as a cofactor for many of the enzymes involved in metabolic processes. In addition to being a cofactor in metabolism of energy-yielding nutrients, manganese also is involved with gluconeogenesis, synthesis of cholesterol, formation of urea, and protection against free radical damage in the body.

It is present in many plant foods, particularly whole grains, and a deficiency of this mineral is highly uncommon. Symptoms of deficiency include impairment of growth and reproductive function, a reduction in bone density, and impaired metabolism of the energy-yielding nutrients. Toxicity might result from an excess of manganese supplements in the diet or through the inhalation of large quantities of manganese in work environments.

Fluoride

Fluoride, like manganese, is also needed in minute quantities. However, this tiny amount is essential to proper mineralization of bones and teeth, and in making teeth more resistant to decay. As such, most of the fluoride is located in the bones and teeth. Fluoride works in conjunction with calcium and phosphorus to form fluorohydroxyapatite. This compound makes teeth more resistant to damage from acids and bacteria. Fluoride is found in almost all soils, water supplies, plants, and animals. It is particularly high in fish and tea. Fluoridated water is the most significant source of fluoride in the United States. Fluoride is absorbed directly in the mouth into the teeth and gums as well as through the intestinal tract. Use of fluoride treatments can also have a positive effect on tooth enamel.[23]

A deficiency in fluoride causes an increase in dental decay and is thought to be related to the development of osteoporosis. However, fluoride supplements have not shown a clinically significant effect on any type of osteoporosis when studied in postmenopausal women.[24] Over-fluoridated water may cause discoloration of the teeth called fluorosis. In the majority of cases of fluorosis only minor dental cosmetic defects occur. In rare instances, brown staining or pitted enamel may develop.[25] Severe toxicity symptoms can include nausea, vomiting, diarrhea, abdominal pain, and nervous system disorders including numbness and tingling.

Chromium

Chromium has several functions in the body that include assisting in the metabolism of carbohydrates and lipids. It works closely with insulin to help glucose intake in the cells and assists in energy release. Although individuals sometimes think that chromium supplements will help in the treatment of type 2 diabetes, the FDA concluded that the existence of a relationship between chromium picolinate intake and reduced risk of either insulin resistance or type 2 diabetes is not likely.[26]

Chromium is found in many plant and animal sources, especially in products such as meat, whole grains, nuts, prunes, dark chocolate, and in some beers and wine. Deficiency symptoms are uncommon but may occur when there is a reduced ability to use glucose normally. No toxicity related symptoms have been reported.

Molybdenum

Molybdenum is also important in many enzymes required in cell processes. Deficiencies of molybdenum do not exist because of its abundance in food products and the minute amount required in the diet (75 micrograms per day). Foods that are rich in molybdenum are legumes, grains, leafy green vegetables, milk, and liver. Toxicity is rare and might only result from exposure to environmental contaminates such as manganese.

Summary of Major and Trace Minerals

Despite the often miniscule amounts required, minerals play a major role in the body's structure and regulatory processes. Both deficiencies and toxicities of trace minerals can be hazardous to health. The use of unrefined foods, whole grains, legumes, fresh fruits and vegetables, low-fat dairy products, fish, lean meats, and poultry in dishes can guarantee adequate mineral consumption. Table 7.4 summarizes the minerals, the amounts required, their functions, deficiency and toxicity symptoms, and their sources.

TABLE 7.4 The Functions, Deficiencies, Toxicities, and Sources of Minerals				
NAME	FUNCTION	DEFICIENCY	TOXICITY	SOURCES
Major Minerals				
Calcium	Major mineral of bones and teeth. Also important in nerve functioning, muscle contraction and relaxation, blood clotting, blood pressure and immune system functions.	Osteoporosis in adults, and growth retardation in children.	Kidney dysfunction; including stone formation, constipation	Milk and milk products fortified soy products, legumes, dark greens, oysters, and small fish with bones.
Phosphorous	Major mineral of bones and teeth. Also important in maintaining acid-base balance in cells, part of the genetic material of cells, and assists in energy metabolism.	Growth retardation and rickets in children, bone pain and muscle weakness.	May cause calcium excretion and calcium loss from the bone.	Milk and milk products, meat, chicken, fish, cola beverages, added to many processed foods.

NAME	FUNCTION	DEFICIENCY	TOXICITY	SOURCES
Major Minerals				
Magnesium	Involved in bone mineralization and bone strength, a cofactor in energy release reactions involved in transport of calcium to the muscles, and for functioning of nerves and muscles.	Growth retardation in children, weakness, muscle twitches, confusion.	Neurologic disturbances	Peanuts, legumes, dark greens, dried fruit, yeast extract, broccoli
Sodium	Closely involved with body's water balance together with potassium and chloride, also in acid-alkaline balance and nerve and muscle function.	Muscle cramps, reduced appetite	High blood pressure in genetically predisposed individuals.	Salt, soy sauce, cured meats, pickles, canned soups, processed foods, cheese.
Major Minerals				
Chloride	Plays a part in acid-base balance; formation of gastric juice.	Growth retardation in children, muscle cramps, mental apathy, loss of appetite.	High blood pressure in genetically predisposed individuals	Same as those of sodium.
Potassium	Electrolyte mineral, plays a major part in water balance and acid-alkaline regulation. Maintaining healthy heart function with sodium. Closely related with sodium and chloride levels.	Muscular weakness, paralysis	Muscular weakness, cardiac arrest	Meats, milk, many fruits and vegetables, whole grains
Sulfur	Involved in make-up of biotin and thiamin, part of several amino acids, helps liver to detoxify substances	none reported	none reported	Protein-rich foods
Trace Minerals				
Iron	Component of hemoglobin, myoglobin, and enzymes	Iron-deficiency anemia, weakness, impaired immune function	Acute: shock, death; Chronic: liver damage, cardiac failure	Meat, eggs, legumes, whole grains, green leafy vegetables

(Continued)

TABLE 7.4 The Functions, Deficiencies, Toxicities, and Sources of Minerals (*Continued*)

NAME	FUNCTION	DEFICIENCY	TOXICITY	SOURCES
Trace Minerals				
Zinc	Part of some enzymes and the hormone insulin, helps in the formation of protein and genetic material, immune reactions, transportation of vitamin A, taste perception, wound healing, sperm production, normal fetal development	Growth failure in children, dermatitis, delayed sexual development, loss of taste, poor wound healing	Fever, GI distress, lack of coordination, anemia, dizziness, progression of atherosclerosis, kidney failure	Protein-containing foods, grains, vegetables
Iodine	Component of thyroid hormones	Enlarged thyroid (goiter)	Iodide goiter	Marine fish and shellfish, dairy products, iodized salts
Copper	Involved in hemoglobin formation, part of many enzymes	Anemia, abnormalities of the bone	GI distress, liver damage	Organ meats, seafood, nuts, seeds, whole grains, drinking water
Manganese	Cofactor for several enzymes, helps in energy metabolism, urea synthesis, growth, and reproduction	None reported	None reported from diet intake	Whole grain products, tea, coffee, cloves, fruits, dried fruit, vegetables
Fluoride	Maintenance of tooth and bone structure	Tooth decay	Acute: GI distress; Chronic: tooth mottling, skeletal deformation	Drinking water, tea, seafood
Chromium	Associated with insulin, involved with energy release from glucose	Abnormal glucose metabolism	Possible skin eruptions	Meat, unrefined grains, vegetable oils
Molybdenum	Cofactor in many enzymes	None reported	None reported from diet intake	Legumes, grains, leafy green vegetables, milk, liver

Water: The Most Essential Nutrient

Water is the most abundant and most essential nutrient in the body. More than 60% of body weight is made up of water. Water deficiency can develop quickly, and one can only survive a few days without it. Water has numerous functions in the body and is found both within and outside the cells. Some of the more important roles of water include:

- Transporting nutrients in the body and eliminating waste products
- Serving as a medium for chemical reactions
- Contributing to energy formation

- Regulating body temperature
- Serving as a solvent for minerals and vitamins
- Acting as a lubricant and shock absorber
- Maintaining acid-base balance and blood volume

Water Balance

Water must be maintained at specific amounts for the body to be in balance. Water balance is ideal when the water consumed is equal to the water excreted. Sources of water are actual fluids and foods consumed, as well as from water metabolized in the body. The best sources of fluids are water, milk, and some juices, which provide water as well as valuable nutrients to the diet. Fluids that contain alcohol and caffeine can actually deprive the body of water, acting as diuretics. Many sodas and sweetened beverages, such as iced tea, contain caffeine. Sweetened fruit drinks, sports beverages, and caffeine-free sodas provide the body with water, but add empty calories to the diet. Some foods have much higher amounts of water than others and contribute more to fluid intake. Figure 7.2 shows a sampling of foods and their water content. Water is excreted through the kidneys (in urine), the skin (in sweat), the lungs (in vapor), and in the feces. The majority of water is lost in the urine and in perspiration.

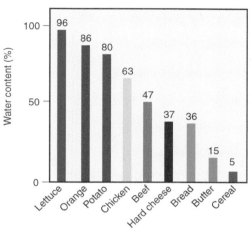

FIGURE 7.2 Water Content of Various Foods

Disturbances in Water Balance: Dehydration and Water Intoxication

Disturbances in water balance can have major consequences in the body. **Dehydration** is excessive water loss in comparison to the amount of water consumed. Initial signs of dehydration may be as simple as thirst, and may progress rapidly to weakness, exhaustion, delirium, and death. Initial warning signs, in addition to thirst and fatigue, may include headache and dark urine with a strong odor. As the percentage of body water lost increases, the severity of symptoms also increases. Results of the Nationwide Food Consumption Surveys indicate that a portion of the American public may be chronically dehydrated as a result of a poor thirst mechanism, dissatisfaction with the taste of water, common consumption of the diuretics caffeine and alcohol, and participation in exercise.[27] Other factors that may increase the risk of dehydration, and increase water needs include fever, prolonged diarrhea and vomiting, surgery and blood loss, pregnancy and lactation, and exposure to extreme environmental temperatures.

Individuals at particular risk for dehydration include infants, the elderly, and athletes. Infants tend to lose fluid rapidly through the skin while the elderly fail to take in adequate amounts of water. Athletes should be aware that optimal performance during exercise requires proper fluid balance. Progressive dehydration during exercise results in poor performance and increases the risk of potentially life-threatening heat injury such as stroke.[28] Chefs are also at risk for dehydration due to high activity levels on the job, heat extremes in the kitchen, and overconsumption of caffeine-containing beverages. A constant supply of drinking water in the kitchen is advisable to maintain physical well-being and productivity.

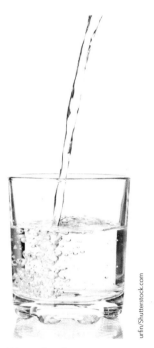

Water is often classified as the most important and essential nutrient in the body.

Overhydration, or water intoxication, may occur when fluid balance is disrupted through the intake of more fluids than the body excretes. Drinking large quantities of water does not cause overhydration when the major organs (kidneys and heart, for example) function normally. For overhydration to occur in an adult with normal kidney function, an intake of two or more gallons of water a day, on a continual basis, would be necessary. Overhydration is rarely caused by the oral consumption of liquids, as one would have to exceed a 15 to 20 liter intake per day. Intravenous feedings that are administered too quickly can cause overhydration.

Overhydration generally causes low sodium levels in body fluids found outside of the cells, and a condition known as **hyponatremia**. Sodium is essential for maintaining blood pressure and the functioning of nerves and muscles. If sodium levels fall in the fluid outside the cells, water enters the cell to restore a balanced concentration of sodium and water, both inside and outside of the cell. Excess water causes cells to swell and produce a condition termed edema. Although most of the body's cells can handle this swelling, brain cells cannot, due to the confines of the skull. Most symptoms of hyponatremia result from swelling in the brain. Symptoms may include loss of appetite, nausea and vomiting, and headaches. Left untreated, confusion and convulsions may occur, and severe cases may result in a coma.

Fluid Needs

Average water recommendations are based on the number of calories consumed. An average of 1 to 1.5 milliliters of water per calorie consumed is estimated. Individuals who consume 2,200 calories per day need 2,200 to 3,300 milliliters of water per day, which is approximately 9 to 13 cups of water. Metric conversions are found on the website. Another method of determining fluid needs is based on kilograms of body weight. The typical ranges used are 25–40 milliliters of water per kilogram of body weight. Conditions that increase fluid needs are summarized in Table 7.5.

TABLE 7.5 Water Needs May be Increased by Many Factors
▪ Age (the very young or elderly)
▪ Dietary Factors (such as an increased intake of fiber, protein, sugar, and or salt)
▪ Extremes of temperature
▪ Forced-air environments (such as airplanes or sealed buildings)
▪ Medical conditions (such as diabetes, prolonged diarrhea, vomiting, fever, blood loss, burns, or surgery)
▪ Medications (especially those that deplete water, such as diuretics)
▪ Physical Activity
▪ Pregnancy and Lactation

Culinary Corner
Phytochemicals

What are phytochemicals and how do they fit into a diet? Phytochemicals are nonnutrients derived from a plant source. Nonnutrients are not considered essential to a healthy body. There are over 2,000 phytochemicals in various plants. Nonnutrients are known to provide color and flavor, and to promote the growth and health of plants. These amazing nonnutrients are also thought to have positive health effects that cannot be explained by their vitamin, mineral, and fiber content alone. Figure 7.3 shows the chemical compounds in foods with known phytochemical composition.

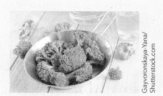

FIGURE 7.3A Broccoli sprouts contain an abundance of sulforaphane.

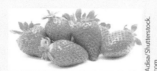

FIGURE 7.3B The ellagic acid of strawberries is a phenolic acid.

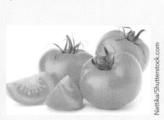

FIGURE 7.3C Citrus fruits provide limonene.

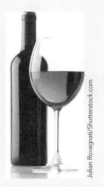

FIGURE 7.3E The phytochemicals of grapes, red wine, and peanuts include resveratrol.

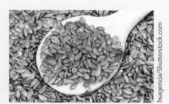

FIGURE 7.3F Tomatoes are famous for their abundant lycopene.

FIGURE 7.3G Flaxseed is the richest source of lignans.

FIGURE 7.3D The flavonoids in black tea may protect against heart disease, whereas those in green tea may defend against cancer.

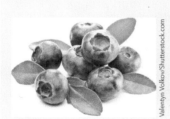

FIGURE 7.3H Blueberries are a rich source of flavonoids.

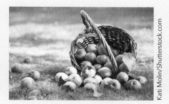

FIGURE 7.3I An apple a day—rich in flavonoids.

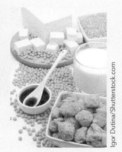

FIGURE 7.3J The phytosterols genistein and diadzein are found in soybeans.

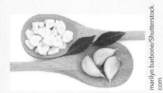

FIGURE 7.3K Garlic, with its abundant allicin, may lower blood cholesterol and protect against stomach cancer.

FIGURE 7.3 Examples of Phytochemicals in Foods

Phytochemicals provide antioxidant activity, simulate hormones, and alter blood constituents that offer protection against certain diseases. Plant pigments, such as lycopene (which helps make tomatoes red), anthocyanins (which give blueberries their blue color), and beta-carotene (which gives carrots their deep yellow color), are phytochemicals that act as antioxidants in the body. Foods high in phytochemicals that help protect against various types of cancers include the sulfur-containing cruciferous vegetables cabbage, broccoli, cauliflower, and brussel sprouts. Unfortunately, many of the foods with high phytochemical content are not as frequently consumed as others. Table 7.6 provides examples of phytochemicals, their food sources, and their potential contribution in disease prevention.

Strong controversies arise over the use of individual phytochemical supplements in lieu of ingesting phytochemicals in food sources. There is no solid evidence that individual phytochemicals extracted from foods benefit health.[29] The effectiveness of phytochemicals appears to depend on the presence of other phytochemicals and compounds in foods.[30]

TABLE 7.6 Examples of Phytochemicals, Their Food Sources, and Possible Effects on the Body		
Phytochemical Name	Phytochemical Function	Top 5 Food Sources
Carotenoids (beta-carotene, lutein, lycopene)	Include over 600 yellow, orange, and red pigments*. Have antioxidant* properties and are associated with a reduced risk of heart disease, and certain types of cancer.	Pumpkin, carrots, dark leafy greens, tomatoes, papaya
Chlorophyll	Include many green pigments. Helps detoxify* cancer-causing agents and may speed up wound healing.	Spinach, parsley, green beans, arugula, sugar snap peas
Curcumin	Bright yellow pigment* found in the spice turmeric*. Has antioxidant* properties and anti-inflammatory* properties. May play a role in cancer prevention.	Turmeric is the only food source
Fiber	A component of plant based foods that cannot be digested by the human digestive tract. May help reduce risk of heart disease, and certain cancers. Also important for regulating blood sugar levels and may help reduce cholesterol levels. Helps prevent constipation.	Beans, oats, bulgur, leafy greens, prunes

Phytochemical Name	Phytochemical Function	Top 5 Food Sources
Flavonoids (anthocyanidins, flavanols, flavones)	A large family of compounds that includes Have antioxidant* and anti-inflammatory* properties. Helps maintain a healthy heart and urinary tract.	Berries, tea, dark chocolate, citrus foods, cranberries
Resveratrol	May help protect the heart from artery damage. May help protect against some cancers.	Grapes, grape juice, peanuts
Soy Isoflavones	May help reduce LDL cholesterol* levels. May decrease the risk of certain types of cancer.	Tofu, miso, soybeans (edamame), tempeh, soy milk

Source: *Antioxidant: A substance in the body that prevents damage to cells; *Anti-inflammatory: Helps reduce inflammation in the body; *Detoxify: To destroy the toxic properties of a substance; *LDL cholesterol: The "harmful" cholesterol; *Turmeric: A bright yellow spice often used in Southeast Asian cooking.

Phytochemicals tend to be heat and light stable because of their chemical properties, and are not easily destroyed by cooking or storage. Phytochemicals contribute to sensory characteristics in foods and help provide protection from a variety of diseases. Most phytochemicals are not stored and are excreted from the body within a few days of ingestion. Regular consumption of fruits and vegetables ensures that the body has a constant supply of phytochemicals. The brighter the color of a food, the greater the phytochemical composition. Tomatoes that have a robust red color, for example, have a high concentration of the phytochemical lycopene. Cooking vegetables with a small amount of fat such as olive oil also increases the body's absorption of some phytochemicals.[31]

References

1   J. P. Bonjour and S. New, "Nutritional Aspects of Bone Health," Royal Society of Chemistry 2003, Cambridge, England.
2   National Osteoporosis Society, Key Facts and Figures 2010. http://www.nos.org.uk/page.aspx?pid=234&srcid=183
3   M. Elliott, "Taking Control of Osteoporosis to Cut Down on Risk of Fracture," *Nursing Older People* 23 (2011): 30–35.
4   M. Svivastara, "Osteoporosis in Elderly: Prevention and Treatment." *Clinics in Geriatric Medicine* 18 (2002): 529–555.
5   B. P. Lukert, "Influences of Nutritional Factor in Calcium Regulating Hormones and Bone Loss," *Calcified Tissue International* 40 (1987): 357.
6   M. Kristensen et al., "Short-Term Effects on Bone Turnover on Replacing Milk with Cola Beverages: A 10-day Interventional Study in Young Men," *Osteoporosis International* 16 (2005): 1803–1808.
7   E. Ma et al., "High Dietary Intake of Magnesium May Decrease Risk of Colorectal Cancer in Japanese Men," *The Journal of Nutrition* 140 (2010): 779–785.
8   http://health.gov/dietaryguidelines/2015/guidelines/executive-summary/
9   Harvard Public Health NOW, *Dean Symposium, Salt and The American Diet*, Office of Communications, Harvard School of Public Health, Boston, MA, 2001.
10 L. J. Appel, "A Clinical Trial of The Effects of Dietary Patterns on Blood Pressure," *New England Journal of Medicine* 336 (1997): 1117–1124.

11   K. M. Kolasa, "Dietary Approaches to Stop Hypertension (DASH) in Clinical Practice: A Primary Care Experience," *Clinical Cardiology* Suppl. 111 (1999): 16–22.

12   F. M. Sacks, "Effects on Blood Pressure of Reduced Dietary Sodium and The Dietary Approaches to Stop Hypertension (DASH) Diet." DASH-Sodium Collaborative Research Group, *New England Journal of Medicine* 344 (2001): 3–10.

13   C. N. Armah, "L-a-Glycerophosphocholine Contributes to Meat's Enhancement of Nonheme Iron Absorption," *The Journal of Nutrition* 138 (2008): 873–877.

14   World Health Organization. Micronutrient Deficiencies. http://www.who.int/nutrition/topics/ida/en/

15   "Iron Deficiency in the U.S. 1999–2000." *Morbidity and Mortality Weekly Report* 51 (2002): 897.

16   R. J. D. Moy, "Prevalence, Consequences and Prevention of Childhood Nutritional Iron-deficiency: A Child Public Health Perspective," *Clinical and Laboratory Haematology* 28 (2006): 291–298.

17   Iron Deficiency Anemia, Medline Plus, National Library of Medicine, http://www.rlm/nih.gov/medlineplus/ency/article/000584.htm

18   A. Klug, "The Discovery of Zinc Fingers and Their Applications in Gene Regulation and Genome Manipulation." *Annual Review of Biochemistry* 79 (2010): 213–231.

19   N. Wijesekara, "Zinc, A Regulator of Islet Function and Glucose Homeostasis," *Diabetes, Obesity, and Metabolism* 11 (2009): 202–214.

20   N. Masoodpoor and R. Darakshan, "Impact of Zinc Supplementation on Growth: A Double-Blind Randomized Trial Among Urban Iranian Schoolchildren," *Pediatrics* 121 (2008): S111–S111.

21   World Health Organization 2004, "Nutrition, Micronutrient Deficiencies," International Council of Control of Iodine Deficiency Disorders. www.who.dk/eprise/main/WHO/Progs/NUT/Deficiency.

22   M. Andersson et al., "Current Global Iodine Status and Progress Over the Last Decade Towards the Elimination of Iodine Deficiency," *Bulletin of the World Health Organization* 83 (2005): 518–525.

23   R. S. Austin et al., "The Effect of Increasing Sodium Fluoride Concentrations on Erosion and Attrition of Enamel and Dentine In Vitro," *Journal of Dentistry* 38 (2010): 782–787.

24   D. Haguenauer et al., "Anabolic Agents to Treat Osteoporosis in Older People: Is There Still Place for Fluoride?" Journal of the American Geriatrics Society 49 (2001): 1387–1389.

25   W. Brown, "Flurosis: Is It Really A Problem?" *Journal of the American Dental Association* 133 (2002): 1405–1407.

26   P. R. Trumbo and K. C. Ellwood, "Chromium Picolinate Intake and Risk of Type 2 Diabetes: An Evidence-Based Review by the United States Food and Drug Administration," *Nutrition Reviews* 64 (2006): 357–363.

27   S. Kleiner, "Water: An Essential But Overlooked Nutrient," *Journal of the Academy of Nutrition and Dietetics* 99 (1999): 200–206.

28   Nutrition and Athletic Performance: "Position of the Academy of Nutrition and Dietetics, Dietitians of Canada, and the American College of Sports Medicine," *Journal of The Academy of Nutrition and Dietetics* 100 (2000): 1543–1556.

29   J. Gingsburg, G. M. Prelevic, "Lack of Significant Hormonal Effects and Controlled Trials of Phytoestrogens," *New England Journal of Medicine* 355 (2000): 163–164.

30   T. Hollon, "Isoflavonoids: Always Healthy?" *The Scientist* 14 (2000): 21.

31   J. E. Brown, *Nutrition Now*, 3rd ed. Belmont, CA. Wadsworth/Thompson Learning, 2002.

Put It into Practice

Define the Term

Review the Culinary Corner "Phytochemicals" and provide the definition of a phytochemical. Make a list of your ten favorite foods, (these should be whole foods or beverages). Use Table 7.6, Examples of Phytochemicals, Their Food Sources, and Possible Effects on the Body, to determine if any of your favorite foods contain phytochemicals. If so, record which phytochemicals they contain and their effects on the body.

Myth vs. Fact

Determine whether the following statement is a myth or fact, and then support your position with evidence from three research articles that you have selected on the topic. *Statement: "If you don't like water, just drink energy drinks."*
　　For each research article, summarize each component below.
　　　　A. Abstract
　　　　B. Methods
　　　　C. Results
　　　　D. Discussion
　　　　E. Conclusion

The Menu

Develop four snack recipes that contain at least two of the major minerals and two of the trace minerals that are outlined in Table 7.4 in the text. List the two specific minerals found in each snack recipe. Each recipe must include the number of servings, an ingredient list, and the method of preparation. A nutrient analysis program must include the amount of calories, protein, carbohydrate, total fat, and the amount of the chosen minerals per serving.

Website Review

Navigate the DASH Diet Eating Plan website through the following link: http://www.dashdietoregon.org/why. Explain what DASH stands for. Click on the "Why the DASH Diet" tab and then click on "DASH Evidence." Summarize the DASH evidence studies and explain the study results. Click on the "Make DASH Work for You" tab on the home page, then click on "Meals," and then "Flavors." List ten salt free seasoning and cooking tips to enhance flavor. How, in your opinion, can this information impacts college age students. List three ways a chef or dietitian could use the information from this website in the workplace.

Build Your Career Toolbox

Ninety nine percent of calcium is stored in the bones. 1200 mg is the approximate equivalent of four cups of milk. As we grow, we need calcium in our diets to contribute to the formation of bone. Unfortunately, calcium intake is declining in children and most teens consume less than 1000 mg of calcium per day. Develop a job description for a public school system "Nutrition Educator." Include salary range, education, and experience requirements. This person is responsible for developing the nutrition education curriculum in the school district and for encouraging the intake of milk and dairy products in the school lunch program.

Hector's Case Study: DASH Diet and Hypertension

Hector is a 53-year-old man who was recently diagnosed with hypertension after a blood pressure reading of 154/95 mmHg. Hector had previously been complaining of nausea, fatigue, and increased sweating while at work as a construction foreman.

His cardiologist would like Hector to lower his blood pressure by losing 20 lbs and improving his diet, before prescribing medications. The doctor asked Hector to lower his salt intake and start exercising and return in 2 months. After Hector's second blood pressure reading of 164/99 mmHg and no change in weight, the cardiologist decided to refer him to a dietitian. Hector's diet was evaluated by an RD who recommended him to follow the DASH diet.

Anthropometric Data

Wt: 208 lbs   Ht: 5'10"   BMI: 29.8kg/m^2

Recommendations

Calorie Needs: 2000–2200 (to promote weight loss)
Protein: 75–90 g
Total Fat: 60–66 g
Sodium: <2300 mg
Calcium: 1000–1250 mg
Potassium: 3500–4700 mg

24-hr Recall

Breakfast: Sausage, egg and American cheese (1-oz each) on a biscuit, 16-oz hot chocolate (prepared with water)

Lunch: Grilled chicken bacon, lettuce, and tomato (BLT) sandwich (5-oz grilled chicken seasoned with salt, 2-oz bacon, 2 tbsp Ranch dressing, 1 iceberg lettuce leaf, 1 slice tomato, 3-oz bun), medium-sized French fries, 24-oz diet Coke

Snack: Nature Valley Oats n' Honey granola bar (2 bars in package)

Dinner: 6-oz meatloaf with 1/3 cup gravy, 2 cups mashed potatoes, 12-oz whole milk

Snack: 3-oz cheddar cheese, 2-oz Wheat Thins crackers

Preferences: Hector doesn't have a lot of time to cook or prepare meals, so he likes things that are "quick and easy." He likes salads but thinks they take too long to prepare, and also likes fish, chicken, and beef. He hates Brussels sprouts, sweet potatoes, carrots, apples, nuts, and olives.

Angela's Anemia Case Study

Angela is 15 years old and is not doing well in school. She is frequently absent because of headaches. When she is in class, her teachers notice that she is not concentrating. At home, her parents find her sleeping when she is supposed to be doing her homework. She is irritable with her family and never wants to do anything with them, complaining that she is too tired. Even her friends have noticed that she is moody and that she cannot keep up with their high-energy activities.

Her medical checkup and blood test results for her hemoglobin level were at 10gm/dl, while the normal blood levels for hemoglobin are 12 – 15 gm/dl. Angela was diagnosed with iron deficiency anemia. Her doctor recommended she see a dietitian in order to increase her dietary intake of iron. The dietitian has consulted with you to prepare a new meal plan for Angela which includes iron-rich foods.

Anthropometric Data

Wt: 108lbs   Ht: 5'3"   BMI: 19kg/m^2 (normal)

Dietitian's Recommendations

Calorie needs: 1400–1600
Protein needs: 60–80g
Fat: 25–30% of calories
Carbohydrates: 50–60% of calories
Iron: 15–18mg
Vitamin C: >65mg

Other recommendations: include recommendations on foods that help to increase absorption, as well as which foods to avoid which block the absorption of iron.

24-hr Recall

Breakfast: 1 1/2 cups Corn Flakes , 6oz skim milk, 1 tsp sugar

Lunch (at school): 1 slice cheese pizza, 4oz applesauce, 3oz French fries with 3 TBSP ketchup, 16oz skim milk

Snack: 1 medium banana

Dinner: 3/4 cup macaroni and cheese, 1 cup salad with iceberg lettuce, carrots and 2 TBSP fat free Italian dressing, 12 oz. diet coke

Preferences:

Likes: cold cereal, frozen waffles, fruited yogurt, macaroni and cheese, pasta, boneless chicken, rice, celery and carrots

Dislikes: red meat such as steak but will eat ground beef in spaghetti sauce, raw tomatoes, lima beans, fish, onions.

Study Guide

Student Name _____ **Date** _____

Course Section _____ **Chapter** _____

TERMINOLOGY

Magnesium____	A. An inorganic element that is essential to the functioning of the human body, which must be obtained from foods
Heme____	B. Involved with bones and teeth
Iron____	C. Deficiency may lead to enlarged thyroid (goiter)
Iodine____	D. Involved with water balance
Zinc____	E. Deficiency may lead to tooth decay
Calcium____	F. Is a component of hemoglobin
Sodium____	G. Food sources include peanuts and legumes
Potassium____	H. Deficiency can result in growth failure
Mineral____	I. Plays a part in acid base balance and formation in gastric juices
Non Heme____	J. Toxicity can lead to hypertension
Chloride____	K. The form of iron found in meats, poultry, and fish
Diuretic____	L. Associated with insulin, involved with energy release from glucose
Fluoride____	M. The form of iron found in vegetables, fruits, and grains
Chromium____	N. A substance or drug that increases urinary output

Student Name _____   Date _____

Course Section _____   Chapter _____

MINERAL MENU PLANNING

Featured Mineral:_____

RDA for college age students (19-30 years) _____ *include unit of measure/day

You are the foodservice director of a large university dining facility and you are in charge of planning menus. Create a lunch meal and a snack item with in each column with specific dietary alternatives that provides a good source of your mineral. **Use the DRI- RDA and Chapter 7: Mineral Table 7.4** to summarize the information about your featured mineral. **Your menu must follow the "Choose Your Foods Lists for Meal Planning" (Appendix B).** *See back for menu plan.

This mineral is a: major mineral   trace mineral   (circle correct answer)

Functions in the body:

Deficiency symptoms:

Toxicity symptoms:

Most common food sources:

Student Name _____   Date _____

Course Section _____   Chapter _____

Mineral:_____

circle or underline menu items with the featured mineral

Each meal should have at least one good food source of your mineral.

Food Choice Requirements:

Lunch: 2 starch, 1 dairy, 2 protein, 1 veg, 1 fat

Snack: 1 fruit, 1 protein

LUNCH -Regular	LUNCH -Lacto	LUNCH -Lacto-ovo	LUNCH -Vegan	LUNCH -Gluten Free
SNACK ITEM -Regular	SNACK ITEM -Lacto	SNACK ITEM -Lacto-ovo	SNACK ITEM -Vegan	SNACK ITEM -Gluten Free

Student Name _____   Date _____

Course Section _____   Chapter _____

CASE STUDY DISCUSSION

DASH Diet and Hypertension Case Study: Shake the Salt Habit

Review the sections in Chapter 7 on Sodium and the DASH Diet. After reading the case study, use the information to answer the following questions:

Explain the relationship between sodium and hypertension; include the definition of "salt-sensitive".

Explain what DASH stands for and the rationale for this diet.

Using Table 7.3 DASH Diet; design a one day low sodium menu for Hector that meets all of the requirements of the food groups/ servings per day. Be sure to include his preferences and sodium free flavor enhancers in the menu.

Student Name _____   Date _____

Course Section _____   Chapter _____

CASE STUDY DISCUSSION

Angela's Iron Deficiency Anemia

Review the section in Chapter 7 on Trace Minerals and Table 7.4 "The Functions, Deficiencies, Toxicities and Sources of Minerals." After reviewing the case study, use the information to answer the following:

1. List the major functions of iron in the body.

2. What are the symptoms of iron deficiency?

3. What are the symptoms of iron toxicity?

4. Explain the difference between heme and nonheme iron.

Student Name _____   Date _____

Course Section _____   Chapter _____

PRACTICE TEST

Select the best answer.

1. The primary function(s) of minerals is
   a. energy production
   b. structure and regulation
   c. muscle building
   d. disease prevention

2. Which of the following is a major mineral?
   a. calcium
   b. zinc
   c. fluoride
   d. iodine

3. The most common nutritional deficiency worldwide is
   a. selenium
   b. copper
   c. iron
   d. calcium

4. Diuretics
   a. decrease water loss
   b. increase water loss
   c. have no effect on water balance
   d. cause edema

5. Initial signs of dehydration include
   a. headache and dark colored urine
   b. stomach pains and nausea
   c. diarrhea and vomiting
   d. excessive sweating and muscle cramps

Student Name _____   **Date** _____

Course Section _____   **Chapter** _____

TRUE OR FALSE

_____ Major minerals are found in the body in amounts greater than 5 grams.

_____ The mineral most closely related to osteoporosis is magnesium.

_____ Heme iron is found in plant products while nonheme iron is found in meats, fish and poultry

_____ The mineral most closely linked to hypertension is sodium.

_____ Water loss from the body is mainly through the urine.

List 2 functions and major food sources of the following minerals:

- Calcium_____

- Magnesium_____

- Potassium_____

- Iron_____

- Zinc_____

List 4 functions of water in the body:

- _____

- _____

- _____

- _____

Digestion, Absorption, and Metabolism 8

Culinary Corner: Probiotics and Prebiotics

References

Put It into Practice

Don's Case Study

Study Guide

KEY TERMS

Absorption	Epiglottis	Metabolism
Active transport	Esophagitis	Mouth
Alcohol	Facilitated diffusion	Mucus
Anabolism	Fetal Alcohol Syndrome	Oligosaccharides
Ancillary organs	Gallbladder	Pancreas
Anus	Gallstones	Peristalsis
ATP	Gastric juice	Portal system
Bicarbonate	GERD	Prebiotics
Binge Drinking	GI tract	Probiotics
Bolus	Glycolysis	Pyloric sphincter
Catabolism	Heimlich maneuver	Rectum
Chemical digestion	Ileocecal valve	Saliva
Chyme	Krebs cycle	Salivary glands
Circulatory System	Large intestine	Simple diffusion
Coupled reactions	Liver	Small intestine
Deamination	Lower esophageal sphincter	Swallowing
Diaphragm	Lymphatic system	Trachea
Digestion	Mastication	Villi
Electron Transport Chain	Mechanical digestion	

Introduction

When preparing a recipe it is necessary to include all the ingredients, as the omission of certain ingredients may drastically alter, or even ruin, a product. The body must also have all the essential nutrient ingredients in correct proportions or it will not work efficiently. Every day, approximately 5% of our body weight is replaced by new tissue. Substances in the blood, body fluids, bone cells, taste cells, and skin are replaced. Foods must be broken down into small usable units that can be absorbed into the body and utilized by the cells. **Digestion** is the breaking down of food into its component parts, or nutrients. Rice, for example, a complex carbohydrate, must be broken down in the body to simple sugars or monosacharrides for it to be of use to the body. The proteins found in chicken must be transformed into amino acids, and the fat in olive oil must be converted to fatty acids for the body to absorb the nutrients. Digestion is followed by **absorption** when the component parts of nutrients are carried to the cells. **Metabolism** then permits the cells to use the nutrients for energy, structure, and regulation.

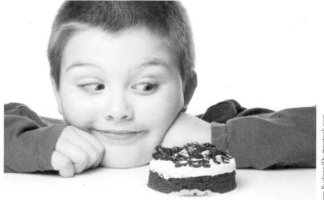

The sensory stimulus of seeing food can start the digestive process.

Digestion actually starts before food enters the body. When the senses of smell, taste, and vision react to sensory stimuli, they produce digestive chemicals and hormonal responses.[1] Walking by a bakery and smelling the wonderful aroma of bread baking can certainly start digestive juices flowing, as can the sight of beautifully prepared, colorful fruits and vegetables.

The processes of digestion, absorption, and metabolism are complex and involve many body systems. The first section of the chapter describes the parts and the functions of the digestive tract and the roles of the ancillary organs that assist in the digestive process. The digestive system as a whole, and the absorption process, are then reviewed.

The Digestive System

The digestive tract (also referred to as the gastrointestinal tract or **GI Tract**) and its component parts include the **mouth, esophagus, stomach, small intestine and large intestine.** (Refer to Figure 8.1 for the components of the

The Digestive System

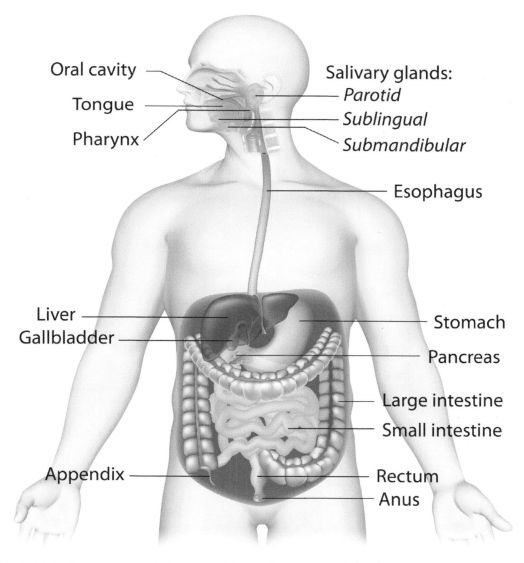

FIGURE 8.1 The gastrointestinal tract and the ancillary organs of the digestive system

Digestive Tract) The GI Tract is a long muscular hollow tube that is approximately 25 feet in length. Two types of digestion occur in the GI Tract. The first, **chemical digestion** occurs throughout the digestive system due to powerful chemical secretions that break down food. These secretions are produced by a variety of organs in response to digestion and include **saliva, gastric juice, mucus, bicarbonate,** enzymes, hormones, and bile.

Saliva is secreted by the salivary glands in the mouth and assists in the initial digestion of carbohydrates. It has multiple functions in the tasting, chewing, and swallowing processes.[2] Gastric juice contains the powerful substance hydrochloric acid. It is secreted by the gastric glands in the stomach to help in the initial breakdown of protein, and in killing foreign bacteria ingested with food. Mucus lines the entire GI Tract and functions to lubricate and protect the lining of the intestinal walls. Bicarbonate is secreted by the pancreas into the small intestine to neutralize the acid of partially digested food coming from the stomach. The food is then further broken down with the aid of enzymes. Enzymes are powerful chemicals that speed up the breakdown of food, as well as other chemical reactions that occur in the body. Hormones are molecules secreted by a variety of glands in response to altered conditions in the body. They act as chemical messengers that signal specific target tissues or organs and restore them to their normal condition. Bile, discussed later in the chapter, is a substance produced by the liver that is needed for fat digestion. The **ancillary organs** (organs that assist in digestion), are responsible for producing many of the powerful secretions needed for digestion. These organs include the **liver, gallbladder, salivary glands,** and **pancreas.** Table 8.1 provides a list of nutrients and a description of how they contribute to the digestion process.

TABLE 8.1 How Macronutrients are Digested and Absorbed				
	Mouth	Stomach	Small Intestine, Pancreas, Liver, and Gallbladder	Large Intestine
Carbohydrates	Digestion initiated due to presence of salivary amylase No action on fiber	Halts in the lower area of stomach due to the presence of hydrochloric acid No action on fiber	Pancreas releases carbohy drase enzymes into the small intestine, cells in intestinal lining complete digestion to monosaccharides for absorption Fiber binds cholesterol and some minerals	Fiber is excreted with feces, some fiber is acted on by intestinal bacteria
Lipids	Digestion of small amount of milk fats due to lipase enzyme produced by the tongue (especially important for nursing infants)	Minimal digestion, fat floats on top and is last to leave the stomach	Liver produces bile and sends to the gallbladder to store, bile is sent to small intestine to emulsify fat. Pancreas secretes lipase enzymes to complete fat breakdown to fatty acids to be absorbed	Small amount carried out with feces
Protein	No digestion	Hydrochloric acid denatures (uncoils) protein strands and activates protease enzyme leaving smaller protein strands	Pancreas releases protease enzymes into the small intestine, cells in intestinal lining complete protein breakdown to amino acids for absorption	Very little, if any, protein is left for excretion

The second type of digestion that occurs in the GI Tract is called **mechanical digestion**. Mechanical digestion is a voluntary process that occurs when food is chewed to break it down into smaller units. Difficulty in chewing, termed impaired **mastication**, can result in difficulty in digesting as well as in absorbing food.[3] **Peristalsis** is another type of mechanical digestion. Peristalsis is a series of involuntary wave-like muscular contractions that break down and push food through the digestive tract from the esophagus to the large intestine. Figure 8.2 provides a diagram of peristalsis in the esophagus. Sphincters, or circular muscles, help to close and open the various sections of the GI Tract and control the flow and exit of food and waste. The four major sphincters or muscular rings are: 1) the **lower esophageal sphincter (LES)**, closes off the stomach from the esophagus, 2) the **pyloric sphincter**, which separates the stomach from the small intestine, 3) the **illeocecal valve**, which separates the small intestine from the large intestine, and 4) the **anus**, which closes off the large intestine and holds waste until it is eliminated.

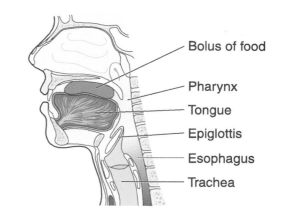

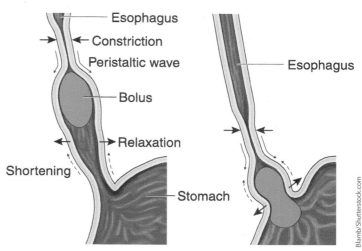

FIGURE 8.2 Peristalsis in the Esophagus

Parts of the Digestive Tract

The digestive tract is made up of a number of organs that work together to effectively break down, process, and distribute nourishment throughout the cells. These organs will be discussed in the following order: the mouth, the esophagus, the stomach, the small intestine, and the large intestine. The ancillary organs that assist digestion will then be reviewed. (Refer to Figure 8.1 for the components of the Digestive Tract)

The Mouth

The mouth is the entry point for food where saliva moistens the food. Saliva contains an enzyme secreted from the salivary glands called salivary amylase. Salivary amylase begins the digestion of the complex carbohydrate, starch. Chewing causes the food to mix with saliva to form a **bolus**. A bolus is a semi-solid mixture of formed food that is swallowed past the **epiglottis**. The epiglottis is made of cartilage and prevents food or fluid from entering the **trachea** (the tube to the lung). Choking occurs when food passes by the epiglottis, enters the trachea, and blocks the airway either partially or completely. (Figure 8.3) When a person is unable to speak or make a sound, it is possible that the airway is completely blocked. In this situation, medical attention is required immediately, unless someone who is qualified to perform the **Heimlich maneuver** (a technique to dislodge the food from the trachea of a choking person) is present.[4]

The tongue allows us to chew and to move food around in the mouth so that the bolus can be formed. Food that is properly chewed and formed into a bolus can then move easily past the epiglottis to the esophagus by the involuntary muscular contraction of **swallowing**.

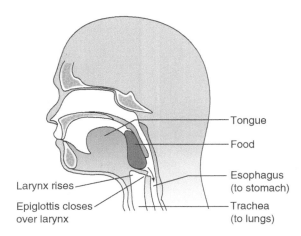

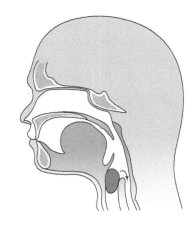

Swallowing. The epiglottis closes over the larynx, blocking entrance to the lungs via the trachea. The arrow shows that food is heading down the esophagus normally.

Choking. A choking person cannot speak or gasp because food lodged in the trachea blocks the passage of air. The arrow points to where the food should have gone to prevent choking.

FIGURE 8.3 Choking occurs when food passes by the epiglottis, enters the trachea, and blocks the airway either partially or completely

The Esophagus

The esophagus is a hollow tube that connects the mouth to the stomach. It consists of strong muscular walls that push food down by a process of wave-like involuntary contractions called peristalsis. When food is not adequately chewed or mixed with saliva, the passage of food becomes difficult, and it is necessary to consume fluids to assist in the process. The esophagus is coated with mucus that protects and lubricates the walls to ease the passage of food. At the end of the esophagus there is a strong muscle called the **diaphragm**. The diaphragm helps to hold the esophagus in place while the bolus enters the stomach.

The Stomach

The stomach is a temporary storage area for food where some digestion of nutrients occurs. When the bolus enters the stomach from the esophagus, it mixes with stomach acid or gastric juice. Gastric juice is made up of approximately 50% water and 50% secretions such as hydrochloric acid, enzymes, and mucus. A valve known as the lower esophageal sphincter closes off the opening of the esophagus to the stomach, once the bolus enters the stomach, to prevent strong gastric secretions from splashing back into the esophagus. Damage and/or discomfort and the initial sensations of "heartburn" take place if the valve does not close. With the help of peristalsis and gastric juices, the bolus is transformed into a semi-liquid known as **chyme**.

The carbohydrates, proteins, and fats in the chyme are transported from the stomach at various rates. Carbohydrate digestion does not occur in the stomach. Carbohydrates are quickly released from the stomach. Proteins are partially digested or denatured in the stomach by hydrochloric acid and are then further broken down by gastric enzymes such as gastric protease. Fat is partially digested in the stomach by gastric enzymes such as gastric lipase. It takes from one to four hours to empty the contents of the stomach, depending on the types of foods and the amounts eaten. Fluids leave the stomach more rapidly than do larger, more solid particles. The partially digested chyme then continues to the small intestine, which is the primary site of digestion.

The Small Intestine

The small intestine is approximately 10 to 12 feet in length and consists of three parts: the duodenum, the jejunum, and the ileum. When chyme enters the small intestine through the pyloric valve, it goes into the duodenum, on through the jejunum, and finally enters the ileum. The digestion of chyme is made possible by secretions from the gallbladder, liver, and pancreas. The small intestine is also the primary site for the absorption of digested nutrients.

The Large Intestine

The chyme that is not absorbed in the small intestine passes through the ileocecal valve to the large intestine, which is approximately 5 feet in length and comprised of the cecum, colon, and rectum. As the chyme passes through the large intestine, it absorbs water and small amounts of minerals. A small amount of vitamin synthesis also occurs here as a result of the bacteria present in the large intestine. Semi-solid waste accumulates in the rectum where strong muscles in the walls hold it until it is time for its release. The anus is a sphincter at the end of the rectum that allows the passage of waste.

Ancillary Organs to the Digestive Tract

The Gallbladder

The gallbladder, an organ located near the digestive tract, assists the digestive process by secreting bile into the small intestine via the common bile duct. Bile is needed for the digestion of fat. Bile is initially made by the liver and stored in the gallbladder until it is needed. An individual can store approximately 2 cups of bile. It is made up of cholesterol, bilirubin, and bile salts. In addition to these components, bile contains immunoglobulins that help maintain a healthy intestinal lining. Disorders and diseases of the gallbladder affect millions of people each year. A common disorder involving the gallbladder is the formation of gallstones, which are typically made of cholesterol, bilirubin, and calcium salts. Gallstones can obstruct the flow of bile out of the gallbladder and cause severe pain. In some instances, inflammation of the gallbladder can occur, making symptoms worse and increasing the potential for complications such as liver damage and inflammation of the pancreas.[5]

The Pancreas

The pancreas, located near the digestive tract, is responsible for secreting bicarbonate via the common bile duct to the small intestine. Bicarbonate is needed to neutralize the acidic chyme that arrives from the stomach. The digestion of food would be difficult if the chyme were not neutralized. The pancreas also secretes powerful enzymes that assist in the breakdown of carbohydrates, proteins, and fats, and produces important hormones needed by other parts of the body. The key hormones insulin and glucagon, which will be discussed in more detail later in the chapter, are produced by the pancreas and are essential in the regulation of glucose in the body. The pancreas produces approximately 1,500 milliliters of secretions, the equivalent of a little more than 6 cups of fluid per day. Aside from the liver, the pancreas is one of the most important organs in digesting and utilizing food.[6]

The Liver

It is estimated that the liver, an organ also located near the digestive tract, has more than 500 vital functions and is the most important organ in the manufacturing and processing of nutrients. The liver is a main storage site for glucose, many vitamins, minerals and fats. It acts as a detoxifying agent for alcohol, drugs, or poisons that enter the body, and is able to regenerate cells unlike any other vital organ.[7] Its ability to regenerate cells has been recognized since mythological times. The liver responds to the injury of its cells and follows a sequential change pattern that involves gene expression, growth factor production, and changes in structure.[8] In addition to its metabolic work, the liver produces a substance called bile that assists in fat digestion.

The Digestive System as a Whole

To explain the digestive system as a whole, let us consider the following scenario. A chef has prepared a wonderful meal that includes grilled salmon with mango fruit salsa, wild rice, grilled asparagus, a French baguette with garlic olive oil, accompanied by a glass of wine and a glass of water. Upon entering his restaurant, you inhale the aromas of his cuisine, which stimulates saliva and gastric juices. The appearance of the meal at the table continues to stimulate both your saliva and your gastric juices. The food is chewed, and with the help of saliva, it is softened into a semi-solid substance called the bolus.

The carbohydrates in the starchy foods (the rice and baguette) are partially broken down with the help of the salivary amylase found in the saliva. The semi-solid bolus then travels down the esophagus past the lower esophageal sphincter into the stomach. The stomach breaks down the food into smaller units and mixes it with gastric juices to form a liquid substance called chyme. The protein found in the salmon is partially broken down by the hydrochloric acid found in the gastric juice and in the gastric enzymes, such as

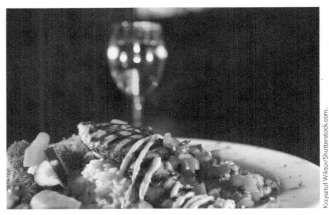

A delicious meal including fish, vegetables, bread, and wine is essentially broken down to an array of amino acids, sugars, fatty acids, vitamins, minerals, and phytochemicals!

gastric protease. The digestion of the carbohydrates (fruit, vegetables, rice, and bread) is halted temporarily in the stomach. Some digestion of the fat, found in the fish and oil, occurs in the stomach with the help of enzymes such as gastric lipase. The water and wine do not need to be digested and are quickly absorbed into the body.

The acidic liquid chyme now enters the small intestine past the pyloric sphincter, and the pancreas releases bicarbonate through the common bile duct to the small intestine, to neutralize the chyme. The broken-down protein from the salmon, the fat from the fish and oil, and the carbohydrates in the rice, bread, vegetables, and fruits complete their digestion in the small intestine. Digestion of the fat in the oil and fish is further helped by bile that is made by the liver and stored in the gallbladder and released into the duodenum. Enzymes from the pancreas complete the breakdown of carbohydrates, fats, and proteins into sugar, fatty acid, and amino acid components. Any chyme not digested or absorbed in the small intestine then passes through the ileocecal valve to the large intestine. Water is absorbed back into the body, and waste such as the fiber found in the asparagus, fruit, and wild rice is accumulated in the rectum and eliminated through the anus. Chefs are essentially chemists who prepare a tasty array of amino acids, sugars, fatty acids, vitamins, minerals, and phytochemicals!

A Common Disorder of the Digestive System: GERD

GERD (Gastroesophageal Reflux Disease) is a relatively common disorder of the digestive system that affects approximately 20% of adults. It is commonly known as heartburn and results from the reflux of gastric and sometimes duodenal contents, including acid into the esophagus. The lower esophageal sphincter normally keeps the stomach's contents in the stomach. When the sphincter loosens or relaxes the stomach contents may irritate the esophagus. The symptoms of reflux include pain and burning in the chest. When symptoms of reflux become chronic, the condition is known as GERD. Untreated GERD may result in more serious conditions such as esophagitis (inflammation of the esophagus), ulceration, scarring, and difficulty swallowing. Medical treatment of GERD includes medications to reduce acid secretion. Lifestyle and nutritional management include:

- Avoiding large, high-fat meals, especially before bedtime.
- Consuming 5–6 smaller meals, spread evenly throughout the day.
- Not smoking or consuming alcohol.
- Avoiding the consumption of chocolate, garlic, caffeine-containing beverages, peppermint, and spearmint.
- Not wearing tight fitting clothes (especially after meals).

- Avoiding vigorous activities after eating.
- Not eating heavily spiced and acidic foods.
- Elevating the head of the bed 4 to 6 inches.[9]

Absorption

Once the three energy-yielding nutrients are broken down into their basic building blocks through digestion—carbohydrates to sugars, proteins to amino acids, and fats to fatty acids—they are ready for absorption in the small intestine. The small intestine is approximately 10 to 12 feet in length and is the primary site for absorption of digested nutrients. Vitamins, minerals, and water that do not require digestion are also absorbed in the small intestine. Millions of molecules pass through the intestinal walls daily and are delivered to the various parts of the body. The large intestine absorbs any remaining water as well as some of the vitamins and minerals.

Anatomy of the Small Intestine

The small intestine has folds in its lining that contain thousands of villi or finger-like projections. Each villus contains hundreds of microscopic hair-like cells called microvilli. The microvilli vastly increase the surface area of absorption of the small intestine and are called the brush border of the small intestine. If we were to spread these projections out flat, they could cover a surface area equal to one-third the size of a football field. The villi are lined with muscles that enable them to be in constant wave-like motion. This movement enhances the ability of the villi to catch and trap the molecules to be absorbed.[10] Figure 8.4 provides a view of the lining of the small intestine.

Types of Absorption

There are three basic ways that nutrients are absorbed into the small intestinal cells of the villi. The first type of absorption is simple diffusion. In this process, molecules such as water and small lipids move freely across the membrane of the intestine into the intestinal cells. Diffusion occurs when a concentrated solution such as soy sauce is added to water and the concentrated salty molecules of the soy sauce diffuse into the less-concentrated water. Nutrients may

INTESTINAL VILLI

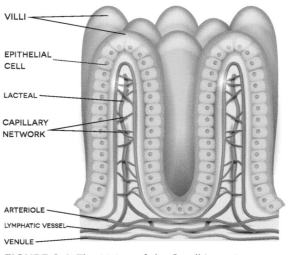

VILLI

EPITHELIAL CELL

LACTEAL

CAPILLARY NETWORK

ARTERIOLE

LYMPHATIC VESSEL

VENULE

Tefi/Shutterstock.com

FIGURE 8.4 The Lining of the Small Intestine

also be absorbed through **facilitated diffusion**, a simple diffusion process in which a "helper molecule" or specific carrier transports molecules over the cell membrane. Water-soluble vitamins require this type of absorption. The third method of absorption, known as **active transport**, allows nutrients to be absorbed into the intestinal cells past the membrane. Nutrients such as glucose and amino acids require the assistance of a specific carrier to be absorbed. These nutrients also need energy to assist in their transport past the intestinal cell membrane.[11] Figure 8.5 illustrates three types of nutrient absorption.

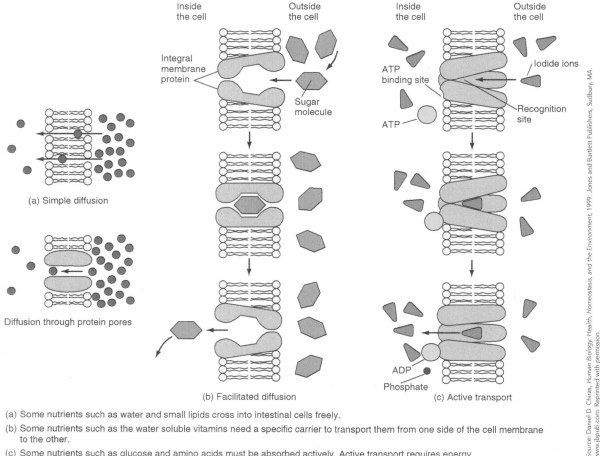

(a) Some nutrients such as water and small lipids cross into intestinal cells freely.

(b) Some nutrients such as the water soluble vitamins need a specific carrier to transport them from one side of the cell membrane to the other.

(c) Some nutrients such as glucose and amino acids must be absorbed actively. Active transport requires energy.

FIGURE 8.5 Three Types of Nutrient Absorption

Source: Daniel D. Chiras, *Human Biology: Health, Homeostasis, and the Environment*, 1999; Jones and Bartlett Publishers, Sudbury, MA. www.jbpub.com. Reprinted with permission.

Delivery Systems of Nutrients

Once the digested molecules are absorbed by the intestinal cells, they must continue to other parts of the body to be used for energy, structure, and the regulation of body processes. There are two main delivery systems, the **portal system**, and the **lymphatic system**. The portal system involves a portion of the **circulatory system** (the bloodstream that is attached to the intestinal tract by a variety of blood vessels), and derives its name from the fact that nutrients are absorbed into the system through the portal (meaning gateway) vein that enters the liver. Nutrients that enter the blood via the portal system include water-soluble nutrients (water, water-soluble vitamins, amino acids, and simple sugars). The liver also serves as a "gatekeeper" for many nutrients, toxins, and foreign substances that may enter the digestive system. Fluid and nutrient delivery occurs through the lymphatic system as well. Fat molecules and fat-soluble vitamins pass through the digestive cells to the vessels of the lymphatic system. Fluids and nutrients transported through the lymphatic system are eventually added to the blood stream.

Metabolism of the Nutrients
Metabolism of Nutrients

Metabolism is the term used to describe the total of all the chemical reactions that occur in the body, including the processes of digestion and absorption. Energy metabolism refers to the chemical reactions that the body performs to obtain and utilize energy from nutrients. Energy can be derived from carbohydrates, fats, and proteins, known as energy-yielding nutrients. The metabolic process begins when the monosaccharide glucose, through a series of chemical reactions, develops ATP (adenosine triphosphate). The entire metabolic process is made up of three primary pathways: Glycolysis, the Krebs Cycle, and the Electron Transport Chain. Carbohydrate metabolism will be discussed first, followed by fat and then protein metabolism.

Carbohydrate Metabolism

Before carbohydrates can be utilized for energy production they must be broken down into glucose, which is their simplest form. Complex carbohydrates must be broken down to monosaccharides through the digestive processes.

Glycolysis

The first process in producing energy from the glucose molecule is called glycolysis. Glycolysis refers to the splitting of the glucose molecule. It is a form of anaerobic energy production, which needs no oxygen to proceed. During glycolysis, the six-carbon glucose molecule is split into two three-carbon molecules known as pyruvate. This metabolic process occurs in the cytoplasm of the cell. Initially a small amount of energy is needed for this breakdown to occur (two ATP molecules). In the formation of the two pyruvate molecules, four ATP molecules are produced, resulting in the release of two ATP molecules (Figure 8.6). This process is a reversible process in which two pyruvate molecules can be utilized to make a glucose molecule when needed.

It is important to remember that the three monosaccharides enter the glycolysis pathway at different stages. Glucose and galactose enter the Glycolytic pathway at the start of the pathway, while fructose enters a bit later. Because of this difference, there is a variation in the metabolism of the monosaccharides. In contrast to fructose, glucose and galactose are subject to two rate-limiting steps that occur in the initial steps of glycolysis. When fructose enters the system, the body is able to utilize this monosaccharide at a faster pace and can convert it to triglycerides that are stored as fat. The brain is slow in responding to this quick influx and still feels the need to consume more carbohydrates. After glycolysis occurs, the pyruvate is irreversibly converted to a compound known as acetyl CoA. This conversion is a transition reaction during which one of the carbon atoms (with it's attached oxygens) is removed from the pyruvate to form carbon dioxide (CO_2). The two remaining carbon molecules then join with a molecule called Coenzyme A (CoA) to form 2 acetyl CoA. The resultant carbon dioxide is released into the blood and travels to the lungs for removal.

Most of the energy metabolism reactions are considered aerobic because they use oxygen throughout the pathway. The glycolysis pathway

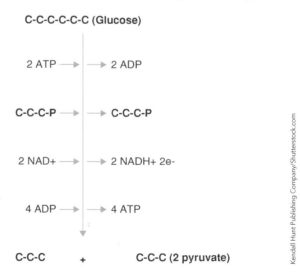

FIGURE 8.6 Overview of Glycolysis
During this process, glucose is broken down into two molecules of PGAL, which are converted to pyruvate. The cell nets two ATP and two NADH molecules.

is an exception because it can be disconnected from the other reactions by converting pyruvate to lactic acid rather than acetyl CoA. If oxygen is in low supply, the pyruvate will take an alternate pathway to form lactic acid. Lactic acid build-up in the muscles causes a burning sensation that can only be relieved by resting the muscle or lowering the intensity of the activity. Lactic acid is transported away from the muscle, through the blood, and to the liver. The liver can then convert the lactic acid back to glucose.

The Krebs Cycle

The second pathway in energy production is called the Krebs Cycle or Citric Acid Cycle (Figure 8.7). This cycle occurs in the powerhouse of the cell known as the mitochondria. It is here that most of the energy derived from the

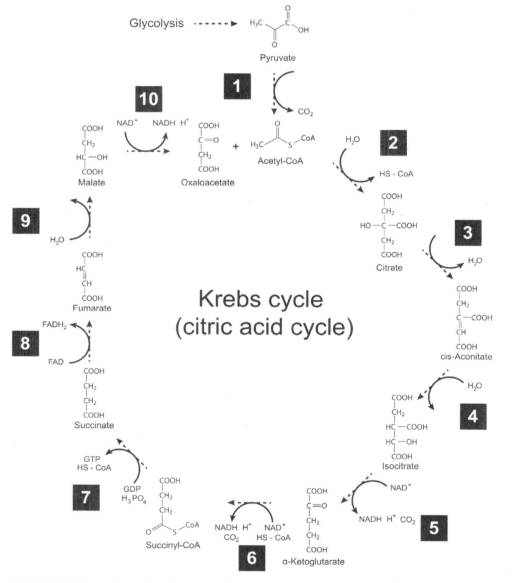

FIGURE 8.7 Overview of the Transition Reaction and the Citric Acid Cycle (a) The transition reaction cleaves off one carbon dioxide and binds the remaining two-carbon compound temporarily to a large molecule called Coenzyme A. The result is a molecule called acetyl-CoA. It then enters the citric acid cycle. (b) Occuring in the matrix of the mitochondrion, the citric acid cycle liberates two carbon dioxides and produces one ATP per pyruvate molecule. Its main products are the high-energy bearing electrons NADH and $FADH_2$, which are then transferred to the electron transport system.

energy-yielding nutrients is produced. The two carbon acetyl CoA formed through the glycolysis pathway go on to enter the Krebs Cycle. The Krebs Cycle is a series of enzymatic steps during which acetyl CoA joins with a 4-carbon molecule to make a 6-carbon molecule. As the cycle continues, one carbon is removed, followed by the removal of a second carbon to form 2 molecules of carbon dioxide. A 4-carbon molecule then remains in the cycle. This 4-carbon molecule goes on to join with another acetyl CoA. This process reoccurs to continue to remove hydrogen atoms and their electrons from the cycle. These electrons are then picked up by coenzymes of the B vitamins riboflavin and niacin and sent to the last pathway known as the Electron Transport Chain. During the Krebs Cycle, one ATP molecule is produced for each pyruvate molecule to generate a total of two additional ATP molecules from the original glucose molecule.

The Electron Transport Chain

The majority of ATP molecules are produced in the last pathway known as the Electron Transport Chain. This stage also occurs in the mitochondria of the cell. Electrons that are released during the first two pathways now enter the Electron Transport Chain, and are picked up and carried along by protein carrier molecules. As the electrons travel along, they lose energy that is used to create ATP (Figure 8.8).

The three pathways ultimately yield 38 ATP molecules for every one glucose molecule. Two molecules are created during glycolysis, two ATP molecules in the Krebs Cycle, and the remaining 34 ATP molecules are generated in the Electron Transport Chain.

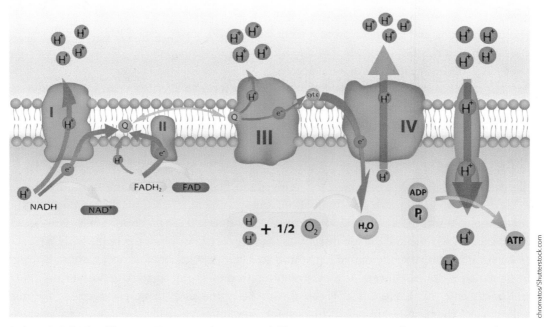

FIGURE 8.8 The Electron Transport System and Chemiosmosis. Located on the inner surface of the mitochondrial inner membrane, the electron transport system produces ATP via chemiosmosis.

Fat Metabolism

Triglycerides are the major form of energy storage in the body. Triglycerides are composed of three fatty acids attached to one glycerol molecule. These fatty acids are made up of hydrocarbon chains ranging in size from 4-to 24-carbon units. When the body uses triglycerides for energy, the fatty acids are removed from the glycerol molecule. Two possibilities now exist for energy production. When energy is needed, the 3-carbon molecule glycerol can be converted quite easily to the 3-carbon molecule pyruvate. The energy pathway continues to produce acetyl CoA as it does in glucose metabolism and further proceeds through the Krebs Cycle and the Electron Transport Chain pathway. If energy is not needed at the time, two glycerol molecules can be converted to glucose because the process of converting glucose to pyruvate is a reversible pathway. The fatty acid chains, on the other hand, enter the metabolic pathway in a different manner. The fatty acid chain is broken down two carbon units at a time by a process known as β-oxidation. During this aerobic reaction, CoA joins to the end of the fatty acid chain. With the removal of a little bit of energy, the last two carbons that are attached to the CoA are removed from the fatty acid chain, to leave the remaining fatty acid chain and a molecule of acetyl CoA. This acetyl CoA now enters the Krebs Cycle as does the acetyl CoA formed from glucose during glycolysis (Figure 8.9). Once acetyl CoA is formed, the reaction cannot form glucose because Acetyl CoA serves only as a forward reaction into the Krebs Cycle. Fatty acids make up approximately 95% of a triglyceride and are therefore a poor source of glucose. Energy derived from triglycerides is useful for building muscle but does not contribute in supplying energy to the brain and the central nervous system. If glucose is present in a small supply (such as during fasting or when on a strict low carbohydrate diet), the body can adapt to some degree.

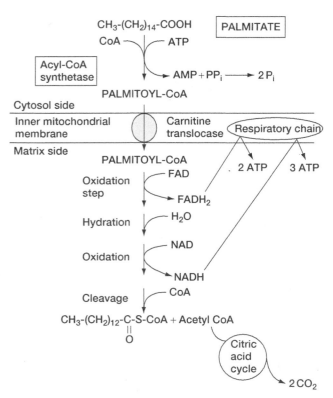

FIGURE 8.9 Conversion of fatty acids to acetyl CoA through β-oxidation

The acetyl CoA fragments formed during β-oxidation will join to form an alternate energy source known as ketones. Ketones can be utilized to a small extent to fuel brain cells and the central nervous system. Unfortunately, as ketone levels rise in the blood, the blood pH lowers and can cause the disruption of all metabolic functions.

Protein Metabolism

Before proteins can be used as an energy source, the nitrogen must be removed from the amino acid by a process that occurs in the liver. This process, known as **deamination**, removes the nitrogen from the amino acid. The remaining nitrogen forms ammonia that is eventually removed through the kidneys. If too much ammonia is produced it may alter the acid-base balance of the blood and cause a disruption of many metabolic processes in the body.

Once deamination is complete, the remaining amino acid component contains only carbon, hydrogen and oxygen. This carbon skeleton can be converted to pyruvate (referred to as glucogenic), to acetyl CoA (known as ketogenic), or can directly enter the Krebs Cycle (Figure 8.10). The amino acids that are converted to pyruvate can also be used to make glucose (hence they are called glucogenic). Proteins can also be used as a source of glucose if carbohydrates are unavailable in the diet.

Fat Storage

All three energy yielding nutrients can be stored in the body as triglycerides. In order to understand this concept, let us review the metabolic pathways for carbohydrates and proteins. Glucose (from carbohydrates) is first converted to pyruvate through glycolysis. Pyruvate is then changed to acetyl Co A, which is an irreversible process. At this point, if energy is not needed by the body, the acetyl CoA is used to make fatty acids and is subsequently stored as fat. The metabolism of energy between fatty acids and acetyl CoA is a reversible step. The ketogenic amino acids in protein are converted to acetyl CoA and are used to make fatty acids that are stored

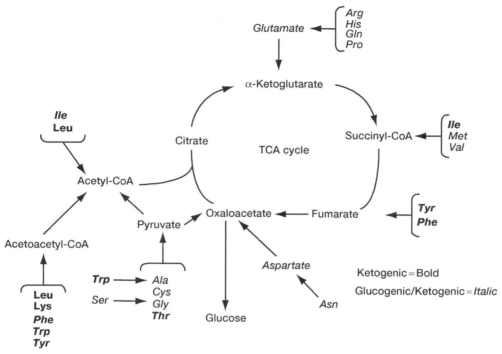

FIGURE 8.10 Use of proteins for energy metabolism

as triglycerides. The remaining nitrogen that has been removed by deamination, can be excreted from the body through the kidneys, or used to make nonessential amino acids through a reaction known as **transamination**.

To fully understand the metabolic pathways, it is necessary to learn how the energy yielding nutrients are converted to other molecules in the pathways. The glycerol obtained from the triglyceride follows a reversible reaction into the glycolysis pathway while the fatty acids follow a reversible pathway to acetyl CoA. Glycerol can be converted into glucose but fatty acids cannot. In the case of amino acids, some will be converted to pyruvate and others to acetyl CoA. Those converted to Acetyl CoA (ketogenic) can

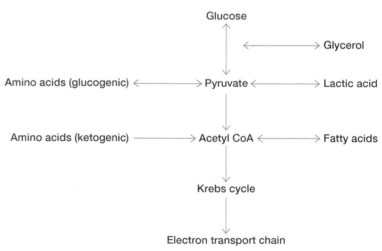

FIGURE 8.11 Fate of the energy yielding nutrients in the metabolic pathway.

be stored as fat when energy is not needed, while those converted to pyruvate (glucogenic) can be utilized to make glucose. Glucogenic amino acids can also be transformed to triglycerides and stored as fat (Figure 8.11).

For a summary of the relationship between the three energy-yielding nutrients in the metabolic pathways, refer to Figure 8.12.

Types of Energy Metabolism

The body performs a variety of chemical and physical reactions to obtain and use energy. Three of the main types are anabolism, catabolism, and coupled reactions. Anabolism is a chemical reaction that requires energy. During anabolism, the basic units of the energy-yielding nutrients, amino acids, glucose, fatty acids, and glycerol are used to

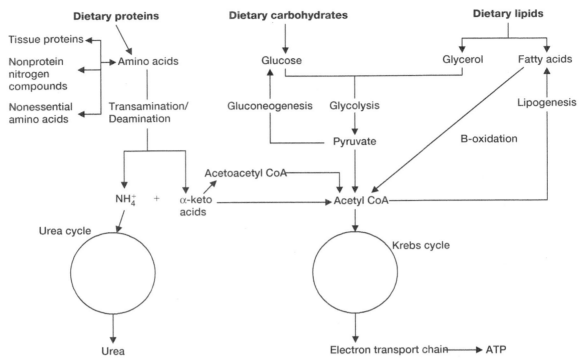

FIGURE 8.12 Summation of the Metabolic Pathways for Carbohydrates, Fats and Proteins.

build larger compounds in the body. The combining of amino acids to form a larger protein compound is an example of **anabolism**. An analogy of anabolism may be made with the preparation of a wedding cake by a pastry chef. The chef combines layers and layers of cake and frosting (molecules of glucose, fatty acids, and glycerol), to form a new and larger compound, and a finished masterpiece. This creation requires a great deal of energy, as does the process of anabolism.

Catabolism is the opposite of anabolism. This reaction yields a release of energy from the breakdown of body compounds. Carbohydrates are broken down to glucose, triglycerides to fatty acids and glycerol, and protein to amino acids. When the body needs energy, it takes these four basic units and breaks them down even farther.

Coupled reactions are pairs of chemical reactions that occur when energy is released from the breakdown of a compound (catabolism) and are used to form another compound (anabolism). ATP (adenosine triphosphate) can be created through catabolism, which captures energy in its bonds for future use. ATP molecules carry the body's energy currency to help build body structures, to maintain and repair the body, and to generate heat as needed. The body is able to convert approximately 50% of consumed food into energy or ATP molecules.

The many factors that affect the metabolism of nutrients will be discussed in Chapter 9 in the sections concerning energy balance, weight, and physical activity. The compound that is discussed next is alcohol. Although not essential, it does provide calories to the diet and must be metabolized by the body. The potential harm that it's excess consumption can cause is also examined.

Alcohol

Introduction

The chemical name for the intoxicating ingredient found in beverages such as beer, wine, and hard liquor is named ethanol or ethyl alcohol. **Alcohol** is a nonessential nutrient that yields 7 calories per gram. Unlike the essential energy-yielding nutrients (carbohydrates, proteins, and lipids), alcohol provides empty calories that do more harm than good.

Alcohol requires no digestion, is quickly absorbed through the intestinal cells to the blood, and reaches the brain minutes after ingestion. Alcohol is classified as a narcotic that has sedative and depressant effects on the brain. Although more than 100 million Americans are said to consume alcohol responsibly, many others imbibe quantities that are far greater than the amount considered to be safe.[12] The Dietary Guidelines propose no more than one drink daily for women and no more than two drinks daily for men. A standard serving or drink (Figure 8.13) contains 14 grams of pure ethanol, which is the equivalent of the following:

- 12 ounces of beer (150 calories)
- 5 ounces of wine (100 calories)
- 1½ ounces of 86-proof distilled spirits (105 calories).

The Dietary Guidelines also suggest that children and adolescents; people of any age who cannot restrict their drinking to moderate levels; women who are or may be pregnant; individuals who plan to drive, operate machinery, or take part in other activities that require attention, skill, or coordination; and those taking prescription or over-the-counter medications that can interact with alcohol should abstain.[13]

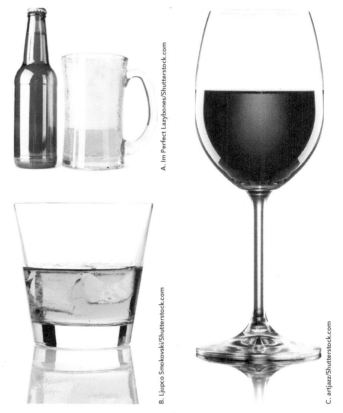

FIGURE 8.13 A Standard Serving or Drink of Alcohol

Physiological Consequences of Alcohol

Alcohol can be directly absorbed into the bloodstream without digestion. On an empty stomach, approximately 20% can be absorbed through the stomach's lining and can reach the brain in one minute. Alcohol that is consumed with or after a meal or snack is not as quickly absorbed. The alcohol dehydrogenase found in the stomach can help to break down up to 20% of alcohol before it reaches the bloodstream. Women produce less alcohol dehydrogenase than do men, so a greater amount of alcohol is able to enter the small intestine and the bloodstream. Men have a higher tolerance to alcohol than women do because of this physiological fact. Once alcohol reaches the small intestine, it is directly and quickly absorbed into the bloodstream and metabolized by the liver. The liver must metabolize alcohol before it can work on the essential nutrients.

The Role of the Liver

The liver metabolizes the majority of alcohol. A small percentage (about 10%) leaves the body through the lungs in the breath and in the urine. The remaining amount passes through the liver, which is considered the "gatekeeper" for nutrients, drugs, and toxins that enter the body. Once alcohol arrives at the liver, it is broken down by the enzyme alcohol dehydrogenase and is metabolized. The liver can process approximately one-half ounce of ethanol per hour, which is the equivalent of one drink. Alcohol consumed in excess of this amount cannot be handled by the liver and is forced to circulate back into the bloodstream, where it can affect all organs—in particular the brain. Table 8.2 outlines the effects of alcohol on the brain.[14] Low food intake, poor general health, low body weight for height, dehydration, and being a female are all factors that may cause an increase in alcohol absorption.

TABLE 8.2 Alcohol's Effects on the Brain

Part of the Brain	Effects
Frontal lobe (most sensitive to alcohol)	Sedative effects, alters reasoning and judgment as it enters the cells
Speech and vision centers	With continued drinking, these centers of the brain become sedated and reasoning becomes even more incapacitated
Large-muscle control centers	With continued drinking, the effect on these centers of the brain result in poor control that is evidenced by staggering and/or weaving when walking
All parts of the brain	With severe intoxication, the conscious brain becomes subdued and the person becomes unconscious
Deepest brain centers that control	At this high blood alcohol level, the brain is anesthetized causing breathing and heart rate cessation, resulting in death

Short-Term Complications of Excessive Alcohol

Binge drinking, considered to be drinking in excess of 4 or 5 drinks consecutively, is common among college-age students across the country. The average number of drinks consumed by college students is 1.5 per week. For binge drinkers in college, the number jumps drastically to 14.5 drinks per week. Nationally, one in five college students is a frequent binge drinker. Binge drinkers account for 68% of all alcohol consumption by students. The majority of alcohol-related problems are caused by binge drinking.[15] Although binge drinking is somewhat socially accepted in college, it increases an individual's chances for alcoholism later in life. The younger a person is when he or she begins to drink alcohol, the greater the risk for alcoholism. Binge drinking can cause death when alcohol saturates the brain and causes the cessation of breathing. It can also cause spasms of the arteries that lead to the heart, and potentially cause a heart attack. Studies show that binge drinking is also associated with impaired memory and difficulty in recognition tasks.[16] The sexual judgment of both men and women has also been found to be affected by alcohol consumption. Intoxicated individuals often exaggerate the meaning of strong dating cues, and ignore ambiguous dating cues.[17]

The Long-Term Effects of Excessive Alcohol Consumption

The long-term effects of alcoholism can be seen in all of the body's systems. Drinking excessively during pregnancy can cause fetal alcohol syndrome, which results in physical and behavioral abnormalities in the fetus. Even small amounts of alcohol are not advised during pregnancy as they may affect the developing fetus in a number of ways. Severe damage to the liver, known as cirrhosis, can also occur from excessive, long-term consumption of alcohol (Figure 8.14).

Alcoholism is believed to be a complex disease with potential complex genetic traits as the cause. As evidenced by studies, alcohol causes some positive short-term effects such as temporary psychological rewarding effects, including reduced inhibitions and feelings of euphoria. The negative consequences to brain systems, the addictive qualities, and the development of increased tolerance far outweigh any of the short-term advantages. New studies are examining specific genes that indicate the propensity of individuals for alcoholism.[18] Table 8.3 provides examples of health and social issues that may be caused or aggravated by alcohol abuse.[19]

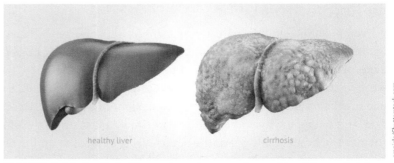

healthy liver   cirrhosis

eranicle/Shutterstock.com

FIGURE 8.14 Realistic illustration of comparison of healthy and sick (cirrhosis) human livers

TABLE 8.3 Alcohol-Related Health and Social Issues	
Problems	**Summary**
1. Social problems	Arguments, strained relationships, work and school absenteeism, and loss of employment all increase with heavy drinking.
2. Legal issues	Committing or being the victim of violence increases with alcohol abuse
3. Medication interactions	More than 150 medications should not be mixed with alcohol. For example, acetaminophen with alcohol may cause liver damage. Antihistamines with alcohol increase the sedative effect.
4. Alcohol-related birth defects	Drinking while pregnant can cause life-long learning and behavior problems for the baby. Fetal alcohol syndrome is a more serious problem with severe physiological, mental, and behavioral problems.
5. Alcohol-related liver disease	Some drinkers may develop alcoholic hepatitis (inflammation of the liver). It can cause death if drinking continues. 10%–20% of heavy drinkers develop cirrhosis, a permanent scarring of the liver, which is irreversible. (Figure 8.10)
6. Heart disease	Moderate consumption may have beneficial effects, but heavy drinking increases the risk of heart disease, hypertension and stroke.
7. Cancer	Long-term heavy drinking may increase the risk for certain types of cancers including cancer of the esophagus, mouth, throat, and larynx, as well as colon and rectal cancer. Women may increase their risk for breast cancer with heavy drinking.
8. Pancreatitis	Long-term heavy drinking may cause inflammation of the pancreas.

Moderate Consumption of Alcohol and the French Paradox

Recent studies show that moderate consumption of alcohol (one to two drinks per day) can help in the prevention of heart disease. These protective effects are attributed to increased plasma levels of high-density lipoprotein and the inhibition of platelet aggregation (the prevention of platelets from clumping together with the potential of forming a thrombus or clot). Although all alcohol has some protective effect against heart disease, wine is said to be the most protective, due to its nonalcoholic phenolic compounds.[20] Red wine, in particular, contains resveratrol and quercitin, which are powerful antioxidants. Grape juice also contains about half the amount of these same compounds.[21]

The protective effects of alcohol may explain what has come to be known as the "French Paradox." Although males in France are at a great risk for diabetes and high cholesterol, and regularly consume large quantities of saturated fat, they display the lowest rate of cardiovascular diseases of all the Western industrialized nations. A regular consumption of wine with meals is considered to be responsible for this "French Paradox."[22]

Cooking with Wine

Wine may be used to flavor soups, sauces, marinades, entrées, and desserts. The quality of the wine used in cooking is very important as is the amount and type of wine. Wines should be of a good quality to accent the flavors of a dish's ingredients. Excessively fruity or sour wines, with a high acidity level, may compromise the taste of a dish. Table 8.4 provides suggestions for wines that might be incorporated to best complement particular dishes.[23, 24] When using wine in cooking, it is important to remember that cooking time, temperature, method of preparation, quantity of product, ingredients used, and type of alcohol all affect the amount of alcohol maintained. The alcohol in table wines, fortified wines, and brandies varies and must be carefully

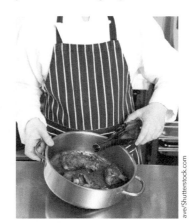

Chefs can create dishes that are enhanced with the addition of wine.

considered. Table wine must be reduced significantly when used in entrées and sauces so that it does not dilute the product. Fortified wines, which include Sherry and Madeira, may be added at the end of the cooking process because they are delicate and require limited reduction. Brandies, on the other hand must be completely "cooked off" due to their high alcohol level, which can overpower, rather than flavor, a sauce.

TABLE 8.4 Culinary Uses of Wine	
Full-Bodied Dry Red Wine (Bordeaux or Cabernet)	
Coq Au Vin	Marinades
Beef	Bourguignon Sauces
Game Ragouts	Bean Dishes
Fish Stews	
Dry White Wine (Sauvignon Blanc or Chardonnay)	
Fish	Chicken
Shellfish	Sauces
Aromatic White Wine (Gewürztraminer, Riesling, Viognier)	
Dishes with Bold and Spicy Flavors	
Fortified Wine (Sherry, Port, Madeira)	
Desserts	Sauces

Culinary Corner
Probiotics and Prebiotics

It is crucial to maintain a balance of beneficial and pathogenic bacteria in the colon. Beneficial bacteria, also known as commensal bacteria, are the good bacteria that are naturally present in the intestinal tract. Pathogenic bacteria are the bad bacteria that can lead to disruption in the gastrointestinal function. Probiotics are live microorganisms, mostly bacteria, that are similar to those found in the human gut. They are referred to as "friendly", or "good" bacteria. Probiotics are found in dietary supplements, milk and milk solids, yogurt, and kefir. Conversely, prebiotics alter the bacterial composition of the gut, by providing a food source to the probiotic to allow it to proliferate. Probiotics and prebiotics have been studied to determine their positive health impacts on disease prevention, namely the reduction of risk of intestinal infectious diseases, cardiovascular disease, non-insulin-dependent diabetes, obesity, osteoporosis, and cancer.[25]

Many microorganisms in the gut are dependent upon the type of bacteria consumed in the diet. There are two groups of bacteria that are most often utilized as probiotics: Lactobacillus and Bifidobacterium. Within each group, there are different species (Lactobacillus acidophilus and Bifidobacterium bifidus) as well as different strains within the species (varieties). In 2001, the Joint Food and Agriculture Organization of the United Nations/World Health Organization Expert Consultation on Evaluation of Health and Nutritional Properties of Probiotics developed guidelines for evaluating probiotics in food. This was done so that substantiation of health claims could be made regarding the use of probiotics.

The proposed guidelines recommend:

- Identification of the genus and species of the probiotic strain
- In-vitro testing to determine the mechanism of the probiotic effect
- Substantiation of the clinical health benefit of probiotic agents with human trials.

Safety assessment of the probiotic strain also needs to be evaluated as to its interaction with other drugs, its metabolic activities in the gut, its potential side effects and potential for toxin production.[26]

There are 3 levels of probiotic action. Level 1 is the "interference" with the growth or the survival of pathogenic microorganisms in the gut lumen. Level 2 is when the probiotic functions to improve the mucosal barrier and the mucosal immune system. Level 3 acts beyond the intestinal tract by affecting the systemic immune system as well as other cell and organ systems, such as the liver and the brain.[27]

Fermented milk has been shown to cause an increase in human intestinal bacterial content. The bacteria are thought to ferment indigestible carbohydrates from food, and to cause an increased production of short-chained fatty acids and a decrease in blood cholesterol levels.[28] Research also shows that probiotics decrease fecal concentrations of enzymes, mutagens, and secondary bile salts that are potentially involved in colon carcinogenesis.[29] The short-chained fatty acids produced during fermentation decrease the pH of the colon contents, which leads to an enhanced growth of normal cells and a suppression of abnormal cells that further reduce the incidence of colon cancer in various population groups.[30] Table 8.5 shows some of the potential benefits of probiotic therapy.

For use in foods, probiotic microorganisms have to be able to survive conditions in the digestive tract and also have the capability to multiply in the intestinal tract.

TABLE 8.5 Potential Benefits of Probiotic Therapy

- Metabolic benefits:
  Lactose digestion
  Lipid metabolism
  Composition/metabolic indicators of intestinal bacteria
- Inflammatory bowel diseases
  Crohn's Disease
  Ulcerative Colitis
- Irritable Bowel Syndrome
- Allergic diseases
  Eczema
  Rhinitis
  Asthma
- Reduction of risk factors of infection
- Infectious diarrhea (acute and antibiotic-associated)
- Urinary tract and vaginal infections
- Traveler's diarrhea
- Necrotizing Enterocolitis (infants)
- Helicobacter Pylori
- Respiratory tract infections (adults and children)
- Ear, nose, and throat infections
- Infectious complications in surgically ill patients

The use of probiotic microorganisms for health benefits, when used as a supplement, should indicate the daily dosage and duration of use as recommended by the manufacturer of each individual strain or product based upon scientific evidence.[31]

In addition to probiotics, a substance known as a prebiotic has been determined to assist in the functioning of the probiotic. A prebiotic is a type of functional food defined as a non-digestible ingredient that beneficially affects the probiotic by stimulating the growth and/or the activity of beneficial microorganisms. This then allows for the colonization of the gastrointestinal tract and improves health at the enteric level.[32] The viability of the intestinal bacteria depends upon substrates such as prebiotics, which are broken down by enzymes to substances including short-chain fatty acids, amino acids, polyamines, growth factors, vitamins, and antioxidants. All of these are important for the health and function of the intestinal mucosa.[33]

Prebiotics can be in the form of neosugars (carbohydrates) such as inulin, soy oligosaccharides, lactulose, raffinose, sorbitol, and xylitol.[34] Oligosaccharides are the sugars most widely studied. They consist of 2 to 20 saccharide units, which are considered short-chain polysaccharides. The oligosaccharide, inulin, occurs naturally in several foods such as leeks, asparagus, chicory, Jerusalem artichokes, garlic, artichokes, onions, wheat, bananas, oats and soybeans. However, these foods contain only trace levels of prebiotic. Functional foods are now being used to supply health benefits beyond basic nutrition and to reduce the risk of disease and provide optimal health.

It has been proven that Bifidobacteria are able to inhibit the growth of pathogenic bacteria; to modulate the immune system; to produce digestive enzymes; to repress the activities of rotaviruses; and to restore the microbial integrity of the intestinal tract microflora, following antibiotic therapy or antibiotic-associated diarrhea. One possible side effect of prebiotic intake is intestinal discomfort from gas production.[35]

Combinations of probiotics and prebiotics are known as synbiotics.[36] A high number of viable probiotic bacteria in the intestines maintains and enhances the presence of a prebiotic.[37, 38] A combination of both probiotic and prebiotic bacteria has shown positive effects in many health disorders. One such study on these benefits showed a reduction of colorectal cancer in rats.[39] Manufacturers are looking for ways to incorporate a prebiotic into foods containing a probiotic to create a synbiotic effect. The inclusion of both a probiotic and a prebiotic has been tried in ice cream. It was found that the addition of microorganisms and inulin did not significantly affect the ice cream's consistency, taste intensity, or homogeneity, although its appearance was more opaque. Scores for flavor were higher due to higher sweetness intensity.[40] Although the results of research on the effects of utilizing probiotics and prebiotics have been promising, more research is needed to determine the effects of their individual and combined uses on a variety of health conditions.

References

1   J. LeBlanc, "Nutritional Implications of Cephalic Phase Thermogenic Responses," *Appetite* 34 (2000): 214–216.

2   A. M. Pedersen, "Saliva and Gastrointestinal Functions of Taste, Mastication, Swallowing and Digestion," *Oral Disease* 8 (2002): 117–129.

3   P. I. N'gom, "Influence of Impaired Mastication on Nutrition," *Journal of Prosthetic Dentistry* 87 (2002): 667–673.

4   H. J. Heimlich and M. H. Uhley, "The Heimlich Maneuver," *Clinical Symposia* 31 (1979): 1–32.

5   L. K. Mahan and S. Escott-Stump, Krause's *Food Nutrition & Diet Therapy*, 9th ed. Philadelphia, PA: WB Saunders Company, 1996.

6   P. Insel, R. E. Turner, and D. Ross, *Discovering Nutrition*, Sudbury, MA: Jones and Bartlett Publishers, 2003.

7   D. Chiras, *Human Biology*, 3rd ed. Sudbury, MA: Jones and Bartlett Publishers, 1999.

8   G. K. Michalopoulos, "Liver Regeneration," *Science* 276 (1997): 60–66.

9   L. K. Mahan and S. Escott-Stump, *Krause's Food Nutrition & Diet Therapy*, 11th ed. Philadelphia, PA: WB Saunders Company, 2000.

10   F. Sizer and Eleanor Whitney. *Nutrition Concepts and Controversies*, 8th ed. Belmont, CA: Thomson Wadsworth Publishing, 2000.

11   D. Chiras, *Human Biology*, 3rd ed. Sudbury, MA: Jones and Bartlett Publishers, 1999.

12   *Moderate Consumption of Distilled Spirits and Other Beverage Alcohol in an Adult Diet for the Food and Nutrition Professional.* Edited by ADA's Knowledge Center. Technical review by the Nutrition Research Dietetic Practice Group of the Academy of Nutrition and Dietetics. Academy of Nutrition and Dietetics, Fact Sheet, 2001.

13   USDA Dietary Guidelines Advisory Committee, *Nutrition and Your Health: Dietary Guidelines for Americans*, 5th ed. Home and Garden Bulletin #232, 2000.

14   F. Sizer and Eleanor Whitney. *Nutrition Concepts and Controversies*, 8th ed. Belmont, CA: Thomson Wadsworth Publishing, 2000.

15   H. Wechsler, B. E. Molnar, A. E. Davenport, and J. S. Baer, "College Alcohol Use: A Full or Empty Glass?" *Journal of American College Health* 47 (1999): 247–252.

16   R. Weissenborn and T. Duka, "Acute Alcohol Effects on Cognitive Functions in Social Drinkers: Their Relationship to Drinking Habits," *Psychopharmacology.* 165 (2003): 306–312.

17   A. Abbey, T. Zawacki, and P. McAuslan, "Alcohol's Effects on Sexual Perception," *Journal of Studies on Alcohol* 6 (2000): 688–697.

18   J. C. Crabbe, "Alcohol and Genetics: New Models," *American Journal of Medical. Genetics* 114 (2001): 969–974.

19   National Institute on Alcohol Abuse and Alcoholism, *Alcohol What You Don't Know Can Harm You, NIH Publication No. 94-4323*, Rockville, Maryland, Revised 2002.

20   J. Belleville, "The French Paradox: Possible Involvement of Ethanol in the Protective Effect Against Cardiovascular Diseases," *Journal of Nutrition* 2 (2002): 173–177.

21   J. Constant, "Alcohol, Ischemic Heart Disease, and the French Paradox," *Coronary Artery Disease* 10 (1997): 645–649.

22   S. Renaud and R. Gueguen, "The French Paradox and Wine Drinking," *Novaritis Foundation Symposium* 216 (1998): 208–217.

23   K. MacNeil, *Cooking with Wine*, 2003, www.cookinglight.com

24   J. Robuchon and the Gastronomic Committee, *Larousse Gastronomique*, The World's Greatest Culinary Encyclopedia, New York, NY: Clarkson Potter Publishers, 2001.25.

25   M. B. Roberfroid, "Prebiotics and Synbiotics: Concepts and Nutritional Properties," *British Journal of Nutrition* 80 (1998): S197–S202.

26   V. Venugopalan, K. A. Shriner, and A. Wong-Beringer, "Regulatory Oversight and Safety of Probiotic Use," *Emerging Infectious Diseases* 16 (2010): 1661–1665.

27   G. T. Rijkers et al., "Guidance for Substantiating the Evidence for Beneficial Effects of Probiotics: Current Status and Recommendations for Future Research," *Journal of Nutrition* 140 (2010): 671S–676S.

28   M. St Onge, T. Farnworth and P. J. H. Jones, "Consumption of Fermented and Nonfermented Dairy Products: Effects on Cholesterol Concentrations and Metabolism," *American Journal of Clinical Nutrition* 71 (2000): 674–681.

29   I. Wollowski, G. Rechkemmer and B. L. Pool-Zobel, "Protective Role of Probiotics and Prebiotics in Colon Cancer," *American Journal of Clinical Nutrition* 73 (2001): 451S–455S.

30   A. Hague, D. J. E. Elder, D. J. Hicks and C. Pareskeva, "Apoptosis in Colorectal Tumor Cells: Induction by the Short Chain Fatty Acids Butyrate, Propionate and Acetate and by the Bile Salt Deoxycholate," *International Journal of Cancer* 60 (1995): 400–406.

31   Food and Agriculture Organization of the United Nations, World health Organization. http://www.who.int/foodsafety/publications/fs_management/en/probiotics.pdf

32   O. Brunser, M. Gotteland, S. Cruchet, G. Figueroa, D. Garrido & P. Steenhout, "Effect of a Milk Formula with Prebiotics on the Intestinal Microbiota of Infants after an Antibiotic Treatment." *Pediatric Research* 59 (2006): 451–456.

33   P. Fric, "Probiotics and Prebiotics-Renaissance of a Therapeutic Principle." *Central European Journal of Medicine* 2 (2007): 237–270.

34   P. J. Jones, "Clinical Nutrition: 7 Functional Foods—More Than Just Nutrition," *Canadian Medical Association Journal* 166 (2002): 1555.

35   S. Kolida and G. R. Gibson, "Prebiotic Capacity of Inulin-Type Fructans," *Journal of Nutrition* 137 (2007): 2503S–2506S.

36   G. R. Gibson and L. J. Fooks, "Probiotics as Modulators of The Gut Flora," *British Journal of Nutrition* 88 (2002): 39–49.

37 R. Mohammadi and A. Mortazavian, "Review Article: Technological Aspects of Prebiotics in Probiotic Fermented Milks." *Food Reviews International* 27 (2011): 192–212.

38 U. Sairanen, L. Piirainen, S. Grasten, T. Tompuri, J. Matto, M. Saarela, and R. Korpela, "The Effect of Probiotic Fermented Milk and Inulin on the Functions and Microecology of the Intestine," *Journal of Dairy Research* 74 (2007): 367–373.

39 A. Klinder, A. Forster, G. Cardeni, A. P. Fermia, and B. L. Pool-Zobel, "Fecal Water Genotoxicity is Predictive of Tumor-preventive Activities by Inulin-like Oligofructoses, Probiotics (Lactobacillus rhamnosus and Bifidobacterium lactis), and Their Symbiotic Combination," *Nutrition Cancer* 49 (2004):144–155.

40 T. Di Criscio, A. Fratianni, R. Mignogna, L. Cinquanta, R. Coppola, E. Sorrentino, and G. Panfili, "Production of functional probiotic, prebiotic, and symbiotic ice creams," *Journal of Dairy Science* 93 (2010): 4555–4564.

Put It into Practice

Define the Term

Review the definition of digestion. Explain the difference between mechanical and chemical digestion and provide an example of each.

Myth vs. Fact

Determine if the following statement is a myth or fact and support your position with evidence from three research articles on the topic. *Statement: "Drinking strong coffee or taking a cold shower can help you sober up quickly."*

For each research article, summarize each component below.

A. Abstract
B. Methods
C. Results
D. Discussion
E. Conclusion

The Menu

You have just consumed a meal of grilled chicken, sautéed spinach in olive oil, wild rice, a sourdough roll, and a glass of sparkling water. Diagram how the digestion of this meal occurs. (Refer to Figure 8.1 and Table 8.1.) List the essential nutrients found in the foods and list where each of the nutrients is digested and absorbed. List the secretions that assist in the digestion of the meal; where they come from; and how do they work. Describe the delivery system through which each of the nutrients in the meal will be absorbed (lymphatic or portal systems).

Website Review

Review the information in the Culinary Corner: "Probiotics and Prebiotics." What is the positive health impact of consuming these good bacteria? List three food sources of each probiotics and prebiotics. View the two WebMD videos through the following links.

http://www.webmd.com/video/good-bacteria

http://www.webmd.com/video/dairy-probiotics

In your opinion, how does this information impact college age students?

Build Your Career Toolbox

Review the "Cooking with Wine" section of the text. Develop a job description for the Executive Chef responsible for training chefs who will be preparing a five star menu. Include salary range, education, and experience requirements. Remember that most of the menu items include wine in their preparation and that it is important not to compromise the flavor of the items by using the wrong type of wine or the wrong quantity. Using the information in the text and Table 8.4, explain how table wine, fortified wine, and brandy are different, and their culinary uses.

Don's Case Study

Don is 33 years old and started drinking alcohol at the age of 14. When he turned 18, he joined the Armed Forces where he spent most of his weekends drinking beer, vodka, and whiskey. When Don got married he said that he wouldn't drink alcohol. That promise did not last long and soon his home became "a total war zone." Don continued to drink daily from the time he got out of work until he went to bed at night. His wife wanted nothing to do with him because he was abusive and violent most of the time. He continued to work in retail management running a grocery store, and this lifestyle continued for the next 15 years. During this time period, he lost their first house in a foreclosure. They had two children, a boy and a girl, but he missed most of their childhood because of his illness of alcoholism. On more than one occasion he admitted that he had a problem, but he felt that he had a good job that paid well and he never drank before work or while he was on the job.

Don woke up one morning feeling very sick. He looked at himself in the mirror and saw that his skin had an orange tint to it. He could not "keep anything down" and vomited continuously for hours. He eventually saw a doctor and was diagnosed with cirrhosis and pancreatitis. Don was referred to a Registered Dietitian for meal planning.

Wt: 145 lbs   Ht: 5'11"   BMI: 20.3 kg/m² (normal)

Dietitian Recommendations
  Calorie Needs: 2000–2200 calories per day
  Protein Needs: 75–85 g/day
  Fat: Goal of 25% calories from fat, <10% calories from saturated fat
  Fiber: 25–30 g/day
  Sodium: <3 g/day (<3000 mg/day)

Other Recommendations: Add lean protein, fruits, and vegetables to every meal (at least five servings per day); avoid high fat foods and begin taking a multivitamin daily with B-vitamins.

24-hr Recall

Breakfast: none

Lunch: 2 slices cheese pizza, 1-oz potato chips

Dinner: 12–20-oz cans of beer nightly

Preferences: orange juice, oatmeal, bagels, eggs, bacon, deli meats such as turkey, ham, roast beef, raw carrots, broccoli, celery, steak, chicken, ground beef, potatoes.

Dislikes: spinach, cooked vegetables, beans, soup, casseroles, apples, bananas

Study Guide

Student Name _____ Date _____

Course Section _____ Chapter _____

TERMINOLOGY

Villi_____	A. The organ that supplies enzymes and bicarbonate to the small intestine to aid digestion
Bolus_____	B. Semi-liquid formed in the stomach by peristalsis and gastric juices
Metabolism_____	C. Circular muscles that close and open to control the flow and disposal of food and wastes
Liver_____	D. Allows the cells to use nutrients for energy, structure, and regulation
Peristalsis_____	E. Line the small intestinal tract and function to increase absorption
Absorption_____	F. The breaking down of food into its component parts, i.e. nutrients
Pancreas_____	G. When the component parts of nutrients are carried to the cells
Digestion_____	H. The involuntary wave-like muscular contractions that push food through the digestive tract
Sphincter_____	I. The most important organ in the manufacturing and processing of nutrients
Chyme_____	J. A semi-solid mixture of formed food that is swallowed

Student Name _____ Date _____

Course Section _____ Chapter _____

JOURNEY THROUGH THE DIGESTIVE TRACT

Use the word bank to fill in the missing words. Each word is only used once.

active transport	carbohydrate	facilitated	jejunum	pyloric
amino acids	chyme	fatty acids	large	re-entering
amylase	composition	fiber	liver	salivary gland
anal	duodenum	gall bladder	lower esophageal	simple
bacteria	emulsify	hormone	monosaccharides	stomach
bicarbonate	energy	hydrochloric	gastric juice	surface area
bile	enzyme	ileocecal	peristalsis	vitamins
bolus	esophagus	ileum	protein	

As food enters the mouth, it is chewed to increase the _____.

The food is mixed with saliva from the _____. The saliva contains the enzyme

salivary _____ that begins chemical digestion of _____.

The chewed food, now termed a _____, is swallowed and then travels down the

_____ by means of _____, a series of muscular contractions.

The entrance of the _____ is separated from the esophagus by the presence of the

_____ sphincter muscle. This muscle is designed to prevent material from

_____ the esophagus.

As the material mixes in the stomach with the aid of _____ acid, it is turned into a

liquid material called _____. This material will remain in the stomach for one to

four hours, depending on the _____ of the meal.

In the stomach, digestion of _____ begins. The material is blocked from entering the small intestine
by the presence of the _____ sphincter.

Once the material enters the small intestine, the acid is neutralized by _____ in the
_____. This liquid also contains the digestive _____ that break down the
_____ yielding nutrients.

Student Name _____   **Date** _____

Course Section _____   **Chapter** _____

The beginning of the small intestine is called the _____. When fat enters the beginning of the small intestine; a _____ is released, this is called cholecystokinin (CCK). This travels through the blood to the _____ where _____ is stored. This substance was originally produced by the _____ and it's job is to _____ fat.

As digestion continues, carbohydrates are broken down into smaller units called _____, fats to _____, and protein to _____. These are absorbed through the intestinal lining by the three possible mechanisms. The mechanisms include; _____ diffusion, _____ diffusion and _____.

Absorption occurs mainly in the middle and lower portions of the small intestine, namely the _____ and the _____. The remaining material is sent through the _____ valve into the _____ intestine.

In the large intestine, _____ feeds on any undigested material and produces_____:

The remaining waste products, which includes indigestible _____ waits for excretion. The voluntary muscle which holds the material in the rectum is called the _____ sphincter.

The journey is now complete!

Student Name _____   Date _____

Course Section _____   Chapter _____

CASE STUDY DISCUSSION

Alcoholism Case Study: Don's Close Call with Cirrhosis

Review the sections in Chapter 8' "The long term effects of excessive alcohol consumption". After reading the case study, use the information to answer the following questions:

1. **Describe Don's relationship with his family and explain the health and social issues that he is facing due to his drinking.**

2. **Name and explain the liver disease that is alcohol-related.**

3. **List 3 dietary and lifestyle recommendations that can help Don.**

Student Name _____   Date _____

Course Section _____   Chapter _____

PRACTICE TEST

Select the best answer.

1. The ability to break down food into its component parts is known as
   a. absorption
   b. digestion
   c. metabolism
   d. peristalsis

2. The process whereby the cells are able to use nutrients for energy, structure and regulation is termed
   a. metabolism
   b. digestion
   c. absorption
   d. all of the above

3. The process of digestion begins when
   a. asensory input is obtained
   b. food enters the mouth
   c. food enters the stomach
   d. food enters the small intestine

4. The lower esophageal sphincter
   a. closes off the stomach from the esophagus
   b. separates the stomach from the small intestine
   c. separates the small intestine from the large intestine
   d. closes off the large intestine

5. The type of alcohol in beer, wine, and hard liquor is
   a. ethanol
   b. hexanol
   c. methanol
   d. xylitol

Student Name _____   Date _____

Course Section _____   Chapter _____

TRUE OR FALSE

_____ A bolus is formed by the movement of the tongue.

_____ Bile is made in the gall bladder.

_____Metabolism is the total of all the chemical reactions that occur in the body.

_____ The Dietary Guidelines recommend no more than one drink for women and 2 drinks for men daily.

_____ Permanent scarring of the liver is seen in cirrhosis.

List the 5 major parts of the Digestive Tract in proper order and one function of each of these parts.

- ▪ _____
- ▪ _____
- ▪ _____
- ▪ _____
- ▪ _____

List 2 tasks that each of the following ancillary organs performs:

- ▪ **Salivary Glands**_____
- ▪ **Gallbladder**_____
- ▪ **Liver**_____
- ▪ **Pancreas**_____

Energy Balance, Weight Control, and Exercise

9

Determining Specific Energy Needs for Sports Activities: Metabolic Equivalents (METs)
References
Put It into Practice
Andrew's Case Study
Brian's Case Study
Study Guide

KEY TERMS

Aerobic	Bulimia Nervosa	Obesity
Amenorrhea	Central obesity	Overfatness
Anaerobic	Eating disorders	Overweight
Anorexia Nervosa	Energy	Physical activity
Appetite	Ergogenic aids	Sarcopenia
Bariatric surgery	Fatfolds	Satiety
Basal metabolic rate (BMR)	Female athlete triad	Subcutaneous fat
Behavior modification	Hamwi method	Target heart rate
Binge eating disorder	Hunger	Thermic effect
Bioelectrical impedance	Ideal body weight	Total energy needs
Body composition	Maximum heart rate	Visceral fat
Body mass index (BMI)	Metabolic Equivalents (METS)	

Introduction: Energy Balance

Energy is the capacity to do work. The energy in food is chemical energy and is measured in kilocalories. When an individual consumes chemical energy, the body converts it to mechanical, electrical, or heat energy. The three major functions of energy in the body are: (1) to maintain our basic bodily functions, otherwise termed **basal metabolic rate (BMR)**; (2) to provide for physical activity; and (3) to process our consumed food. Figure 9.1 shows the percentage of energy needed for each function.

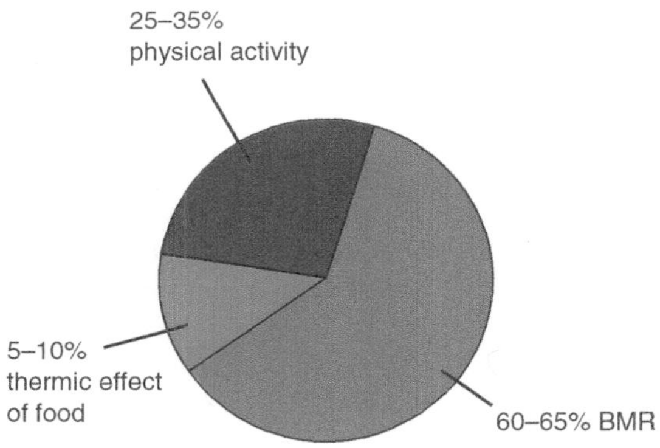

For maintenance of optimal health, weight, and well-being our bodies must be in a state of equilibrium. The energy we consume from food must equal the energy we expend for our three basic energy needs. The body can be compared to a simple food inventory control system. When we deplete a food product from an inventory supply, it is necessary to replace that food to maintain a consistent supply. When there is an excess inventory, we must reduce it to maintain a constant par stock.

FIGURE 9.1 Energy is needed for three major functions.

Basal Metabolic Rate (BMR)

The majority of the energy derived from the food we consume, approximately 60%–65% is used for maintaining our basic body functions. These functions are the sum of all involuntary activities that are necessary to sustain life. They include breathing, blood circulation, temperature maintenance, hormone secretion, nerve activity, and the making of new tissue. There are several factors that can increase or decrease the basal metabolic rate. Table 9.1 lists the variables that affect the BMR.

TABLE 9.1 Factors Affecting the Basal Metabolic Rate
Increases in BMR
High body percentage of lean body mass
Height and weight: Tall, thin people
Growth periods: i.e., childhood, pregnancy
Fever
Stress
Extremes of heat and cold
Decreases in BMR
High body percentage of body fat
Fasting or starvation
Malnutrition
Sleeping
Aging

A number of methods are used to calculate the calorie needs of a BMR. A quick method involves using body weight. The greater the body weight the greater the energy needs for maintaining basal metabolism. Males also require slightly more energy than females. The following equation can be used to calculate metabolic needs. First, convert weight in pounds to weight in kilograms. There are 2.2 kilograms per pound (body weight in pounds / 2.2 = body weight in kilograms). The next equation is gender-specific. For males, use this equation: kilograms of body weight × 1 calorie/kilogram/hour × 24 hours = calories needed per day for BMR. For females, use the following: kilograms of body weight × .9 calorie/kilogram/hour × 24 hours = calories needed per day for BMR.

Examples

1. A male weighs 165 lbs.
   165 divided by 2.2 = 75 kg
   75 kg × 1 calorie/kg/hour × 24 hours = 1,800 calories needed for BMR per day

2. A female weighs 132 lbs.
   132 divided by 2.2 = 60 kg
   60 kg × .9 calories/kg/hour × 24 hours = 1,296 calories

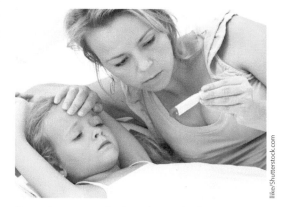

Fever increases the basal metabolic rate.

Physical Activity

The body also requires energy for the voluntary movement of the skeletal muscles and support systems, or **physical activity**. Twenty-five to thirty-five percent of our energy is used for physical activity. The amount of energy we need for physical activity depends on body weight, muscle mass, and the intensity and duration of the activity. An increase in any or all of the aforementioned factors increases the energy needs. A 220-pound male, with a large muscle mass, who runs 3 miles in 20 minutes, needs more energy than a female who weighs 150 pounds and also runs 3 miles in 20 minutes. The male needs more energy due to at least three factors: a larger amount of muscle mass, higher BMR needs, and a greater amount of body weight.

The Thermic Effect of Food

The third function of energy in the body is the **thermic effect** of food, which describes the energy used to process consumed foods. About 10% of our energy intake is dedicated to the thermic effect of food. Since this amount is small, it is not factored in total energy needs. Meals that are high in carbohydrates have a greater thermic effect than high-fat meals.[1]

Total Energy Needs

To determine **total energy needs**, multiply the number of calories needed to maintain the basal metabolic rate by a standard activity factor. Table 9.2 provides energy factors for physical activity.

TABLE 9.2 Energy Factor for Physical Activity	
Activity Level	**Physical Activity Factor**
Confined to bed	1.2
Ambulatory (able to walk), low activity	1.3
Average activity	1.5–1.75
Highly active	2.0

By determining total energy needs, one can approximate the number of calories needed daily to maintain energy balance. Consuming more calories than needed may result in weight gain, while an intake of a lesser amount may result in weight loss. Consider the following example:

To calculate the total energy needed by a woman who weighs 130 lbs. and has an average to high activity level:

1. Determine weight in kilograms:
   130 lbs. divided by 2.2 = 59 kg of body weight

2. Determine the BMR:
   59 kg × .9 cal/kg/hour × 24 hours = 1,274 calories per day to maintain BMR

3. Choose the physical activity factor from Table 9.2:
   Average to high activity = 1.75

4. Determine total energy needs
   BMR × physical activity factor = Total energy needs per day
   1274 × 1.75 = 2,230 calories per day

Assessment of Body Weight, Body Composition, and Overall Health

Energy equilibrium, or balance, refers to an energy intake that is equal to an energy output for the maintenance of a healthy weight. A disruption of energy balance results in either a weight gain or loss. Body weight is made up of fat and lean tissue (including water). It is important to determine a healthy or optimal amount of body fat, lean tissue, and overall body weight to achieve optimal well-being. Health problems may occur if a person has too much or too little body weight and/or body fat. Several methods can be used to assess body weight and composition.

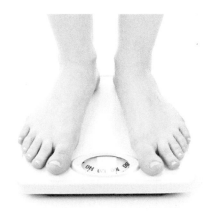

Body weight is made up of fat and lean tissue.

Methods of Assessing Body Weight: Height/Weight Standards

One method of assessing body weight is using anthropometric measures. This method involves measuring the physical characteristics of the body such as height and weight. These measurements are then compared to the standards set for height and weight. Another method of measurement is the Hamwi method of determining ideal body weight (IBW) for height. Ideal body weight is also referred to as relative or desired weight for height (DBW). Individuals weighing more than their desired weight for height are believed to have a greater risk for obesity-related diseases. Appendix D provides a height/weight table for determining IBW and examples of alternative methods. Children's weight is assessed according to the appropriate weight for height at a specific age. Height, weight, and BMI are plotted on a growth chart to monitor a child's progress. Appendix D provides a sample growth chart.

There are equations to determine weight for height standards for both male and female adults.[2] The calculations follow:

- For males: The suggested weight for a male 5 feet tall is 106 pounds. For every inch over 5 feet, add 6 pounds to calculate the ideal body weight for height. If Tom is 5′6″ tall, what is his ideal or relative body weight for height?
  Base Weight + (6″ × 6 lbs.) = Relative or ideal body weight for height 106 + 36 = 142 lbs.
  Tom's ideal body weight is 142 lbs.
- Also add or subtract 10% of ideal body weight to account for small or large frame size and to establish a weight range.
  10% of 142 = 14
  142 – 14 = 128 or 142 + 14 = 156 for an IBW range of 128–156
- For Females: The suggested weight for a female 5 feet tall is 100 pounds. Add 5 pounds for every inch in excess of 5 feet. If Mary is 5 feet 4 inches tall; what is her ideal or relative body weight for height?
  Base weight + (4″ × 5 lbs.) = Relative or ideal weight for height 100 + 20 = 120 lbs.
  To establish a weight range, add or subtract 10% of the calculated ideal or relative body weight.
  10% of 120 = 12
  120 – 12 = 108 or 120 + 12 = 132 for an IBW range of 108–132

Body Mass Index (BMI)

Another anthropometric unit measure is the use of relative weight to height, called body mass index (BMI). A chart that is found in Appendix D can be used to help determine BMI. A mathematical formula can also be used to determine BMI.

$$BMI = \frac{\text{weight in pounds}}{(\text{height inches})^2} \times 703$$

The general classifications in which a BMI falls are listed in Table 9.3.

TABLE 9.3 Body Mass Index (BMI) Ranges	
	BMI
Underweight:	<18.5
Normal:	18.5–24.9
Overweight:	25–29.9
Class 1 Obesity:	30–34.9
Class 2 Obesity:	35–39.9
Class 3 Obesity:	>40

Obesity-related diseases increase when the BMI exceeds 25. The methods of comparing weight for height/weight standards and body mass index do not take into account body composition. A person involved in bodybuilding or football may exceed the acceptable height/weight standards, but may not necessarily have too much body fat. In such cases, it is also beneficial to assess body composition.

Assessing Body Composition: Fat versus Lean

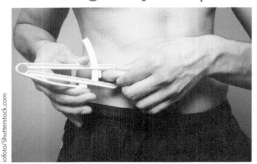

Skinfold calipers are used when determining body fat composition.

Another way to determine if a person is at a healthy weight is to look at body composition or body fat versus lean tissue. One method includes the use of skinfold calipers (a hand-held device that measures the thickness of fat tissue under the skin) to measure fatfolds on the external surface of the body. Areas can be measured at a variety of locations including the back of the arm (triceps), the lower stomach (abdomen), or the back of the lower leg (calf).

These measurements are then compared to standards and an estimate of total body fat is projected. Another method of measurement is bioelectrical impedance, which conducts a harmless amount of electrical charge through the body. Lean tissue and water conduct electrical currents that body fat impedes or stops. Simple hand-held machines or more sophisticated computer-generated machines are used in this method to evaluate body fat. Changes in body water can distort values, as seen in cases of dehydration. A diagram showing how to measure triceps fatfold is provided in Appendix D.

Body composition estimates for the U.S. population are thought to be important in analyzing trends in obesity, sarcopenia (age-associated loss of muscle mass and function), and other weight-related health conditions.[3] Less common methods of determining body composition include calculating the density of lean tissue by underwater weighing, and a technique called dual energy X-ray absorptiometry, which measures total body fat, fat distribution, and bone density. The costs of underwater weighing and energy X-ray absorptiometry are quite high. (Figure 9.2)

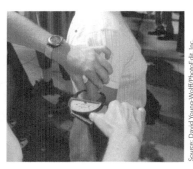

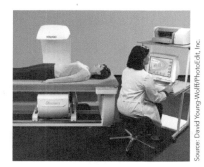

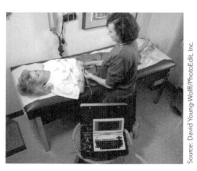

Fatfold measures can yeild accurate results when trained technician measures body fat by using a caliper to gauge the thickness of a fold of skin. Measurements are taken on the back of the arm (over the triceps), below the shoulder blade (subscapular), and in other places (including lower-body sites) and are then compared with standards

Dual energy X-ray absorptiometry (DEXA) employs two low-dose X-rays that differentiate among fat-free soft tissue (lean body mass), fat tissue, and bone tissue, providing a precise measurement of total fat and its distribution in all but extremely obese subjects.

Bioelectrical impedance is simple, painless and accurate when properly administered; the method determines body fatness by measuring conductivity. Lean tissue conducts a mild electric current; fat tissue does not.

FIGURE 9.2 Three methods of determining body composition

Concerns and Causes of Excessive Body Fat and Low Body Fat

Control of Food Intake

Normal eating consists of eating when hungry and continuing to eat until you are satisfied. Sometimes, this means eating healthy foods, but at other times it means eating just for the enjoyment of eating something you like or crave. You may overeat and feel uncomfortable, or you may wish that you had more to eat. Normal eating is a reaction to emotions, to a particular schedule, or to actual hunger, while trusting that the body will balance itself accordingly. Food intake is controlled by both physiological and psychological mechanisms. Three things that influence intake are hunger, satiety, and appetite.

Hunger is the internal signal that stimulates an individual to acquire and to consume food. Chemical messengers or hormones in the brain, especially in the hypothalamus, trigger the need for food. In addition to these triggers, the amount of nutrients circulating in the blood, the type and amount of food just eaten, the amount of circulating sex hormones, and the state of physical and mental disease affect hunger. The physiological internal signal to stop eating is termed satiety. Satiation results when food enters the upper digestive tract and the brain receives messages that the body has received adequate nutrients. Satiety continues to suppress hunger until the body needs more food.

Another factor that affects food consumption is appetite. Appetite, unlike hunger, is psychological and is a learned behavior. Psychological factors that affect food intake include sensory input. Chefs understand the importance of enticing the customer's taste, smell, and visual senses with the dishes they prepare. Even when a person is not very hungry, the smell of fresh-baked bread or the aroma of sautéed garlic and herbs can stimulate appetite. Other psychological factors that affect our appetite include learned preferences and certain aversions to food. Eating frequently takes place at established meal times rather than in response to internal signals of hunger. Food intake is also affected by social and cultural differences. Drugs can increase or decrease the appetite and hence our food intake.

Concerns of Excessive Body Fat or Weight

An estimated 33.8%, or approximately 73 million adult Americans over the age of 20, are classified as obese. The average American adult today is 24 pounds heavier than the average adult was in 1960. Statistics show that 16.9%, or approximately 12.5 million children and teens from the age of 2 to 19 are also qualified as obese.[4] Obesity is the term used to define "overfatness" that has potential adverse health effects and a BMI measure of 30 or higher. Obesity increases the risk for cardiovascular disease, hypertension, and diabetes. Obesity may also increase the chances of arthritis, gallbladder disease, gout, liver malfunction, respiratory problems, sleep apnea, and some cancers. The average medical costs for obesity-related disease in America is 9.1% of all medical costs, which in dollars can be as high as $78.5 billion.[5]

When discussing obesity and "overfatness," it is important to explain two types of fat distribution in the body. Fat that is located deep within the central abdominal area near vital organs is called visceral fat, while fat located in layers beneath the skin that line the entire body is called subcutaneous fat. Individuals with a large amount of visceral fat are said to have central obesity. Central obesity further increases a person's risk for heart disease, stroke, hypertension, and diabetes. Visceral fat is easily mobilized to the bloodstream and can increase lipid levels in the blood, in particular cholesterol-carrying lipids. Subcutaneous fat is less easily mobilized and is less likely to increase lipid levels (Figure 9.3).

Causes of Obesity

When discussing obesity, it is important to remember that energy balance and macronutrient balance or imbalance, play an important role. Obesity results only when energy intake remains higher than the energy expended over an extended period of time.[6] There are many theories on the causes of obesity and no one theory holds true for

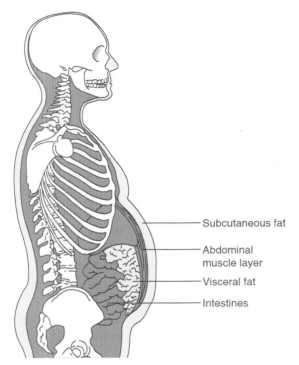

Subcutaneous fat

Abdominal
muscle layer

Visceral fat

Intestines

FIGURE 9.3 A Diagram of Visceral
Fat and Subcutaneous Fat

all cases; however, it is a fact that obesity has become a national epidemic that needs to be addressed. Most theories support the belief that there is a genetic predisposition to obesity for some people. Obesity is a complex issue that involves many factors. Theories of obesity are shown in Table 9.4. One theory is that obese people may lack leptin, a factor found in the body that helps control adiposity. An understanding of leptin, and its associated molecules, may help in the future treatment of this condition.[7] Several key environmental and cultural factors in the past few decades, both active and inadvertent, are also believed to have substantially contributed to overeating. An increase in the availability and the promotion of cheap, energy-dense diets that are high in fat, such as fast foods, and a transition to extremely sedentary lifestyles are major contributors to obesity. Obstacles in addressing obesity include public and corporate ignorance about the effects of energy-dense diets in encouraging passive overeating, and a lack of knowledge about the severe health effects of inactive lifestyles.[8]

An alarming trend in the United States over the past two decades is the increase in the number of overweight and obese children. This trend is of particular concern because of the negative health and psychological effects it has. Characteristics that place children at risk for becoming overweight and obese include excessive dietary intake, lack of physical activity, and sedentary behavior. Family, school, and social environments may also contribute to this problem.[9]

TABLE 9.4 Examples of Obesity Theories	
Theory	Explanation
Enzyme Theory	Obese people may produce more of the enzyme lipoprotein lipase, which may increase fat storage.
Leptin Deficit Theory	Leptin is a hormone produced by fat tissue and is linked to the suppression of appetite. Obese people may lack adequate leptin production.
Set-point Theory	The body may choose a weight at which it wants to be and attempts to remain at that weight despite efforts to change it.
Thermogenesis Theory	Obese people may inherit a regulatory mechanism that slows the rate of fat breakdown and thermogenesis (the release of energy with the breakdown of body fuels).

Many factors have contributed to an increase in obesity over the years. These include:

- A decrease in smoking
- An increase in sedentary occupations
- An increase in two-income households and single-parent households
- Transportation and infrastructure that discourage physical activity
- A decrease in physical education classes and extracurricular sports in schools
- An increase in sedentary forms of entertainment
- Demographic changes

- A decrease in food costs with an increase in food availability
- Changes in food consumption patterns[10]
- A proliferation of packaged foods
- An increase in consumption of sugar sweetened beverages
- Fewer people preparing meals at home

A relatively new area to examine is the role of genetic make-up in relation to weight gain and obesity. Obesity results from interactions between environmental and genetic factors. More than 40 genetic variants have been associated with obesity and fat distribution.[11] The fat mass- and obesity-associated gene (FTO) has been connected to an increased BMI in children and adults in white European populations.[12] The association of this gene and its variants pose an interesting insight into the obesity epidemic. The effect that environment can impose on this gene regulation also needs to be considered.

Treating obesity can be complex, and its prevention may prove to be the real long-term solution. Chefs can assist in this process by developing nutritious menus and recipes for school lunch programs, restaurants, and fast food venues that have mass appeal. The following section discusses the treatment and prevention of obesity.

The Treatment of Obesity: Healthy Management of Weight

There are many weight-loss programs available; however, many of them are not safe or scientifically supported. It is important to emphasize the optimum goal of well-being and health when encouraging weight control for obese people. Stressing the addition of healthy foods, fluids, and improved health-conscious habits, as opposed to the negative concept of restriction, provides a much more positive and long-lasting result. Individuals who attempt to lose weight too quickly often fail to consider the health consequences of the diet regimen they choose. Losing ten pounds in one week by consuming a fad diet such as "the grapefruit-only diet" provides a quick fix but does not change habits or promote health and well-being. The dieter will often gain the weight back quickly because much of the initial weight loss is due to loss of fluid rather than body fat. Muscle is also lost with rapid weight loss. This change in body composition reduces the BMR, making it more difficult for the individual to maintain the weight loss.

A brief list of some of the general products and/or programs available, and the potential problems they pose, follows.

1. Very-low-calorie diets—These diets generally allow less than 800 calories per day and are of the liquid variety. They are often medically supervised and promote a dramatic initial weight loss. The long-term benefits of this type of weight loss are often negative, especially when an exercise component and a change in eating habits are not encouraged.

2. Meal-replacement formulas—Meal replacements are often of a liquid variety and are intended to replace one meal. The other two meals are low-calorie meals. If the user skips meals, or overeats at the next meal, this defeats the purpose.

3. Low-carbohydrate diets—There are many popular low-carbohydrate diets on the market including the Atkins New Diet Revolution, the Calories Don't Count Diet, the Drinking Man's Diet, the Mayo Clinic Diet, the Scarsdale Diet, the Ski Team Diet, and the Zone Diet. All of these diets promote burning fat for energy through the production of ketones. Ketones promote ketosis, suppress appetite, and increase water loss. These diets are often also low in calories, which is the real reason for weight loss. Dramatic initial weight loss is often due to fluid loss, and once an individual resumes eating carbohydrates, weight gain results. Diets that promote high levels of protein and fat, especially saturated fat, may also increase the risk of heart disease and place increased strain on the kidneys and the liver.

4. Novelty diets—There are countless diets that promise quick weight loss fixes. These include diets that promote eating just one type, color, amount, or combination of food at prescribed times of the day. These

are considered fad diets and have no scientific backing. They are often nutritionally inadequate and fail to promote healthy eating or living.

5. Diet medications—There are several prescription medications on the market. Many of these suppress appetite, but may also have adverse effects on the central nervous system and the cardiovascular system. Another type of prescription medication has anti-absorptive properties (prevents or delays absorption of nutrients), however it may have significant gastrointestinal side effects. Over-the-counter medications and herbal remedies do not undergo the evaluation that prescription medications do and have the potential for adverse life-threatening effects.[13]

6. Surgery—In severe cases of obesity, known as extreme obesity (BMI >40), more radical weight-loss procedures are considered. Surgery that is performed to treat obesity is called **bariatric surgery**. Bariatric surgery for weight loss involves reducing the stomach size and bypassing a significant part of the small intestine. The weight loss that ensues is from the restriction of food intake and the malabsorption of nutrients. Another type of procedure involves the placement of a band at the top of the stomach to cause food restriction. These types of radical surgery pose many medical risks and must be carefully evaluated. Registered Dietitians play a vital role in the nutritional management of the patients before and after surgery. Surgical treatment for obesity should only be considered after diet, exercise, and/ or pharmacological methods have been exhausted. In addition a psychological evaluation must be completed prior to surgery.

A Well-Balanced Guide to Weight Management

To achieve and maintain a desirable weight, a lifestyle change is often needed. There are no quick fixes to the problems of being overweight or obese. A good program for healthy living and weight management focuses on three basic concepts:

1. **A nutritionally sound diet** that has no fewer than 1,200 calories per day. Diets that are very restrictive lower the basal metabolic rate, making it harder to lose weight. Diets should be high in fiber, high in fruits and vegetables, moderate in fat, including monounsaturated fat such as olive oil, moderate in protein (with the use of fish and chicken encouraged over red meats), moderate in dairy (with the use of low-fat or fat-free milk products encouraged), and moderate in complex carbohydrates (with whole grains greatly encouraged). The introduction of high-fructose corn syrup in the U.S. has been associated with increased rates of obesity and diabetes. High fructose corn syrup is said to lessen insulin sensitivity and to increase visceral adiposity in obese adults.[14] This result, however, has not been conclusively supported.[15] Working the glycemic index into the diet appears to have an impact on weight management. Short-term studies suggest that low-glycemic-index carbohydrates and fiber intake can delay hunger and decrease subsequent energy intake in contrast to an intake of high-glycemic-index foods.[16]

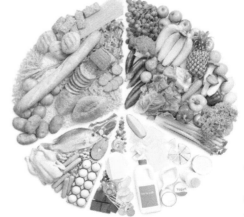

A nutritionally sound diet should be part of a good weight management program.

2. **An exercise program** is encouraged at least 3–5 times per week for approximately 30 minutes or more per session. A combination of different exercises is best to promote weight loss and eventual weight maintenance. It should be

stressed, however, that any exercise is beneficial. In relation to the FTO gene mentioned previously, it has been shown that living a physically active lifestyle is associated with a 40% reduction in the genetic predisposition to common obesity.[17] The contributions of exercise will be discussed in greater detail later in the chapter.

3. **Behavior modification** involves changing negative behaviors that lead to unhealthy eating and lifestyle habits, and possible weight gain. Choosing the largest portion size at a fast food restaurant and eating it in the car, or snacking while watching television, often distorts our awareness of how much we actually consume. Walking or riding a bike rather than driving to a destination also provides a chance for exercise. According to a Conference Board Report, more than 40% of U.S. companies currently have obesity reduction or wellness programs, and an additional 24% plan to start such programs. It is estimated that for every $1 invested in these programs, the return on that investment is between $0 and $5.[18]

Using recipes that are creative, moderate in fat, and full of flavor enhancers can counter the concept of "dieting" as being restrictive, boring, and tasteless.

Concerns of Low Body Fat or Weight

Inadequate energy intake results in too little body fat and inadequate weight. Although obesity is the main concern in the United States, individuals in other parts of the world suffer from being underweight and having deficient body fat. Overly thin people have little nutritional reserves and lose body tissue when they need to fight infection or disease. A person who is thin has a difficult time fighting wasting diseases such as cancer and HIV, which deplete the body nutritionally. Poor nutritional status can compromise the immune system and cause the defense system to decline.

Causes of Low Body Fat or Weight

Deficient energy intake that does not meet nutritional needs may be due to poverty, famine, disease, or the inability to acquire an adequate food supply. Millions of people suffer from undernutrition and starvation. Approximately five million Americans with low body fat and weight are victims of self-inflicted diseases known as **eating disorders**. Eating disorders are classified as disturbances in eating behavior that jeopardize physical and psychological health. A discussion of three classifications of eating disorders follows.

Anorexia Nervosa

Anorexia means "without appetite" and nervosa signifies of "nervous origin." The eating disorder anorexia nervosa is characterized by the refusal to maintain a minimally normal body weight in the context of age, sex development trajectory, and physical health. Self-starvation is imposed, and a distorted perception of body weight and shape occurs. People who suffer from anorexia nervosa have a relentless pursuit of thinness. It is typically seen in teenage girls and young women and affects approximately .5%–1% of this segment in the United States. Anorexia Nervosa is believed to have both psychosocial and biological origins. The malnutrition that ensues can affect almost all organs of the body, and medical complications can be severe.

Heart complications account for 50% of the reported deaths. Treatment includes medications, psychotherapy, and family therapy.[19] Hospitalization is sometimes necessary and may promote lasting changes. A multidisciplinary team approach consisting of clinical and nutritional approaches, individual and group psychotherapy, family therapy, occupational therapy, body therapy, and pharmacotherapy is considered best. Table 9.5 lists symptoms and diagnostic criteria for Anorexia Nervosa.[20]

TABLE 9.5 DSM V Diagnostic Criteria for Anorexia Nervosa (AN)
A person with anorexia nervosa demonstrates the following:
A. Restriction of energy intake relative to requirements, leading to a significant low body weight in the context of age, sex, development trajectory, and physical health. *Significantly low weight* is defined as a weight that is less than that minimally normal or, for children and adolescents, less than that minimally expected.
B. Intense fear of gaining weight or of becoming fat, or persistent behavior that interferes with weight gain, even though at a significantly low weight.
C. Disturbance in the way in which one's body weight or shape is experienced, undue influence of body weight or shape on self-evaluation, persistent lack of recognition of the seriousness of the current low body weight.

Reprinted with permission from the Diagnostic and Statistical Manual of Mental Disorders, Fifth Edition, Copyright © 2013. American Psychiatric Association. All Rights Reserved.

Bulimia Nervosa

Bulimia nervosa is a condition that involves recurring episodes of binge eating that are combined with a morbid fear of becoming fat. The binging is typically followed by self-induced vomiting or purging. It has been estimated that 1.1%–4.2% of females have bulimia nervosa during their lifetime. People with bulimia usually weigh within their range for height. Like people with anorexia, bulimics fear gaining weight, have a desire to lose weight, and are intensely dissatisfied with their bodies. Table 9.6 lists the symptoms and diagnostic criteria for Bulimia Nervosa (BN).

TABLE 9.6 Symptoms and Diagnostic Criteria for Bulimia Nervosa
A person with bulimia nervosa demonstrates the following:
A. Recurrent episodes of binge eating. An episode of binge eating is characterized by both of the following:
1. Eating, in a discrete period of time (e.g., within any 2-hour period) an amount of food that is definitely larger than what most individuals would eat in a similar period of time under similar circumstances.
2. A sense of lack of control over eating during the episode (e.g., a feeling that one cannot stop eating or control what or how much one is eating).
B. Recurrent inappropriate compensatory behaviors in order to prevent weight gain, such as self-induced vomiting; misuse of laxatives, diuretics, or other medications; fasting; or excessive exercise.
C. The binge eating and inappropriate compensatory behaviors both occur, on average at least once a week for 3 months.
D. Self-evaluation is unduly influenced by body shape and weight.
E. The disturbance does not occur exclusively during episodes of anorexia nervosa.

Reprinted with permission from the Diagnostic and Statistical Manual of Mental Disorders, Fifth Edition, (Copyright © 2013). American Psychiatric Association. All Rights Reserved. Published Exclusively

Another eating disorder known as **binge-eating disorder** involves binge eating and the fear of becoming fat, but does not involve vomiting or purging. Symptoms experienced in this disorder include frequent out of control eating, eating much more rapidly than normal, eating until feeling uncomfortable, eating alone, and feelings of self-disgust and shame. Binge eating disorder (BED) became a formal diagnosis in the new Diagnostic and Statistical Manual of Mental Disorders (DSM V) that was recently published. The new criteria require that the episodes of consumption of unusably large amounts of food, accompanied by a strong sense of lack of control, occur a minimum of 1 time per week for 3 months. Treatment for binge eating disorder and bulimia nervosa is similar and includes many of the strategies used with anorexia nervosa.[21, 22, 23]

Female Athlete Triad

The **female athlete triad** is a condition that can be seen in female athletes and dancers who consume insufficient calories for their level of activity and stage of growth. The features are **amenorrhea** (cessation of menstruation), and osteoporosis in the face of inadequate caloric intake. Calorie intake can be inadequate due to disordered eating, or simply due to calorie intake not matching the energy requirements of high levels of physical activity. Although it can occur in any sport, it is most frequently seen in athletes who participate in events that emphasize thinness such as gymnastics, ballet, and diving. If undetected, it can cause irreversible bone loss and even death. Treatment should consist of a team approach that includes the patient, a nurse practitioner, a dietitian, a psychologist, and/or a psychiatrist, the patient's family, coaches, and trainers.[24] Male athletes and dancers can also develop eating disorders as a result of the pressure of achieving body weight. One may observe this condition in wrestlers who are attempting to make weight in the lowest weight class.

Exercise is often extreme and at an obsessive level in people suffering from disordered eating. However, exercise, when practiced safely, is key to optimal health and weight control. The benefits of nutrition and the role it plays in exercise and sports will be discussed next.

The Role of Exercise in Maintaining Optimal Weight and Health

Health Benefits of Exercise

We thrive on movement because it can bring pleasure and stimulate creativity. Movement has physiological benefits such as stimulating blood flow and psychological effects that include relieving tension and promoting well-being. Studies have shown that exercise is helpful in treating and preventing many disorders and diseases as well. The following list provides examples of the contributions of exercise to positive health:

- Heart Disease—Research suggests that exercise may raise HDL, the "good" cholesterol in the bloodstream, which may help reverse established diseases, as well as prevent disease.
- Stroke—Exercise helps to prevent strokes, and restore function after a stroke.
- Hypertension (HTN)—Exercise helps to lower mild to moderate HTN, as part of nondrug therapy. It also helps to control hypertension in people on drug therapy.
- Diabetes—Exercise can prevent or delay vascular complications, help control blood sugar, and may reduce the need for insulin.
- Arthritis—Exercise increases joint flexibility and range of motion.
- Osteoporosis—Weight-bearing exercise may help improve bone density, thereby preventing and reversing bone loss.
- Cancer—Exercise may reduce the risk for certain cancers including colon and breast cancer.
- Depression—Exercise increases the sense of well-being, promotes a positive self-image, and decreases stress, thereby reducing depression and anxiety.
- Excess body weight—Exercise helps promote healthy body weight, as well as decrease in body fat percentages.[25]

Exercise and Aging

On average, people who are physically active outlive those who are inactive. Exercise helps to maintain the functional independence of older adults and enhances the quality of life for people of all ages. Despite these positive findings, only about 23% of adults in the United States report regular physical activity using the larger muscle groups in movement for twenty minutes or longer, three or more days per week. The number drops to 15% for those who exercise five or more days per week, for thirty minutes or longer. Almost 50% of Americans do not participate in any regular physical activity.

The highest risk of death and disability is found among those who do not participate in regular physical activity.

Exercise throughout the Lifespan

Physical activity guidelines, as outlined by the Department of Health and Human Services (DHHS), state that adults should do either 150 minutes of moderate-intensity exercise or 75 minutes of vigorous-intensity exercise weekly. Muscle-strengthening activities should be performed two or more days per week. Increasing the time or level of activity each week provides additional health benefits. The DHHS states that some activity is better than none, and walking or using stairs throughout the day is effective exercise.[26] Exercise and the many benefits it provides are important throughout the lifespan. For children and adolescents, it is important for cardiorespiratory function, blood pressure control, and weight management. A physically active lifestyle adopted early in life may continue into adulthood. Parents, educators, and healthcare providers need to be positive role models in promoting exercise. Unfortunately, children today are less active than what is recommended, and their activity level declines as they progress to adolescence. Studies show that 25% of U.S. children spend four hours or more watching television daily and that basal metabolic rate drops lower when watching television rather than when participating in normal sitting activities. Schools must also continue to include physical activity in the school day. Programs that incorporate physical education in the curriculum have been effective in changing the attitudes, behaviors, and overall physical fitness of students.[27]

Physical Fitness: Aerobic and Anaerobic Activity

Exercise can help individuals feel better, look better, and work more efficiently. Any exercise is good, including activities such as pleasure walking, stair climbing, gardening, yard work, housework, and dancing. The key, even if it is exercising for just a few minutes, is to get started. Exercise should have a combination of **aerobic** activity (where oxygen is needed for the activity), and **anaerobic** activity (which does not require oxygen). Because oxygen is needed to break down fat for energy, aerobic exercise is also termed "fat" burning. Aerobic activity strengthens the heart and lungs, and improves muscle conditioning by making heart and lung muscles work harder than normal to deliver oxygen to the tissues. Anaerobic activity, on the other hand, strengthens muscles and improves flexibility, bone density, and muscle endurance. Table 9.7 provides examples of activities and the percentage of each energy

TABLE 9.7 Examples of Activities and the Percentage of each Energy System used During the Activity.

Sport	AnaeroBic		Aerobic
	Atp-Pcr & Glycolysis	Glycolysis & Oxidative	Oxidative
Basketball	60	20	20
Fencing	90	10	0
Field Events	90	10	0
Golf Swing	95	5	0
Gymnastics	80	15	5
Hockey	50	20	30
Rowing	20	30	50
Running (distance)	10	20	70
Skiing	33	33	33
Soccer	50	20	30
Swimming (distance)	10	20	70
Swimming (50m freestyle)*	40	55	5
Tennis	70	20	10
Volleyball	80	5	15

Taken from Foss ML and Keteyian S. (1998) *The Physiological Basis of Exercise & Sport 6th Edition.*
*Stager JM and Tanner DA. (2005) *Swimming: 2nd Edition.*

system used during the activity. For example, basketball is primarily an anaerobic form of activity (60%) from the phosphocreatine/glycolysis steps in energy metabolism. The remaining 40% is split between a crossover from anaerobic to aerobic energy metabolism (20%), and then finally to full aerobic in the Kreb's Cycle (20%).

Repeated actions are cumulative in their effects. A single activity does not always burn a huge number of calories, but when added to others, a significant amount of energy can be expended and can contribute to weight control. Calories burned in exercise will vary depending on weight and basal metabolic rate. The more an individual weighs the more calories he/she burns. When two individuals run at the same pace, the one with the higher weight will burn more calories per hour. Table 9.8 lists the calories burned per hour in common physical activities by a person who weighs 150 pounds.[28]

TABLE 9.8 Energy Expenditure Chart	
Sedentary Activities	**Calories Burned per Hour**
Lying down or sleeping	90
Sitting quietly	84
Sitting and writing, card playing, etc.	114
MODERATE ACTIVITIES	
Bicycling (5 mph)	174
Canoeing (2.5 mph)	174
Dancing (ballroom)	210
Golf (carrying clubs)	324
Horseback riding (sitting to trot)	246
Light housework	246
Swimming (crawl, 20 yds/min)	288
Tennis (doubles)	312
Volleyball (recreational)	264
VIGOROUS ACTIVITIES	
Aerobic dancing	546
Basketball	450
Bicycling (13 mph)	612
Circuit weight training	756
Football (touch, vigorous)	498
Ice skating (9 mph)	384
Racquetball	588
Roller skating (9 mph)	384
Jogging (10 minute mile, 6 mph)	654
Swimming (crawl, 45 yds/min)	522
Tennis (singles)	450
X-country skiing (5 mph)	690

Starting a Safe Exercise Program

The most important thing in starting an exercise program is choosing an activity that you enjoy. If you are not fit or have not exercised recently, it is best to start with a less strenuous activity such as walking. Once you exercise regularly, you may choose to participate in activities that are more strenuous for longer periods of time. Also, consider whether you like to exercise alone or with someone. If exercising alone is more appealing to you, activities such as walking, running, biking, and swimming may be best. If you prefer to exercise with others, team sports or exercise classes may be more satisfying. It is important to remember to exercise at a comfortable pace initially. You should be able to keep up a conversation while jogging or walking briskly. If you have any difficulty breathing, faintness, or prolonged weakness during or after exercising, you are exercising too hard and should cut back on the intensity and/ or the length of the activity.

To improve the fitness of the heart and lungs, it is important to determine how hard to exercise by keeping track of your heart rate. **Maximum heart rate** (100%) is the fastest your heart can beat. Exercise that exceeds 75% of your heart rate may not be beneficial unless you are very fit, while exercise below 50% does little conditioning for the heart or lungs. Maintaining between 50% and 75% of your maximum heart rate is most beneficial, and is termed **target heart rate**. When starting an exercise program, it is best to start at the lower end of the range and to gradually increase as you become more fit. Maximum heart rate is closely determined by taking the number 220 minus your age. Table 9.9 provides general guidelines for your target heart rate.

TABLE 9.9 Maximum and Target Heart Rates		
Age	Target HR Zone 50%–75% Average	Max HR 100%
20 years	100–150 beats per min.	200
25 years	98–146 beats per min.	195
30 years	95–142 beats per min.	190
35 years	93–138 beats per min.	185
40 years	90–135 beats per min.	180
45 years	88–131 beats per min.	175
50 years	85–127 beats per min.	170
55 years	83–123 beats per min.	165
60 years	80–120 beats per min.	160
65 years	78–116 beats per min.	155
70 years	75–113 beats per min.	150

Follow these steps to take your heart rate during exercise:

1. Place the tips of your first two fingers lightly on the blood vessels of your neck (the carotid arteries are located to the left or right of the Adam's apple) **or** place the tips of your first two fingers lightly on the inside of your wrist, just below the base of your thumb.

2. Feel for a regular pulse.

3. Count your pulse for ten seconds and multiply by six.

4. This total is your heart rate in beats per minute. Compare your heart rate to your target heart rate.

Steps for a Safe Exercise Program

A safe exercise program should contain several elements:

1. Warm up for 5 minutes. Start exercising slowly to give the body a chance to limber up and to get the heart and lungs ready for exercise that is more vigorous.
   This step may also include stretching exercises, depending on the activity.

2. Exercise within your target heart rate for 30–60 minutes.

3. Cool down for 5 minutes. Slow down gradually to allow your body to relax and your heart rate to return to normal. Cool-down time may include stretching, depending on the activity.

To achieve optimal results, it is best to exercise three to four times per week or every other day.[29] Key points to remember are that exercise should not be painful or exhausting. When you push yourself too hard or too long, your common sense should tell you to stop. Exercise should, first and foremost, be enjoyable and make you feel better!

Sports nutrition is an exciting field that is continually growing. Chefs can assist both amateur and professional athletes to achieve their physical and health goals by providing menus that promote optimal performance. The Culinary Corner explores this special field and the specific nutritional concerns of the athlete.

Culinary Corner
Sports Nutrition

The beneficial effects of good nutrition on exercise performance have been clearly documented for the past twenty years. Chefs continue to play an important role in planning meals and menus to fit the needs of athletes. Chefs who combine culinary techniques with sound nutrition knowledge certainly have the edge! Job opportunities for culinary professionals in this area include Olympic training facilities, health clubs, spas, and college and professional sports team training sites. What an athlete eats can affect health, body weight and composition, recovery time, and overall performance. The specific nutrient needs of athletes include energy, protein, vitamins, minerals, and water.

Energy

The energy needs of the athlete are a priority. It is essential to achieve energy balance to promote the maintenance of lean tissue, immune and reproductive function, and peak performance. The majority of energy (55%–58%) is derived from carbohydrates. Athletes need approximately 6–10 grams of carbohydrates per kilogram of body weight. Higher carbohydrate diets that exceed 60% are also advocated. Complex carbohydrates such as whole grains should be consumed to derive additional benefits. Healthy unsaturated fats also contribute about 25%–30% of the diet. When determining energy needs, it is important to consider variables such as body size, weight and body composition goals, the sport being performed, and the gender of the athlete.

Protein

The protein needs of athletes exceed the recommended average for individuals, due to micro damage to muscle fibers and the need to gain lean tissue mass. The typical range for protein requirements is 1.2–1.7 grams of protein/kilogram of body weight. Athletes involved in endurance sports such as running have needs on the lower end of the range, while athletes who participate in more resistance-based exercises, such as bodybuilders, place in the higher range. When energy intake is insufficient from carbohydrate and fat sources, protein must be used for energy. When energy intake is exceeded, the protein does not add extra muscle but is stored as fat.[30] Consuming large quantities of protein is not effective for strength athletes and may be associated with some health risks.[31] A diet rich in animal and plant protein provides athletes with all the amino acids needed.

Vitamins and Minerals

The current DRIs for vitamins and minerals should be adequate to meet the needs of most athletes. Those who restrict their energy intake, eliminate one or more food groups from their diet,

(Continued)

or consume high carbohydrates are at risk. The minerals that are most frequently deficient in the diet of athletes, especially in females, are calcium, iron, and zinc. Factors that may contribute to this deficiency include a low intake of animal products and dairy products. Female athletes commonly show iron depletion due to excessive loss of iron through sweat, feces, urine, and menstrual blood. If iron deficiency is detected, nutritional intervention and iron supplementation should be started.

Fluid Needs

Fluid balance is essential for an athlete's optimal performance. When dehydration progresses, exercise performance is impaired. Athletes must remain well hydrated before, during, and after exercise. The fluid of choice for exercise is water, although beverages that contain carbohydrates in concentrations of 4%–8% can also be beneficial for intense exercise that lasts longer than one hour. Electrolytes, such as sodium and potassium, are not needed in beverages if they are already consumed in the diet. A small amount of sodium, .5 grams to .7 grams per liter is only recommended when exercise lasts longer than one hour. Table 9.10 provides the recommended fluid amounts for athletes.

TABLE 9.10 Fluid Needs for the Athlete	
Before Exercise	Generous amounts of fluids in the 24 hours before the session: 400–600 ml (13–20 oz.)2–3 hours before the session
During Exercise	150–350 ml (6–12 oz.) of fluid in 15–20 minute intervals
After Exercise	Consumption of fluids at 150% of what is lost in body weight For example, 1 lb. of body weight loss after exercise needs 24 oz. of fluid.

Ergogenic Aids

No discussion of sports nutrition would be complete without the mention of ergogenic aids. Ergogenic aids claim to increase work output or performance and are the basis for a multimillion dollar business. One of the more popular ergogenic aids is branched-chain amino acids (BCAA). The branched-chain amino acids include the essential amino acids leucine, isoleucine, and valine. These three amino acids can be obtained in many forms including whole foods, protein supplements, solutions containing protein hydrolysates (produced from purified protein sources such as casein), and also in free amino acid form. BCAAs make up about 15% of the amino acids present in foods. The average protein intake may be up to 126 grams of protein, which would equal 19 grams of BCAA.

Athletes typically have a greater amount of these amino acids, due to a higher caloric intake that equates to a higher protein intake. BCAA as a fuel source for exercise is not necessarily valid but many athletes do feel that these delay the onset of fatigue. BCAAs also have an anti-catabolic effect during and after exercise.[32] Manufacturers of ergogenic aids list product ingredients but may often make unfounded claims. When choosing an ergogenic aid, it is important to pay attention to the claim, the quality of the evidence provided, and the health consequences of the claim. Table 9.11 lists the common ergogenic aids used by athletes and the concerns linked to their use.[33] Culinary professionals with a sound nutritional background can positively address the nutritional needs and concerns of athletes.

TABLE 9.11 Ergogenic Aids				
Ergogenic Aids	Action	Research on Ergogenic Effects	Side Effects	Legality
Alcohol	Decreases anxiety	No benefits	Significant	Banned for shooting events
Amphetamines	Improves concentration, decreases fatigue and appetite	Mixed, some positive	Significant, dangerous	Illegal
Anabolic steroids	Increases strength, lean muscle mass and motivation	Positive	Significant, dangerous	Illegal
Androstenediol	Same as steroids	Limited, refutes	Unknown	Banned by IOC
Androstenedione	Same as steroids	Refutes, no benefits	Significant	Banned by IOC NCAA
Antioxidants	Decreases muscle breakdown	Mixed, no clear benefits	Mild at high doses	Legal
Arginine, ornithine, lysine	Stimulates growth hormone release	No benefit	None at doses used	Legal
Aspartates	Increases free fatty acid use, sparing muscle glycogen	Mixed, some positive benefits	Mild at high doses	Legal
Aspirin	Decreases pain with muscle fatigue and muscle breakdown	No benefit	Mild	Legal
Avena sativa	Increases steroid production	Limited, refutes	None	Legal
Bee pollen	Increases strength and endurance	Refutes, no benefits	Allergic reaction	Legal
Beta blockers	Decreases anxiety	Positive effect on fine motor control, negative effect on aerobic capacity	Significant	Banned by IOC
Beta$_2$ antagonists	Increases lean muscle mass	Mixed, no benefit from inhaled formulations	Mild	Banned by IOC, legal when prescribed
Blood doping	Increases aerobic capacity	Supports	Significant, dangerous	Illegal
Boron	Increases endogenous steroid production	Refutes, no benefit	Mild at high doses	Legal
Branched-chain amino acids	Decreases mental fatigue	Mixed, negative	Mild at high doses	Legal

(Continued)

TABLE 9.11 Ergogenic Aids (Continued)

Ergogenic Aids	Action	Research on Ergogenic Effects	Side Effects	Legality
Caffeine	Increases muscle contractility and aerobic endurance, enhances fat metabolism	Supports	Mild	Legal to urine level of 12–15 µg per mL
Calcium	Increases muscle contractility, enhances glycogen metabolism	Refutes, no benefit	Mild at high doses	Legal
Carbohydrates	Increases endurance, decreases fatigue	Supports	Mild at high doses	Legal
Carnitine	Increases fat metabolism	Refutes	None	Legal
Choline	Increases endurance	Mixed, inconclusive	None	Legal
Chromium	Increases lean mass	Refutes, no benefit unless prior deficiency	Safe to 400 µg daily, potentially dangerous above this level	Legal
Chrysin	Inhibits aromatase, increases endogenous steroids	Limited, refutes	None	Legal
Cocaine	Stimulates CNS, delays fatigue	Mixed	Significant, dangerous	Illegal
Coenzyme Q_{10} (ubiquinone)	Delays fatigue, acts as antioxidant	Refutes, no benefit	None	Legal
Coenzyme Q_{12}	Increases aerobic capacity, speeds muscle repair	Refutes, no benefit	None	Legal
Creatine	Increases muscle energy, endurance, strength and lean muscle mass	Supports, insufficient data on long-term use	Mild	Legal
DHEA	Increases endogenous steroid production	No benefit in healthy athletes	Potentially dangerous	Banned by IOC, some other organizations
Diuretics	Decreases body mass	Limited benefit	Potentially dangerous	Banned by IOC
Ephedrine, other Sympathomimetics	Stimulates CNS, increases energy, delays fatigue, stimulates weight loss	No benefit	Potentially dangerous	Banned by IOC, some other organizations

Ergogenic Aids	Action	Research on Ergogenic Effects	Side Effects	Legality
Ephedrine plus caffeine	Increases energy, stimulates weight loss	Supports	Potentially dangerous, fatal at high doses	Banned by IOC, some other organizations
Erythropoietin	Increases aerobic capacity	Supports	Significant, dangerous	Illegal
Fat supplements	Increases endurance	Refutes	Mild	Legal
Fluids	Increases endurance	Supports	Mild	Legal
Folic acid	Increases aerobic capacity	Refutes	None	Legal
GHB	Stimulates growth hormone release and muscle growth	Limited, refutes	Significant, dose-related; abuse potential	Illegal
Ginseng	Increases endurance, enhances muscle recovery	Limited, refutes, no benefit	Mild, abuse syndrome reported	Legal
Glucosamine	Serves as NSAID alternative, enhances recovery	Limited, may have limited NSAID abilities	None	Legal
Glutamine	Boosts immunity and growth hormone levels	May boost immunity, no other benefits	None	Legal
Glycerol	Improves hydration and endurance	Limited, supports	Mild	Legal (oral)
Guarana (herbal caffeine)	Same as caffeine			
HMB	Decreases muscle breakdown, enhances recovery	Limited, some strength benefits	None	Legal
Human growth hormone	Anabolic effect on muscle growth, increases fat metabolism	Refutes, limited ergogenic benefits	Significant, dangerous	Illegal
Inosine	Enhances energy production, improves aerobic capacity	Refutes, no benefit	Mild	Legal
Iron	Increases aerobic capacity	No benefit unless preexisting deficiency	Mild, toxic at high doses	Legal

(Continued)

TABLE 9.11 Ergogenic Aids (*Continued*)

Ergogenic Aids	Action	Research on Ergogenic Effects	Side Effects	Legality
Leucine	Decreases muscle breakdown and spare muscle glycogen stores	Limited, no ergogenic effect	None	Legal
Ma huang (herbal ephedrine)	Same as ephedrine			
Magnesium	Enhances muscle growth	No benefit unless preexisting deficiency	Mild at high doses	Legal
Marijuana	Decreases anxiety	Refutes, negative effect	Significant, dangerous	Illegal
Multivitamins	Increases energy, endurance and aerobic capacity, enhances recovery	No benefit unless preexisting deficiency	None at RDA, some toxicities at high doses	Legal
Narcotics	Increases endurance by suppressing pain, decreases anxiety	Mixed, negative	Significant, dangerous	Illegal
Niacin	Increases energy and endurance	No benefit unless preexisting deficiency	Mild at high doses	Legal
Oxygen	Increases aerobic capacity, enhances recovery	No benefit if given before or after activity	Mild	Legal
Phosphates	Increases ATP production, energy & muscle endurance	Mixed, negative	Mild at high doses	Legal
Phytosterols	Stimulates release of endogenous steroids and growth hormone	Refutes, no benefit	Little data, allergic reaction possible	Legal
Protein	Optimizes muscular growth and repair	Supports, increased need for protein with activity	None unless underlying medical condition	Legal
Pycnogenol	Boosts antioxidant levels, enhances recovery	Supports, dietary sources offer same benefit	None	Legal
Pyruvate	Increases lean body mass	Limited research, benefit only in specific cases	None	Legal

Ergogenic Aids	Action	Research on Ergogenic Effects	Side Effects	Legality
D-Ribose	Increases cellular ATP and muscle power	No human research	None known	Legal
Selenium	Enhances antioxidant functions	Limited, no benefit	Mild at high doses	Legal
Sodium bicarbonate	Buffers lactic acid production, delays fatigue	Supports	Mild, dangerous at high doses	Legal
Strychnine	Unknown	No research on ergogenic benefits	Significant, dangerous	Legal
Tribulus terrestris	Increases endogenous steroid production	Refutes	Potentially dangerous at high doses	Legal
Tryptophan	Decreases pain perception, increases endurance	Mixed, no benefit in trained athletes	Mild, potentially dangerous	Legal
Vanadyl sulfate	Increases glycogen synthesis, enhances muscle recovery	Refutes, no benefit in healthy individuals	Mild	Legal
Vitamin B_1 (thiamin)	Enhances energy production, increases aerobic capacity, improves concentration	No benefit unless preexisting deficiency	None	Legal
Vitamin B_2 (riboflavin)	Increases aerobic endurance	No benefit unless preexisting deficiency	None	Legal
Vitamin B_6 (pyridoxine)	Enhances muscle growth, decreases anxiety	No benefit unless preexisting deficiency	Mild at high doses	Legal
Vitamin B_{12} (cyanocobalamin)	Enhances muscle growth	No benefit unless preexisting deficiency	None	Legal
Vitamin B_{15} (dimethylglycine)	Increases muscle energy production	Mixed, negative	None proven, but concerns raised	Legal
Vitamin C	Acts as antioxidant, increases aerobic capacity & energy production	No benefit unless preexisting deficiency	Mild at high doses	Legal
Vitamin E	Acts as antioxidant, improves aerobic capacity	Mixed, some positive	Mild	Legal

(Continued)

TABLE 9.11 Ergogenic Aids (*Continued*)

Ergogenic Aids	Action	Research on Ergogenic Effects	Side Effects	Legality
Yohimbine	Increases endogenous steroid production	Refutes, no benefit	Mild	Legal
Zinc	Enhances muscle growth, increases aerobic capacity	Limited, negative	Mild	Legal

IOC = International Olympic Committee; NCAA = National Collegiate Athletic Association; CNS = central nervous system; DHEA = dehydroepiandrosterone; GHB = gamma-hydroxybutyrate; NSAID = nonsteroidal anti-inflammatory drug; HMB = calcium betahydroxy beta-methylbutyrate; RDA = recommended daily allowance; ATP = adenosine triphosphate.
Source: Reprinted from "Ergogenic Aids: Counseling the Athlete" which appeared in American Family Physician, volume 63(5), March 1, 2001. Copyright © American Academy of Family Physicians. All rights reserved. Reprinted with permission.

Determining Specific Energy Needs for Sports Activities: Metabolic Equivalents (METs)

The intensity of an exercise or action can be categorized by a formula called Metabolic Equivalents of Task (METs) or Metabolic Equivalent Units. METs starts at the energy expressed while at rest, which is 1. METs can range from 1 MET for resting/sleeping/meditating and go up to 23 METs for running at 14 mph (4.3 minutes per mile).[34, 35] One MET could also be expressed as the amount of oxygen consumed:

- 1 MET = 3.5 ml/kg/min of oxygen consumption.

Since METs remain relatively constant for particular activities but are used against the basal metabolic rate (BMR), one can accurately predict the calories expended during an activity or even for the whole day, once the BMR is known. A copy of the 2011 estimated MET values of different activities (also known as the Compendium of Physical Activities tables) along with the 2000 and 1993 Compendia references can be found at this website: https://sites.google.com/site/compendiumofphysicalactivities/compendia. A sample of METs is found in Table 9.12.[36]

TABLE 9.12 A Sample of METs taken from the 2011 Compendium of Physical Activities

Code	Mets	Major heading	Specific Activities
01018	3.5	Bicycling	Bicycling, leisure, 5.5 mph
02003	3.8	Conditioning exercise	Activity-promoting video game (Wii Fit), moderate effort (e.g., aerobic resistance)
02048	5.0	Conditioning exercise	Elliptical trainer, moderate effort
08120	5.0	Lawn and garden	Mowing lawn, walk, power mower, moderate or vigorous effort
02054	3.5	Conditioning exercise	Resistance (weight) training, multiple exercises, 8–15 repetions at varied resistance
12050	9.8	Running	Running, 6 mph (10 min/mile)
02065	9.0	Conditioning exercise	Stair-treadmill ergometer, general
15055	6.5	Sports	Basketball, general

Code	Mets	Major heading	Specific Activities
02105	3.0	Conditioning exercise	Pilates, general
02160	4.0	Conditioning exercise	Yoga, power
03021	7.3	Dancing	Aerobic, high-impact
05049	3.5	Home activities	Cooking or food preparation, moderate effort
07020	1.3	Inactivity quiet/light	Sitting quietly and watching television
15720	3.0	Sports	Volleyball, non-competitive, 6–9 member team, general

To calculate caloric needs using METs, employ the following:

First, evaluate the calories expended <u>during a single event</u> by determining:

1. the basal metabolic rate (as you did in the beginning of this chapter)

2. the intensity of the event by assigning a MET Value

3. how long the event lasted, in units of hours.

Then use this formula:

(BMR / 24) × (MET Value of event) × (Duration of event, expressed in HOURS)

Example:

Mike plays soccer at a competitive level (10 METs) for 45 minutes (3/4 hour). BMR is approximately 1,800 kcals per day.

(1800 kcals / 24) × (10 METs) × (3/4 hour) = kcals Expended during activity

or

(75 kcals) × (10) × (.75) = 562.5 kcals expended during this activity

In this example, 562.5 kcals represents the total calories burned during 45 minutes of soccer play.

Culinary professionals with a sound nutritional background can positively address the nutritional needs and the concerns of athletes. By efficiently calculating nutrient needs for daily activities and sports, a chef can be a major contributor in promoting the development of peak performance of an athlete.

References

1   E. Whitney and S. Rolfes, *Understanding Nutrition*, 7th ed. St. Paul, MN: West Publishing Company, 1996.

2   R. Lee and D. Nieman, *Nutritional Assessment*, 3rd ed. New York, NY: McGraw Hill, 2003.

3   W. C. Chumlea, et al., "Body Composition Estimates from NHANES III Bioelectrical Impedance Data," *International Journal Obesity Related Metabolic Disorders* 26 (12), (2002): 1596–1609.

4   C. L. Ogden, C. D. Fryar, M. D. Carroll, and K. M. Flegal, "Mean Body Weight, Height, and Body Mass Index, United States 1960–2002," www.cdc.gov/nchs/data/ad/ad347.pdf

5   A. Finkelstein, J. D. Trogdon, J. W. Cohen, and W. Dietz, "Annual Medical Spending Attributable To Obesity: Payer-And Service-Specific Estimates," *Health Affairs* 28 (2009): 822–831.

6   O. Ziegler, et al., "Physiopathology of Obesity. Dietary Factors and Regulation of Energy Balance," *Annual Endocrinology* (Paris) 61 Suppl 6 (2000): 12–23.

7   Y. Suresh, "Leptin, The Fat Controller," *Journal Association Physicians India* 46 (6) (1998): 538–544.

8   A. M. Prentice, "Overeating: The Health Risks," *Obesity Research* 9 Suppl 4 (2001): 234S–238S.

9   K. K. Davison and L. L. Birch, "Childhood Overweight: A Contextual Model and Recommendations for Future Research," *Obesity Review* 2 (3), (2001): 159–171.

10 R. A. Forshee, M. L. Storey, D. B. Allison, W. H. Glinsmann, G. L. Hein, D. R. Lineback, S. A. Miller, T. A. Nicklas, G. A. Weaver and J. S. White, "A Critical Examination of the Evidence Relating High Fructose Corn Syrup and Weight Gain," *Critical Reviews in Food Science and Nutrition* 47 (2007): 561–582.

11 B. M. Herrera, S. Keildson, C. M. Lindgren, "Genetics and Epigenetics of Obesity," *Maturitas* 69 (2011): 41–49.

12 T.M. Frayling, N.J. Timpson, M. N. Weedon, E. Zeggini, R.M. Freathy, C.M. Lindgren, et al., "A Common Variant in the FTO Gene is Associated with Body Mass Index and Predisposes to Childhood and Adult Obesity," *Science* 316 (2007): 889–894.

13 C. Haller and J. B. Schwartz, "Pharmacologic Agents for Weight Reduction," *Journal Gend Specif Med* 5(5), (Sep–Oct, 2002): 16–21.

14 M. Lafontan, "The Role of Sugar Intake in Beverages on Overweight and Health," *Nutrition Today*, Nov/Dec 2010 Supplement, Vol. 45, S13–S17.

15 L. C. Dolan, S. M. Potter, G. A. Burdock, "Evidence-Based Review on the Effect of Normal Dietary Consumption of **Fructose** on Development of Hyperlipidemia and **Obesity** in Healthy, Normal Weight Individuals," *Critical Reviews in Food Science & Nutrition* 50 (2010): 53–84.

16 S. B. Roberts, "Glycemic Index and Satiety," *Nutrition in Clinical Care* 6 (2003): 20–26.

17 L. Shengxu, J. H. Zhao, J. Luan, U. Ekelund, R. N. Luben, K. Khaw, N. J. Wareham, R. J. F. Loos, "Physical Activity Attenuates the Genetic Predisposition to Obesity in 20,000 Men and Women from EPIC-Norfolk Prospective Population Study," *PLOS Medicine* 7 (2010): 1–9.

18 M. Scott, "Obesity More Costly to U.S. Companies than Smoking, Alcoholism," Workforce Management 2008. http://www.workforce.com/section/00/article/25/46/91.html

19 M. B. Tamburrino and R. A. McGinnis, "Anorexia Nervosa. A Review," *Panminerva Medicine* 44 (4), (Dec 2002): 301–311.

20 D. Matusevich, et al., "Hospitalization of Patients with Anorexia Nervosa: A Therapeutic Proposal," *Eating Weight Disorders* 7 (3), (2002): 196–201.

21 M. Spearing, *Eating Disorders: Facts about Eating Disorders and the Search for Solutions*, NIH Pub No 01–2901, 2001.

22 APA DSM 5 website: http://www.dsm5.org/Pages/Default.aspx

23 S Goyal, et. al., "Revisiting Classification of Eating Disorders-toward Diagnostic and Statistical Manual of Mental Disorders-5 and International Statistical Classification of Diseases and Related Health Problems-11", Indian Journal of Psychological Medicine, 34 (2012): 290–296.

24 R. W. Kleposki, "The Female Athlete Triad: A Terrible Trio, Implications for Primary Care," *Journal American Academy Nurse Practitioners* 14 (2002): 26–31.

25 H. Elrick, "Exercise—The Best Prescription," *The Physician and Sports Medicine* 24 (2), (1996).

26 U.S. Department of Health and Human Services (DHHS). "Physical activity guidelines for Americans," 2008. www.health.gov/PAGuidelines/factsheetprof.aspx

27 U.S. Department of Health and Human Services, Healthy People 2010, 2nd ed., Chapter 22, *Physical Activity and Fitness*, Washington DC: Government Printing Office, 2000.

28 U.S. Department of Health and Human Services, Public Health Services, *Exercise and Your Heart: A Guide to Physical Activity*, NIH Publication Number 93–1677, August 1993.

29 W. McArdle, F. Katch, and V. Katch, *Exercise Physiology: Energy, Nutrition and Human Performance*, 2nd ed. Philadelphia PA: Lea and Febiger, 1986.

30 "Nutrition and Athletic Performance—Position of The Academy of Nutrition and Dietetics, Dietitians of Canada, and The American College of Sports Medicine," *Journal of The Academy of Nutrition and Dietetics* 100 (2000): 1543–1556.

31 P. W. Lemon, "Protein and Amino Acid Needs of the Strength Athlete," *International Journal Sport Nutrition* 1 (1991): 127–145.

32 M. Gleeson, "Interrelationship Between Physical Activity and Branched-Chain Amino Acids," *Journal of Nutrition* 135 (2005): 1591S–1595S.

33 F. Sizer and E. Whitney, *Nutrition Concepts and Controversies*, 9th ed. Belmont CA: Wadsworth/Thomas Learning, 2003.

34 M. Dunford, A. J. Doyle, *Nutrition for Sport and Exercise*, 1st ed., Thomson Wadsworth Publishing 2008.

35 B. E. Ainsworth, W. L. Haskell, A. S. Leon, D. R. Jacobs Jr., H. J. Montoye, J. F. Sallis, R. S. Paffenbarger Jr., "Compendium of physical activities: Classification of Energy Costs of Human Physical Activities," Medical & Science in Sports & Exercise 25 (1993): 71–80.

36 Compendium of Physical Activities. https://sites.google.com/site/compendiumofphysicalactivities/compendia

Put It into Practice

Define the Term

Review the definition of ergogenic aids. Using Table 9.11, Ergogenic Aids, choose five ergogenic aids and identify why an athlete may be taking these supplements. List the action, research, side effects, legality, and your concerns about their use.

Myth vs. Fact

Determine if the following statement is a myth or fact and support your position with evidence from three research articles on this topic. *Statement: "Elite athletes need a high-protein diet."*

For each research article, summarize each component below.

- A. Abstract
- B. Methods
- C. Results
- D. Discussion
- E. Conclusion

The Menu

Develop a 1-day vegetarian meal plan for an athlete. The menu must include breakfast, lunch, dinner, and two snacks. The menu plan should be rich in complex carbohydrates, moderate in protein, and moderate in fats. The fats suggested should be unsaturated fats. Review the vegetarian pyramid in the healthy US Vegetarian Meal Pattern in Chapter 2.

Website Review

Navigate the WebMD website's information on Healthy Eating and Diet through the following link: http://www.webmd.com/diet/20050105/americas-fittest-fattest-cities

View the slideshow entitled: "The Fattest and Fittest States in America." List two areas that the fattest states and the fittest states have in common. In your opinion, discuss how this information impacts college age students. How can a chef or dietitian use the information from the slide show in the workplace.

Build Your Career Toolbox

Review the section in the text entitled "Physical Fitness: Aerobic and Anaerobic Activity—Starting a Safe Exercise Program" and the Culinary Corner: Sports Nutrition. Using Table 9.7, explain the difference between anaerobic and aerobic activity. Explain the difference between maximum heart rate and target heart rate. List five employment opportunities for culinary professionals in sports nutrition.

Andrew's Case Study

Andrew is a 23-year-old male who has recently seen a sports RD to evaluate his current eating practices. He attends a CrossFit gym 6 days a week (usually spending 2–3 hrs per workout) and has been following a Paleo diet for about a year. Recently, his workout partner was hospitalized for acute kidney failure, which his doctors told him was likely due to his excessive exercise, in addition to a high protein diet and inadequate fluid intake. Andrew would like to make sure he is meeting his energy and fluid needs and getting enough protein to fuel his weight lifting and muscle-building exercises. He had been following a Paleo diet since he had heard it would help build muscle faster but after talking to the dietitian he is willing to increase carbohydrates and decrease his protein intake.

Ht: 5'11"   Wt: 174 lbs   BMI: 24.3 kg/m²
Typical weight loss during workout: 1.5 lbs

Recommendations

Calorie Needs: 2850–3300
Protein: 118–135 g
Carbohydrates: 430–500 g
Fat: 80–95 g
Total Fluid: ~175 oz/5250 mL (from beverages: about 140 oz/4200 mL)

Include instructions on hydrating and eating before, during, and post-workouts

24-hr diet recall

Breakfast: Egg white omelet (3 egg whites, 1/2 cup broccoli, 2 tbsp chopped tomatoes), Paleo protein shake (50-g protein powder, 1 cup raw spinach, 1 cup strawberries, 1 cup ice, 4-oz unsweetened almond milk)

Snack: 2 boiled eggs, 1 medium orange, 16-oz water

Lunch: 6-oz grilled, skinless chicken breast (coated with 1 tbsp coconut oil), 1 cup mango-avocado salsa (2/3 cup mango, 1/3 avocado, 2 tbsp diced red onion, 1 tsp cilantro, 2 tsp coconut oil, lime juice, dash salt, and black pepper), 12-oz water

Snack (post-workout): Paleo protein shake (50-g protein powder, 1 cup raw spinach, 1 cup strawberries, 1 cup ice, 4-oz unsweetened almond milk)

Dinner: 8-oz broiled ribeye steak seasoned with salt and pepper, 2 cups salad (1½ cup Romaine lettuce, 1/4 cup diced tomatoes, 1/4 cup sliced cucumbers) with 1 tbsp apple cider vinegar and 2 tsp olive oil, 12-oz water

Snack: 1 large apple sliced with 4 tbsp natural peanut butter

Preferences: Andrew loves meats, fruits, and peanut butter; but dislikes potatoes, yogurt, bananas, and asparagus.

Brian's Case Study

Brian is a 27-year-old male who has been running for about a year and is planning to begin training for a marathon that is to take place in 12 weeks. He currently runs about 25 miles per week, but he recently joined a team and will be gradually increasing his mileage up to about 60–70 miles per week. He knows that he'll have to eat more to support his activity, but he's not sure how and what he should be eating. He has been told that he should have a lot of carbs so he's been focusing on getting carbs and lean meats into his diet. He's also concerned because he's started to get really tired in the afternoon when he runs in the morning even though he sleeps from 7 to 9 hrs per night.

Current running schedule
> *Monday, Tuesday, Friday:* 4–6 miles at a pace of 7.5 mph (METs = 12.5)
> *Wednesday:* swim 45 minutes (METs = 8)
> *Thursday:* yoga 1.25 hrs (METs = 6)
> *Saturday:* rest
> *Sunday:* 7–9 miles at a pace of 7 mph (METs = 11.5)

He met with a dietitian who gave him some initial pointers and calorie/protein goals. It seemed that he probably wasn't eating quite enough to support his activity so she has encouraged him to increase his fat intake, but she thought it would be helpful to have you show him what meals and snacks should look like. She thought you could come up with a menu with three meals and three snacks that would meet his nutrition needs on days that he runs in the morning before work.

Wt: 175 lbs   Ht: 6'3"   BMI: 21.9 kg/m² (normal weight)
No recent weight change

Dietitian Recommendations
> *Calorie Needs:* 3000–3300
> *Protein Needs:* 95–105
> *CHO:* 60%–65% calories from CHO
> *Fat:* 25%–35% calories from fat
> *Fiber:* 35–45 g/day
> *Sodium:* 3500–4500 mg/day

Other Recommendations: Try eating three meals and three snacks daily; avoid high fiber and high fat foods before running; breakfast should have at least 500-600 calories, snacks should have 300-400 calories each; Of note, he has said that there are a few foods that he can eat before running (a Clif bar or a banana with toast or oatmeal with a few blueberries), and he avoids dairy and nut butters before he runs because they give him a stomach ache.

24-hr Recall

Pre-Run: 1 Chocolate Chip Clif Bar, 6-ozs orange Gatorade

Breakfast (post-run): 1 whole-wheat bagel (3.5 oz) with 2 tbsp peanut butter, 1 banana, 1 tbsp honey; 12-oz latte with nonfat milk and 2 packets of Equal

Snack: 6-oz plain fat-free Greek yogurt with 1/2 cup chopped strawberries, 1 tbsp honey

Lunch: 2 slices of whole wheat bread, 2-oz fat-free turkey, 1-oz shredded lettuce, 1-oz Swiss cheese, 1 tbsp mustard, 1 pickle, 1 small steamed sweet potato + a pinch of salt, 1 green apple, 8 almonds

Dinner: 6-oz whole-wheat pasta (cooked with salt) with 3/4 cup fat-free marinara sauce, 1/2 cup steamed zucchini, 1 tbsp chopped basil, 1 tbsp Parmesan cheese, 4-oz grilled chicken breast, 5-oz red wine

Snack: 2 cups 99% fat-free popcorn, 12 chocolate chips, 8-oz green tea

Preferences: Allergic to kiwis and pineapple; doesn't drink much milk and doesn't like bell peppers, watermelon, fried foods, rice, breakfast cereals, pork, many desserts; likes peanut butter (hasn't tried other nut butters), bananas, grilled chicken, fish

Study Guide

Student Name _____   Date _____

Course Section _____   Chapter _____

TERMINOLOGY

Hunger___	A. An eating disorder characterized by the refusal to maintain a minimally normal body weight
Anthropometrics___	B. An internal signal that stimulates a person to acquire and consume food
Anorexia Nervosa___	C. A term used to define overfatness with potential adverse health effects and a BMI of over 30
Satiety___	D. The type of activity which strengthens muscles and improves flexibility, bone density, and muscle endurance
Anaerobic___	E. A method to assess body weight using physical characteristics, such as height and weight
Visceral___	F. Activities such as jogging and swimming where oxygen is required
Aerobic___	G. A condition that involves recurring episodes of binge eating that are combined with a morbid fear of becoming fat, often followed by self-induced vomiting
Bulimia Nervosa___	H. A feeling of satisfaction and a signal to stop eating.
Obesity___	I. Fat which is located deep within the central abdominal area

Student Name _____ Date _____

Course Section _____ Chapter _____

ANTHROPOMETRIC MEASURES FOR ADULTS

Use the anthropometric formulas on back.

1. Height: _____

2. Current Actual Weight: _____

3. IBW: _____

4. IBW Range:_____

5. %IBW:_____

6. Body Fat %: _____
   (Bioelectrical Impedance Device)

7. Body Mass Index (BMI):_____
   (Bioelectrical Impedance Device)

8. Basal Metabolic Rate (BMR):_____

9. Total Energy Needs (TEE):_____

10. In the space below interpret your measurements according to the standards in your book.

FORMULAS ON BACK.

-Hamwi Method for Ideal Body Weight (IBW) for adults

   Male: 106# for the first 5 feet (60 inches) add 6# for every inch over

   Female: 100# for the first 5 feet, add 5# for every additional inch

-IBW Range

   Add 10% to your IBW

   Subtract 10% from your IBW

-%IBW

   Actual weight $\times$ 100 = %IBW

-Basal Metabolic Rate (BMR)

   Males: Kg of actual body weight $\times$ 24 $\times$ 1

   Females: Kg of actual body weight $\times$ 24 $\times$ .9

-Total Energy Expenditure (TEE)

   BMR $\times$ Activity Factor

   Activity Factors-- Chapter 9, Table 9.2

Student Name _____   Date _____

Course Section _____   Chapter _____

CASE STUDY DISCUSSION

Anaerobic Sports Nutrition Case Study: Andrew's High Protein Intake

Review the sections in Chapter 9, Culinary Corner; "Sports Nutrition". After reading the case study, use the information to answer the following questions:

1. What are some considerations when determining energy needs for an athlete?

2. What is the typical range for protein requirements for athletes and why?

3. Calculate Andrew's protein needs: his weight is: 174 pounds, the dietitian recommends 1.7 grams of protein per kilogram.

4. What is the best choice of fluid during exercise? Review Table 9.10 and summarize fluid needs before, during and after exercise for Andrew.

Student Name _____   Date _____

Course Section _____   Chapter _____

CASE STUDY DISCUSSION

Brian's Case Study: Calories Expended with METs

Review the sections in Chapter 9, "Determining Specific Energy Needs for Sports Activities: Metabolic Equivalents (METs)". After reading the case study, use the information to answer the following questions:

Using the example in the text, calculate Brian's calories expended during his activities below:

Running for one hour (METs = 12.5) _____ calories expended

Swimming 45 minutes (METs = 8) _____ calories expended

Yoga 1.25 hours (METs = 6) _____ calories expended

1. Calculate his BMR_____

2. Use the formula: (BMR / 24) × (MET value) × (Duration of event, expressed in hours)

Student Name _____   Date _____

Course Section _____   Chapter _____

PRACTICE TEST

Select the best answer.

1. Basal metabolic rate is
   a. the minimum amount of energy needed to sustain life
   b. the maximum amount of energy to lose weight
   c. includes the digestive process
   d. includes aerobic activities

2. Physical activity refers to
   a. the involuntary movement of the skeletal muscles and support systems
   b. the voluntary movement of the skeletal muscles and support systems
   c. both the involuntary and voluntary movements of the skeletal muscles and support systems
   d. neither the involuntary nor voluntary movements of the skeletal muscles and support systems

3. 25-35% of energy consumed goes toward
   a. basal metabolic rate
   b. digestion
   c. physical activity
   d. thermic effect of food

4. Anthropometric measurements include all of the following except
   a. body mass index
   b. blood tests
   c. height and weight
   d. waist to hip measurements

5. According to the Hamwi Method, the ideal body weight (IBW) for an adult female 5'4" tall is
   a. 100 pounds
   b. 110 pounds
   c. 120 pounds
   d. 140 pounds

Student Name _____ **Date** _____

Course Section _____ **Chapter** _____

TRUE OR FALSE

_____ Energy is the capacity to do work.

_____ Appetite is a learned behavior.

_____ Aerobic exercise is considered to be fat burning exercise.

_____ Beverages containing 4 %-8 % carbohydrate may be beneficial for an exercise program that lasts for more than one hour.

_____ Visceral fat is located just under the surface of the skin and is associated with increased disease risk.

1. Determine the Basal Metabolic Rate (BMR) and the Total Energy Needs (TEE) in calories per day for an adult male who weighs 190 pounds with a physical activity factor of 1.5. (show your work)

2. Determine the Basal Metabolic Rate(BMR) and the Total Energy Needs (TEE) in calories per day for an adult female who weighs 140 pounds with a physical activity factor of 1.75. (show your work)

Nutrition and the Lifespan

10

KEY TERMS

AAP	Childhood	Extrusion reflex
Accutane	Competitive foods	Fetus
ADHD	Complementary foods	Food intolerances
Adolescence	Congregate Dining Program	Food sensitivities
Adulthood	Constipation	Free radicals
Allergic reactions	Critical periods	Gestational diabetes
Autism spectrum disorder	Dental caries	Heartburn
Breastfeeding	Embryo	Hemorrhoids

Infancy
Meals on Wheels
Menopause
Menstruation
Morning sickness
Myoglobin

Older adult
Osteoarthritis
Placenta
Pregnancy
Puberty
Retin-A

Sebaceous gland
SIDS
SNAP
Stillborn
WIC
Zygote

Introduction

The Importance of Nutrition throughout the Life Stages

This chapter addresses the stages of human development and the accompanying nutritional needs for these stages. Human development can be described as the changes that occur in the body and mind during each segment of life. These changes and their effects on nutritional and food requirements are discussed at length, throughout this chapter.

Foods that provide the six essential nutrients are required throughout the lifespan, although the body uses these nutrients at varying rates and levels of efficiency throughout the life stages. Calcium and iron, for example, are leading nutrients that are needed throughout life, yet their rate of absorption is greatest during periods when they are most needed by the body. Adequate intake of vitamin D is needed for the absorption of calcium. Dairy products (milk, yogurt, cheese) and foods that are fortified with calcium and vitamin D are especially valuable choices during growth periods (pregnancy, lactation, infancy, childhood, and adolescence), when bone structure is increasing. Calcium is important for the bone health of women of all ages. It is especially valuable in protecting the bones of pregnant women with developing babies who need large amounts of this nutrient.

Foods high in iron, such as meats, egg yolks, and plant sources (fortified cereals, beans, lentils, tofu and cooked spinach), are valuable choices during growth periods, because blood volume increases and more red blood cells are required. Young women, in particular, have increased iron needs that put them at risk for iron-deficiency anemia due to monthly losses caused by **menstruation**. Plant-based foods are often nutrient rich and can provide a substantial amount of both calcium and iron, if consumed "strategically" and in sufficient quantities. Absorption of iron from plant sources can be improved when consumed in conjunction with a vitamin C-containing food at the same meal or snack. An example of such a combination would be vegetarian bean chili topped with chopped, fresh tomatoes. Table 10.1 offers suggestions for menu items that provide calcium and iron. Culinarians can play an important role in promoting health during every stage of the lifespan by preparing healthy foods in restaurants; by creating recipes using nutrient rich ingredients; and by teaching food preparation techniques.

TABLE 10.1 Some Examples of Foods Providing Calcium and Iron	
Foods Providing Calcium	**Examples of Culinary Use**
Milk	Fruit smoothies, puddings, sauces
Yogurt	Fruit smoothies, yogurt cheese, dip for fruit kebabs, tzatziki, filling in fruit tarts, chicken salad, layered bean dips
Cheeses, especially reduced-fat varieties, includes string cheese	Toppings for snacks, in salads, sandwiches, and in casseroles as a meat alternative
Cottage or ricotta cheese	In quiche, casseroles, with pasta
Tofu	Stir-fries with vegetables over rice, soft tofu can substitute for milk in pudding and ice cream
Legumes/beans, lentils	Stews, chili, soups, loafs, dips, quesadillas, side dishes. Include vitamin C-rich ingredients for better absorption of iron

Pumpkin seeds	In trail mix with nuts, seeds, in baked products
Soybean nuts	Snack
Lean red meats, fish, shellfish, poultry	In recommended portion size (2–4 oz.) roasted with vegetables, grilled as kebabs with vegetables
	In small amounts in stews with grains
Whole eggs	As breakfast or dinner omelets, as sandwich fillings, as "benedicts," quiches or frittatas, boiled as a snack
Enriched breakfast cereal	As breakfast or snack
Enriched rice, quinoa	Side dish, base for "minimal meat" dishes, hot or cold salads
Cooked spinach	Side dish, loaves, scrod Florentine, include vitamin C-rich ingredient(s) for better absorption of iron

The Beginning of Life

Pregnancy

Preparing for a Healthy Pregnancy

From childhood, the female body develops to provide the environment necessary for a new life to begin. Experts urge women to do two things in preparation for **pregnancy**. The first recommendation is that all women should consume nutrient-dense diets featuring fruits and vegetables, especially those that are high in the B vitamin folic acid. A 400 microgram supplement of folic acid is recommended for all women of childbearing age.[1],[2] Oranges and grapefruit and their juices, dark-green leafy vegetables such as spinach, and many kinds of beans are high in this nutrient. Folic acid can help prevent specific, serious birth defects. Since 1996 the Food and Drug Administration (FDA) has mandated the addition of folic acid in a variety of grain products due to its contribution in the prevention of birth defects. Folic acid is critical for at least a month prior to conception and during the early weeks of pregnancy. Unfortunately many women are not aware of the pregnancy until after the end of the first month.[3] The second suggestion is the maintenance of a healthy weight before pregnancy. Being either underweight or overweight can complicate a woman's pregnancy or interfere with the baby's growth and development.[4]

The Stages of Pregnancy

A pregnancy begins when the male sperm fertilizes the female egg/ovum. In a normal pregnancy, three stages follow according to a very specific schedule (shown in Table 10.2). This figure illustrates the cycle from the prenatal period to the period immediately after birth, known as the postnatal period.

The Zygote Stage

Pregnancy begins with the zygote stage, the two-week period after fertilization when three very important developments occur. First, the egg/ovum is implanted in the wall of the woman's uterus. Then the **placenta**, a growing baby's lifeline to the mother, starts to form. Lastly, the division of the zygote into the three layers (the ectoderm, the mesoderm, and the endoderm) takes place, to form what will be the baby's major organs. If a mother's body is malnourished or damaged by drug abuse, the zygote may be lost because implantation fails or an abnormal development of the zygote occurs.

The Embryo Stage

The period from week three through week eight of pregnancy is the embryo stage when major organs of the body, the nervous system, the heart, and the gastrointestinal system begin to form. In addition, fingers and toes become defined.

TABLE 10.2 Stages of Pregnancy		
Stages	**Development**	**Weeks**
Zygote	The period after fertilization: Implantation; placenta formation; organ differentiation	1–2
Embryo	A period of development including major organ formation	3–8
Fetal Stage	The period of the greatest development of the fetus: Continuing development of organ systems; steady increase in length; steady increase in weight until the last month when the rate of gain increases	9–40
Postnatal Stage	The period immediately after birth: Major organ development continues throughout the first year of life	41–44

Critical periods occur during the embryo and fetal stages. These are periods of growth in major organ systems that require specific nutrients. Lack of a nutrient may result in irreversible damage to the developing infant.

Critical periods occur at a particular time during pregnancy when specific nutrients are required for the development of the major organ systems. The lack of even one of these nutrients, when it is required, can lead to the abnormal development of an organ's structure or of its function after birth. Since a woman may not know that she is pregnant well into the embryo stage, all women of childbearing age are urged to consume nutrient rich foods to avoid damage that can occur at these early stages.

The Fetal Stage

The third stage of development is the fetal stage, the period from week nine until the end of a normal pregnancy (about forty weeks). From week nine, the developing baby is referred to as a **fetus** and the weeks of pregnancy are referred to as trimesters. These trimesters consist of three thirteen-week segments. Periods of rapid growth in weight and length along with the continuing development of organ systems occur during the third trimester.

Weight Gain in Pregnancy

A pregnant woman gains weight due to increases in her body tissue and the growth of the fetus. One of the most important changes in the mother's body is the production of the placenta, a lifeline that carries nutrients and oxygen to the fetus and removes the waste excreted by the fetus. A healthy placenta is dependent upon the nutritional condition of the mother's body and is absolutely necessary for the normal development of the fetus. Figure 10.1 illustrates the relationship of the mother and the baby through the placenta. Other contributions to the weight gain of a pregnant woman include increases in fluid and fat in her body, and the actual weight of the baby. While a pregnant woman may gain 30 pounds or more, the typical 7 1/2 pound newborn may represent only one-quarter of the total increase in weight.[4]

The Amount and Rate of Weight Gain

The weight gain of a pregnant woman, including the rate of gain, is the measure used by health professionals to determine the health and well-being of the fetus. Guidelines have been established for women in a variety of weight categories since not all women are at ideal weight or BMI standards. Weight levels that are too low or too high may result in complications at birth. Babies may be born too soon or may be too small to survive if the mother is underweight. Mothers who are overweight may develop **gestational diabetes** or experience a difficult labor and delivery. A woman of "normal weight" should gain 24 to 35 pounds while a goal of 28 to 40 pounds is suggested for underweight women. Table 10.3 summarizes these recommendations along with those for overweight and obese women who are advised to gain fewer pounds. Weight loss during pregnancy is not encouraged.

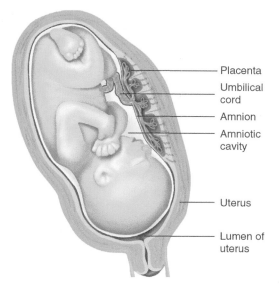

FIGURE 10.1 The Placenta

This organ, made from maternal and fetal tissue, helps to nourish the developing fetus and to remove wastes. It also produces important hormones.

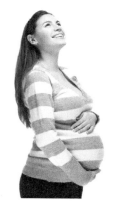

The weight gain of a pregnant woman, including the rate of gain, is the measure used by health professionals to determine the health and well-being of the fetus.

The rate of the recommended weight gain should follow the pattern described in Table 10.3. For a woman of normal weight, 3 1/2 pounds in the first trimester and less than 1 pound per week for the remainder of the pregnancy is recommended. This table also identifies the appropriate rates of weight gain for women in all weight categories. The 2009 recommendations were updated for the first time in 20 years and special attention was paid to the dramatic increase in the number of pregnant women who are overweight at the time of conception.[5]

TABLE 10.3 2009 IOM Recommendations for Rate and Amount of Weight Gain During Pregnancy, Based on Pre-pregnancy BMI			
Pre-Pregnancy BMI	BMI	Total Weight Gain (LBS.)	Rates of Weight Gain* 2nd and 3rd Trimester (LBS./Week)
Underweight	<18.5	28–40	1(1.0–1.3)
Normal Weight	18.5–24.9	25–35	1(0.8–1.0)
Overweight	25.0–29.9	15–25	.6(0.5–0.7)
Obese	>30	11–20	.5(0.4–0.6)

*Calculations assume a 1.1–4.4 lbs. weight gain in the first trimester

Energy Needs and Leading Nutrients

In spite of all the changes that occur in the mother's body and in the fetus, a relatively small number of additional calories are recommended for a pregnant woman (340 additional calories during the second trimester and 452 for the third trimester). Women with special needs, those at low weight levels, pregnant teenagers, or those who are very active will probably need more calories to reach an appropriate weight. The additional calories needed during pregnancy should be derived from foods that provide the nutrients for which increases are recommended. Figure 10.2 presents nutrient comparisons for non-pregnant, pregnant, and breastfeeding women. Folate and iron are the nutrients that account for the greatest increases in recommendations during pregnancy. These nutrients are especially important in producing the cell tissue required for growth. They also contribute to the production of additional blood cells that are necessary in the 50% blood supply increase of pregnant women.

There are three other reasons that iron is required in larger amounts during pregnancy: (1) the fetus needs to store iron for the first 4–6 months of life, (2) the mother loses iron through blood loss at delivery and immediately afterwards, and (3) few women have adequate iron stores before pregnancy. Pregnant women should consume bean dishes, oranges and dark-green leafy vegetables to help meet the required iron and folate intake. Iron and folate fortified foods such as breads and cereals are also good sources. The 400 microgram folic acid supplement recommendation for women of child-bearing age increases to 600 micrograms during pregnancy. Since it is unlikely that women will be able to consume enough iron-rich food to fully meet pregnancy needs, a supplement of 30 mg is usually recommended during the second and third trimesters. Smaller, but also important, increases in other vitamins and minerals are also needed in pregnancy as indicated in Figure 10.2.[6]

Calcium: A Special Case

Another leading nutrient that is important during pregnancy is calcium. The recommendation for this mineral does not increase, because calcium is used more efficiently during this period and can therefore adequately accommodate a woman's increased needs. Since a woman's body absorbs two times the usual amount of calcium during pregnancy, she can store enough of this mineral to make it available for the development of the bones and teeth of the fetus in the last weeks of her pregnancy. While a large amount of additional calcium is not recommended, a pregnant woman needs to achieve a dietary intake that meets the recommendation of 1,000 mg (equal to 3 servings from the dairy group). A "smoothie" made with milk or yogurt and fruit can increase calcium and is an enjoyable meal or snack for pregnant women.

All nutrients are necessary in the diet of a pregnant woman, even though the calorie increase is small. The USDA ChooseMyPlate Health and Nutrition Guide for Pregnant and Breast feeding Women is helpful in planning the amount and types of food needed. Additional servings from the meat and beans group are needed in the second and third trimester.

Concerns during Pregnancy

Teen pregnancy

Teen pregnancy is a great concern because the young mother has nutritional needs for her own growth and development, in addition to those of her baby. Since the high nutrient demands of both mother and baby are often unmet, babies of teen mothers are more likely to be **stillborn**, premature, of low birth weight, or at risk of dying during the first year of life. Previously, teen girls were advised

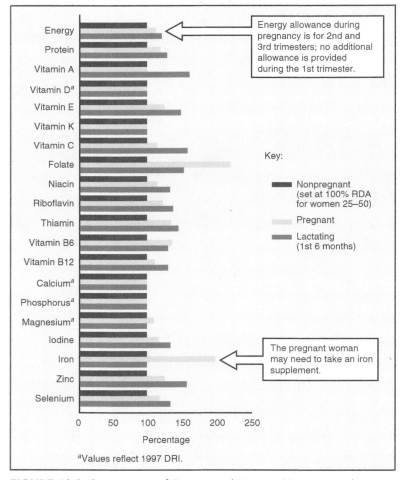

FIGURE 10.2 Comparison of Energy and Nutrient Recommendations for Non-pregnant, Pregnant, and Lactating Women

to gain extra weight. However, the 2009 IOM recommendation is that teen girls should follow adult guidelines based on their pre-pregnancy weights. The consumption of a fourth serving of high calcium/dairy foods is recommended.

Medical Considerations

Gestational Diabetes

Gestational diabetes is a medical condition in women who do not have diabetes before pregnancy, but who develop abnormal blood sugar control at around the twentieth week of pregnancy. Women who have this problem are frequently overweight and this additional weight may cause insulin resistance. Although they will not have diabetes immediately after the baby is born, they have an increased risk of developing type 2 diabetes later in life. Women are urged to achieve a healthy weight and to exercise regularly to decrease this risk. If blood sugar levels are not well controlled during pregnancy, the baby can be born excessively large and can have difficulty breathing.

Common Discomforts

Morning sickness, heartburn, constipation, and hemorrhoids are commonly experienced by pregnant women and can sometimes be helped by some simple nutritional interventions. The problem of morning sickness may be due to hormonal changes in pregnancy and often occurs for only a brief period. Eating small frequent meals can aid in the relief of both nausea and heartburn for some women. Heartburn results from acid backup from the mother's stomach to the esophagus, due to pressure from the fetus. To alleviate constipation and hemorrhoids (swollen veins in the rectum that can result from straining at bowel movements), an increase in the consumption of high-fiber foods, such as bran cereals, beans, fruits, and vegetables, and at least 8 glasses of non-caffeinated fluids is advised. Regular exercise can also help to relieve constipation.[7]

Food Safety

Consumption of some foods presents a risk for the developing fetus and/or the breastfed infant. Certain organisms can cross the placenta to the fetus. Infection can result in miscarriages, stillbirths, premature labor or severe complications for the baby.

Table 10.4 lists some of these foods and the risks with consumption.[8, 9, 10, 11]

TABLE 10.4 Harmful Substances to Avoid		
Harmful Substance	**When to Avoid Foods**	**Foods to Avoid and or Precautions**
Listeria bacteria	Pregnancy Can be transmitted to developing fetus even if the mother is not showing symptoms	FOODS TO AVOID ■ Hot dogs, luncheon meats, and deli meats unless reheated to steaming hot ■ Refrigerated pâté, meat spreads from a meat counter, or smoked seafood found in the refrigerated section of a food store ■ Salads made in the store such as ham salad, chicken salad, egg salad, tuna salad, or seafood salad ■ Raw (unpasteurized) milk ■ Soft cheese such as feta, queso blanco, queso fresco, Brie, Camembert cheeses, blue-veined cheeses, and Panela, unless made with pasteurized milk

(Continued)

TABLE 10.4 Harmful Substances to Avoid (*Continued*)		
Harmful Substance	When to Avoid Foods	Foods to Avoid and or Precautions
Mercury	Pregnancy and Breastfeeding The mercury can harm the developing nervous system in an unborn child or young child.	FOODS TO AVOID - Shark, swordfish, king mackerel, or tilefish due to high levels of mercury. Depending on where it was raised, farm-raised salmon, especially the skin, may contain high levels of mercury. - **No more than 12 oz. a week** (2 average meals) of fish and shellfish that are lower in mercury. Shrimp, canned light tuna, salmon, pollock. - "White" tuna (albacore) has more mercury than canned light tuna. So, when choosing fish and shellfish, include only up to 6 oz. per week of white tuna.
Toxoplasma gondii: (a parasite)	Pregnancy Infection during pregnancy can be passed on to developing fetus	PRECAUTIONS - Wash hands with soap and water after touching soil, sand, raw meat, or unwashed vegetables. - Cook meat completely. The internal temperature of the meat should reach 160°F. Chicken and turkey need to be cooked to a higher temperature. Do not sample meat until it is cooked. - Freeze meat for several days before cooking to greatly reduce the chance of infection. - Wash all cutting boards and knives with hot soapy water after each use. - Wash and/or peel all fruits and vegetables before eating.

Growth Stages

Breastfeeding

The American Academy of Pediatrics (AAP) recommends breastfeeding as the most nutritionally sound method of feeding an infant. Milk that is produced in the mother's breast is perfectly designed for a human infant. Breastfeeding provides the infant with a strong immune system and has been found to further the emotional bonding between mother and child. Research indicates that breastfed infants who are nursed longer in infancy have greater intellectual abilities than those not receiving this benefit. Breast milk contains omega-3 fatty acids if the mother consumes foods that provide these. Breast milk also contains probiotics. There is no food preparation needed when the baby is hungry, and the milk is already at the perfect temperature. It is also an economical feeding choice. Making food choices that meet the nutrient needs for breastfeeding are of great importance in supporting the mother's body.

There are also personal benefits for the mother who chooses to breastfeed her baby. The uterus of women who breastfeed contracts more rapidly in recovery from pregnancy and iron is better conserved because of a delay in the menstrual cycle, which usually does not resume for some months. This time without menstruation can prolong intervals between pregnancies and allows the mother's body time to restore itself. Breastfeeding is also said to reduce the risk for sudden infant death syndrome (SIDS). A mother has the option of providing breast milk for her baby when she is away by pumping breast milk and storing it safely for future feeding. Many women who return to work outside the home prolong breastfeeding in this way.

Energy Needs and Leading Nutrients

The energy requirement for a woman who is breastfeeding is greater than the amount needed during pregnancy. In addition to the calories usually required an approximate increase of 450–550 additional calories is needed. It is assumed that 330 calories (first six months) to 400 calories (second six months) of this requirement will come from food and 150 calories will be drawn from some of the fat that has been stored in the mother's body during pregnancy. The USDA ChooseMyPlate for breastfeeding women recommends nutrient-dense choices from each food group. Special attention must be given to the many nutrient needs of breastfeeding women.

Although the mother's diet is usually found to affect the quantity of breast milk rather than its quality, a mother can increase the level of beneficial omega-3 fatty acids in her breast milk by consuming low mercury oily fish (salmon or chunk light tuna) or by taking fish oil supplements that are not contaminated with mercury. Some fatty fish contain mercury that can be harmful to the young infant. (See Table 10.4)

The quality of the milk may also be affected if the mother's diet is low in the fat-soluble vitamins A, D and E. A 150% increase of these vitamins is needed by women who are breastfeeding. Culinary professionals can offer menu suggestions and recipes that include deep-colored vegetables and other such sources of vitamin A, and healthy plant oils, nuts, and seeds that provide vitamin E. While the calcium level in breast milk will not change with a mother's low-calcium diet, her own calcium supply will be reduced if her intake is inadequate. An additional recommendation for women who breastfeed, is the consumption of a minimum of two quarts of water daily. Finally, special consideration must be given to women who are vegetarians. It is especially important to plan an adequate intake of nutrients such as protein, calcium, and vitamin B_{12}, which are frequently lacking with this style of eating. The challenge to meet the needs of vegetarian women is greatest for "vegans" who do not consume food from animal sources. Such individuals may require supplements to achieve a desirable nutrition intake.

Food Behaviors

In addition to the personal reasons that women who breastfeed select certain foods, time and convenience may be a consideration of major importance. Breastfeeding requires that the mother spend a large amount of time and energy nourishing her baby while she recovers from her pregnancy. She needs rest when the baby sleeps and will benefit from assistance with food preparation and other household responsibilities. Visitors might be advised to bring food gifts that provide the new mother with a "real meal" during this time of adjustment in caring for a baby. Culinary advice about nutritious foods that are easy to prepare can provide valuable help to a new mom who is breastfeeding.

Infancy

Infancy (the period from birth to the first birthday) is when the most rapid growth and development in the body's major organ systems occur. During this period, an excellent nutritional environment must be provided. Birth weight is tripled and a child's length increases by about 50% during this first year of life.

Feeding the Infant

Over the years, feeding recommendations for infants have changed based on available on-going research. Currently, it is recommended that for the first 4–6 months of life, a baby should consume only breast milk or a commercial formula. The decision concerning how to feed an infant should be made by the parents after examining the pros and cons of breastfeeding and commercial infant formula feeding.

The Nutrients in Breast Milk and Infant Formula

The nutrients in breast milk and the body's use of these nutrients provide the best choice for infant feeding. For mothers who elect not to breastfeed, the Nutrition Committee of the American Academy of Pediatrics (AAP) has developed standards for formula to help manufacturers provide compositions that are as similar to breast milk as possible. However, formula is often less digestible and less beneficial for infants than is breast milk due to differences in the composition of the carbohydrate, protein, and fat in formulas.

The carbohydrates, proteins, and fats in breast milk are specifically suited for an infant. The carbohydrate lactose in breast milk is a sugar that is easily digested by the baby. Other unique substances are also present in breast milk and serve to protect the baby from bacteria that may be harmful. Breast milk also contains a modest level of protein and a high proportion of whey protein to casein protein. Whey protein is easier for an infant to digest.

The fat content in breast milk is very high (55%), because fat is important both for energy and for the quality of the fatty acids it provides. Body organs, including the central nervous system, utilize fatty acids as they develop. The availability of omega-3 fatty acids can support brain and nervous system development and improve vision. These fatty acids are already present in breast milk and, in recent years, they have been added to infant formulas. Researchers have found slightly higher levels of intelligence in adults who were breastfed as infants and believe that omega-3s may be responsible for this.[12] Probiotics or "good bacteria" are also found in breast milk. Although infant formula companies have recently begun to add probiotics to infant formula in an effort to provide a product that more closely resembles breast milk, ultimately, breast milk remains the ideal choice for infants.

Breast milk contains about 10 times more cholesterol (a substance valuable to the developing nervous system), than infant formula. Formula contains less cholesterol because vegetable oils are used to supply fat in these products. Even though the total amounts of other nutrients in breast milk are lower than those in formula, those in breast milk are better absorbed. Even though the iron level in human milk is low, 50% or more of it can be absorbed in the early months of life as compared to the less than 5% absorbed from formula. Breast milk contains lower amounts of Vitamin D as compared to infant formula.

Infants should not be fed cow's milk to drink during the first six months of life because the form of its dominant protein, casein, can cause bleeding in the immature gastrointestinal tracts of babies. Iron-deficiency anemia can also occur due to intestinal bleeding. The anemia can be made worse by the high calcium and low vitamin C levels in cow's milk that interfere with the absorption of iron from the diet. Cow's milk forms curds that are too difficult to be digested in the immature gastrointestinal tract of an infant. Beginning at about 7-8 months of age, infants may safely be offered cheese and yogurt. From 6-12 months of age, small amounts of cow's milk will not cause harm, however, cow's milk is low in iron and its introduction into the diet as a primary beverage should be delayed until the infant is taking a significant variety of food. In a small percentage of susceptible infants, allergic reactions may result from the abnormal absorption of the proteins in cow's milk[13]. The transition from formula or breast milk to cow's milk occurs at about one year of age, when the infant is eating a broad range of foods that supply multiple nutrients. Whole milk is recommended up until the age of two at which time low-fat or nonfat milk is an acceptable option.

Solid Foods for Baby

Pediatricians recommend that solid foods, also known as complementary foods, should be added to an infant's diet at 4–6 months of age, when the baby's nutrient needs cannot be met by breast milk alone, and when the baby is developmentally ready to eat solid foods. Solids may be added gradually as the baby develops the muscular control that allows food to be taken from a spoon. One of the indications that an infant is ready to start solids is the loss of the extrusion reflex (an automatic thrust of the tongue when food is placed in the infant's mouth with a spoon). When this reflex disappears, at the age of about 4 months, food will reach the back of the mouth and swallowing can occur. Before consuming small amounts of solid foods, a baby should also be able to sit in a high chair and indicate dissatisfaction by turning the head away or pushing the spoon away. Suggested "first" foods for babies include iron-fortified infant cereal and strained vegetables and fruit. The order in which fruits and vegetables are introduced is not important.[14] A few weeks after introducing cereals, vegetables, and fruits, food sources of protein should be added. Meats contain iron and zinc, which are two important minerals during rapid growth stages. At about 7–9 months of age, babies can usually move food around the mouth more efficiently and may be served more coarsely prepared mixtures. Commercial baby foods offer a wide variety of choices for infants at different stages of the first year. Selections of commercial infant foods should be carefully evaluated as to their high carbohydrate and low protein contents. Single ingredient meats contain more protein than mixed dinners and can be combined with vegetables if the baby needs time to become accustomed to the stronger taste of meats. Table 10.5 presents a suggested progression of foods, based on infant development of feeding skills.

TABLE 10.5 Infant Feeding Skills and Recommended Foods		
Age (Months)	**Feeding Skill**	**Appropriate Foods Added to the Diet**
0–4	Turns head toward any object that brushes cheek. Initially swallows using back of tongue; gradually begins to swallow using front of tongue as well. Strong reflex (extrusion) to push food out during the first 2–3 months.	Feed breast milk or infant formula.
4–6	Extrusion reflex diminishes, and the ability to swallow non-liquid foods develops. Indicates a desire for food by opening the mouth and leaning forward. Indicates satiety or disinterest by turning away and leaning back. Begins chewing action. Brings hand to mouth. Grasps objects with palm of hand (palmar grasp).	Begin iron-fortified cereal mixed with breast milk, formula, or water. Begin pureed vegetables and fruits.
	Sits erect with minimal support at 6 months.	
6–8	Able to feed self finger foods. Begins to practice drinking from cup	Offer meats many times if, necessary, as the flavor is strong. Begin simple finger foods such as infant crackers or toast. Begin yogurt, and pureed or mashed foods such as hummus, avocado and sweet potato.
		Offer additional finger foods such as French toast sticks, toast, crackers Begin textured vegetables and fruits. Begin water from cup so infant can practice cup-drinking.

(Continued)

TABLE 10.5 Infant Feeding Skills and Recommended Foods (*Continued*)		
Age (Months)	Feeding Skill	Appropriate Foods Added to the Diet
8–10	Reaches for and grabs food and spoon. Sits unsupported. Develops pincer (finger to thumb) grasp.	Able to hold own bottle. Begin pieces of soft, cooked vegetables and fruit Gradually begin finely-cut meats, fish, casseroles, cheese, eggs, and legumes.
10–12	Begins to master spoon, but still spills some.	Include breads and whole grain foods in addition to infant cereal.[a] Include at least 2 servings/day of fruits and 2 servings of vegetables.[a] Include 2 servings/day of meat, fish, poultry, eggs, or legumes.[a]

[a]Serving sizes for infants and young children are smaller than those for an adult. For example, a serving might be 1/2 slice of bread instead of 1, or 1/4 cup rice instead of 1/2 cup.
Note: Because each stage of development builds on the previous stages, the foods from an earlier stage continue to be included in later stages.

Commercial baby food labels provide valuable information for parents. However, the labels cannot include the calories from fat, grams of saturated fat, monounsaturated fat, polyunsaturated fat, or milligrams of cholesterol. This practice is designed to avoid the elimination of needed fats in infant diets by well-meaning parents.

Honey and corn syrup are omitted during the first year of life because of the risk of botulism. "Chokable" foods such as popcorn, whole grapes, beans, nuts, and hot dogs should also be avoided. To prevent choking, infants should not eat peanut butter from a spoon, since the consistency of this food can create a "plug" that interferes with breathing if it blocks the airway.[15] When consumed in excessive quantities, juices—particularly apple juice—can interfere with the infant's consumption of a nutritious diet. Parents assume that 100% fruit juices are nutritious choices but many infants enjoy the sweet taste and the ease of drinking these from a bottle and they consume overly large amounts. Both The Institute of Medicine (IOM) and The American Academy of Pediatrics (AAP) recommend against feeding juice to infants.[16, 17]

Home Preparation of Baby Food

Some parents prepare their own baby foods and find that it can be a simple, nutritious, and more economical method of infant feeding than using commercial foods. The major caution for those preparing foods for infants at home is the need to follow precise sanitation procedures to reduce the risk of infection or food-borne illness in extremely vulnerable infants. Table 10.6 contains tips for preparing baby food at home.

TABLE 10.6 Preparation of Baby Foods at Home
■ Select high-quality fruits, vegetables, grains, legumes and meats
■ Prepare without salt or sugar for infants from 4–8 months. After 4–8 months, minimal amounts of salt, flavoring herbs (such as thyme), and spices (such as cinnamon) can be used.
■ Apply sanitation procedures to food preparation (work area, utensils, storage containers, temperatures)
■ Steam fruits and vegetables or cook in minimal amounts of water
■ Purée or strain using a food processor or blender to the texture appropriate for the infant's stage of readiness for solids
■ Moisten foods with cooking water, milk, or water
■ Prepare individual portions to allow heating single servings and to limit the bacterial content of the food
■ Previously frozen portions should be thawed in the refrigerator or reheated to a low temperature

Energy Needs and Leading Nutrients

Because of the high growth rate during infancy, energy requirements are greater per kilogram of body weight at this time than at any other time during the lifespan. An infant needs about 100 calories per kilogram of weight as compared to an adult man who requires only about 35 calories per kilogram. Protein is always the most important nutrient during high-growth periods. An infant, for example, should have 13–14 grams of protein per day. The protein in breast milk is best utilized by the human infant.

Vitamin and mineral needs increase as the infant grows. The need for vitamin D is 10 times greater in infants per kilogram of body weight than in adult males. All infants should be given a vitamin D supplement beginning in the first few days of life. Supplementation should continue through the first year of life for both breastfed infants and formula-fed infants. Infants who are dark-skinned, are breastfed, or who have limited exposure to sunlight are at particular risk of vitamin D deficiency and might need a higher dose. The AAP revised a 2003 Policy Statement on vitamin D in 2008, doubling the recommended dose and expanding the recommendation to formula fed infants.[18] During the second 6 months of the first year, iron and fluoride supplements are recommended by the AAP for both breastfed and formula-fed infants. Table 10.7 summarizes the recommendations for supplement use during the first year of life.

TABLE 10.7 Supplements for Full-term Infants

	Vitamin D[a]	Iron[b]	Fluoride[c]
Breastfed infants			
Birth to six months of age	✓		
Six months to one year	✓	✓	✓
Formula-fed infants			
Birth to six months of age	✓		
Six months to one year		✓	✓

[a]Vitamin D supplements are recommended for all infants, especially breastfed infants, those whose mothers are vitamin D deficient or those who do not receive adequate exposure to sunlight and infants with darker skin.
[b]Infants 4–6 months of age need additional iron, preferably in the form of iron-fortified cereal for both breastfed and formula-fed infants and iron-fortified infant formula for formula-fed infants.
[c]At 6 months of age, breastfed infants and formula-fed infants who receive ready-to-use formulas (these are prepared with water low in fluoride) or formula mixed with water that contains little or no fluoride (less than 0.3 ppm) need supplements.
Source: Adapted from American Academy of Pediatrics, Pediatric Nutrition Handbook, 6th ed., ed. R.E. Kleinman (Elk Grove Village, IL: American Academy of Pediatrics, 2009).

Vitamin K, which is integral to normal blood clotting, is produced in the gastrointestinal tract by bacteria. Newborn babies are born without these bacteria because they have not consumed food, and are usually given an injection of Vitamin K to protect them against excessive bleeding. After breast or formula feeding, bacteria grow and produce vitamin K.

How the Body Uses Nutrients for Growth

During the first 6 months of life many calories are utilized for growth and the continuing development of organ systems. In the second 6 months, more calories are used because of the increased activity of the infant who learns to turn over, crawl, and walk. Figure 10.3 shows how a baby from 0–12 months of age uses energy in food. Babies have high water needs because water makes up a large percentage of their body weight, both within and outside the body cells. Water can be easily lost and the baby can become dehydrated if the infant is not regularly fed.

Food Behaviors

Appetite Regulation

Most infants learn to breastfeed instinctively and trigger the mother's body to produce more milk. From the first days of life babies have their own "style" of eating. Parents are urged to accommodate a baby's feeding needs to encourage the baby to develop a sense of satisfaction when fed. Parents are also advised to avoid pressuring formula-fed babies to finish the contents of a bottle or a serving of solid food if the appetite appears to be satisfied. Infants are born with the ability to know when they are hungry and full. If a parent continues to feed an infant who has indicated that he or she if full, overeating may be encouraged.

Competitive Foods

Foods that provide calories but few nutrients are commonly known as "empty-calorie" foods. These foods can act as competitive foods in the diet, especially for infants and young children who have small stomachs. Frequent consumption of competitive foods leaves little room in the diet for more nutritious foods. Some examples of competitive foods are listed in Table 10.8, along with more nutrient-rich choices. It is important for parents and caregivers to carefully consider diet quality, beginning at infancy. Food preferences are "learned." Children learn to prefer certain foods based on how early and how frequently they are given those foods to eat. Research has shown that the food preferences children show by the age of 4 are still present at the age of 8.[19] Culinary professionals can develop recipes for healthier food products for children such as "granola bars" using a nut butter as a base with ingredients such as toasted wheat germ; whole-grain cereal; chopped nuts; seeds; maple syrup or honey; chopped, dried fruits; skim milk powder, etc.

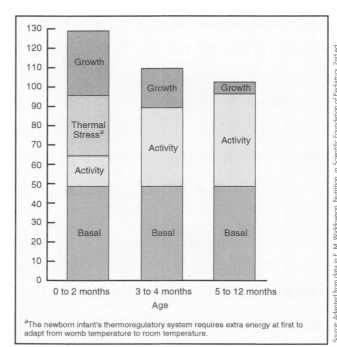

Source: Adapted from data in E. M. Widdowson, Nutrition, in *Scientific Foundation of Pediatrics, 2nd ed* (Baltimore: University Park Press, 1981), pp. 41–53, as cited by M. Gracey and F. Falkner, *Nutritional Needs and Assessment of Normal Growth* (New York: Raven Press, 1985), pp. 23–40.

[a]The newborn infant's thermoregulatory system requires extra energy at first to adapt from womb temperature to room temperature.

FIGURE 10.3 Energy needs of infants in the first year. Infant energy needs vary according to age and weight. As the infant grows older and larger, the growth rate diminishes, and the activity level increases.

TABLE 10.8 Competitive vs. Nutrient-Rich Foods	
Competitive (Empty-Calorie) Foods	**Nutrient-Rich Foods**
Apple Juice and other low-nutrient juices	Whole fruit, orange juice, mango juice
White potato French fries	Baked sweet potato "fries"
Soda, Koolaid, Hi-C, Capri Sun & other "juice" drinks	Milk or flavored milk, almond milk, coconut milk, or smoothie made with fruit and yogurt or milk
Refined-grain products such as crackers, pretzels	Whole-grain crackers or pretzels, peeled, thinly sliced fruits
Commercial chicken nuggets	White breast, chicken pieces with whole-grain coating, baked in olive oil
Donuts, cookies, pastries	Fresh fruit and desserts made with fruit, whole grains, nut butters and minimal sugar

Medical Conditions

Some infants are allergic to protein or other substances in formula, or on rare occasions, are allergic to protein or other substances in breast milk. Allergic reactions involve the immune system and may lead to severe, immediate or delayed reactions that can be life-threatening. The most common infant food allergies are to milk, egg whites, and soy protein.

There is however no evidence that most infants need to stay away from these foods during the first year of life.[20] Parents may find that allergies to some foods diminish or disappear by the first or second birthday, while allergies to other foods are likely to persist into adulthood.

Food intolerances and food sensitivities are not food allergies and do not involve the immune system. Symptoms of these conditions may vary from stomach or head pain to respiratory distress. When infants and children cannot tolerate formula because of allergies or intolerances, there are alternative formula preparations available to provide the required calories and nutrients.

Harmful Influences during the Beginning of Life

The use of any drug including nicotine, alcohol, herbal, over-the-counter, and prescription presents the possibility of serious problems for the fetus and later, for the infant. Smoking for example interferes with the normal development and functioning of the placenta and makes it less efficient in nourishing the fetus and in waste removal. The babies of breast-feeding mothers who smoke compromise the protection from **sudden infant death syndrome (SIDS)** that is provided in breast milk.[21]

The U.S. Surgeon General recommends abstention from alcohol during pregnancy because it can cause permanent mental and physical problems in a child. Even if a woman stops drinking alcohol during pregnancy, her baby may have a low birth weight because of the effects of the alcohol previously consumed on her nutritional status. High alcohol consumption may decrease appetite, reduce food intake, and use valuable nutrients as the body metabolizes the alcohol. Fetal Alcohol Syndrome is a term used to describe a variety of permanent mental and physical abnormalities found in infants of women with high alcohol intake. These abnormalities would not have occurred if the mother had not consumed alcohol.[22]

Cocaine use during pregnancy can lead to life-long learning problems for the children of mothers who use this drug. A reduced ability to concentrate and limitations in attention span are examples of these effects. The amount of cocaine that a mother uses during pregnancy determines the extent of a child's difficulties.[23, 24] In a study of more than 11,000 women, the use of drugs during pregnancy was found to cause emotional problems in children.[25]

Herbs and herbal preparations are included in substances that should be avoided without medical approval. Some of the herbal preparations that have been identified as potentially harmful during pregnancy are listed in Table 10.9. Since there is concern about testing any drug on pregnant women, many herbals have not been investigated, and women should consult with their medical care-givers about the effects of these substances before assuming that they are safe. The intake of herbal teas should be limited to two cups per day, using filtered teabags.[26]

TABLE 10.9 Some Potentially Harmful Herbals for Pregnant Women	
Aloe vera	Anise
Black or blue cohosh	Borage
Comfrey	Dandelion leaf
Ephedra, Ma Huang	Feverfew
Ginkgo	Ginseng
Juniper	Kava
Raspberry leaf	Saw palmetto

Source: Belew, C. Herbs and the childbearing woman. Guidelines for midwives. *J Nurse Midwifery* 1999; 44:231–52. Reprinted with permission.

Childhood

Childhood (the period between the first and the eleventh birthday) is a time of steady physical and mental development that occurs at a slower rate than the growth that takes place in the first year of life. By the end of the first year, a child's growth rate slows. It should then progress consistently, with most children growing 5 inches between the ages of 1 and 2 years old. After age 2, height increases should be approximately 2 1/2 inches per year, and weight gains should be 5–6 pounds per year until adolescence is reached. Health professionals monitor a child's weight throughout childhood and consider it an important indicator of nutritional status. As muscles grow stronger and bones lengthen, physical skills increase and allow children to participate in increasingly active play and in sports activities.

Energy Needs and Leading Nutrients

From a basic need of approximately 1,000 calories at the age of one, the energy requirement of a child increases by about 100 calories per year (a three-year-old would need about 1,300 calories).

The USDA provides recommendations for energy for young children based on age and activity level on their ChooseMyPlate.gov website. (see Table 10.10)

Because of their ongoing growth, children's protein needs increase from about 16 grams per day for one- to three-year-olds to about 28 grams per day for seven- to eleven-year-olds. Growth needs are best met when complete protein is provided daily. Children can make up for periods of poor nutrition if adequate diets are subsequently provided and if severe deficiencies did not exist in early development.

Vitamin and mineral requirements increase with body size and most can be met with a well-planned diet. The need for fluoride supplements occurs when the local water supply is not fluoridated, and an iron supplement is sometimes necessary when a diet consistently provides less than 10 mg of iron/day. Servings shown in the USDA ChooseMyPlate for children ages 6–11, are presented in age-appropriate servings, and provide a basic plan for healthy eating for young children.

Calorie and nutrient recommendations for children are organized by age groups or school grade levels. The amount of food recommended varies with each age group and serving sizes increase proportionately. The USDA ChooseMyPlate.gov website can be used to determine recommended meal patterns for children. Detailed information on age-related development, food behaviors. and promotion of healthy food habits is also included. [27]

In addition, Table 10.11 presents a guide for planning meals and snacks for preschool and elementary school age children based on the feeding patterns of prescribed school lunch - programs. These guidelines include serving sizes that vary for different preschool age groups, and for elementary school grade-level students. These recommendations were developed by the U.S. Department of Agriculture for use in school feeding settings and can also be used as a guide for parents to plan balanced meals at home. The USDA website includes comprehensive information on school nutrition guidelines and new initiatives.[28]

Since a child may receive one-third of his/her daily nutrient intake during the school day, the type of food served in school is of great significance. As you consider the guidelines in Table 10.8, use your culinary knowledge and skills to imagine how you could plan creative and taste-pleasing menu items that achieve these standards. Parental concerns about the quality of food served to children at school make culinary nutritionists in educational settings especially desirable.

TABLE 10.10 Estimate of Energy Needs for Preschool Children

Boys				Girls			
Physical Activity Age	Less than 30 minutes a day	30 to 60 minutes a day	More than 60 minutes a day	Physical Activity Age	Less than 30 minutes a day	30 to 60 minutes a day	More than 60 minutes a day
2	1000	1000	1000	2	1000	1000	1000
3	1200	1400	1400	3	1000	1200	1400
4	1200	1400	1600	4	1200	1400	1400
5	1200	1400	1600	5	1200	1400	1600

TABLE 10.11 Guide for Meal Plans for Children School Lunch Patterns for Different Ages				
Food Group	Preschool (Grade)		Grade School	
	1–2	3–4	K–3	4–6
Meat or meat alternate				
1 serving:				
Lean meat, poultry, or fish	1 oz.	1 ½ oz.	1 ½ oz.	2 oz.
Cheese	1 oz.	1 ½ oz.	1 ½ oz.	oz.
Large egg(s)	½	¾	¾	1
Cooked dry beans or peas	¼ cup	³/₈ cup	³/₈ cup	½ cup
Peanut butter	2 tbsp	3 tbsp	3 tbsp	4 tbsp
Vegetable and/or fruit				
2 or more servings, both to total	½ cup	½ cup	½ cup	¾ cup
Bread or bread alternate				
Servings	5 per week	8 per week	8 per week	8 per week
Milk				
1 serving of fluid milk	¾ cup	¾ cup	1 cup	1 cup

Source: U.S. Department of Agriculture, 2000.

School Lunch Programs

As a result of concerns about childhood obesity, changes are occurring concerning the quality of foods served in the school food lunch program, as is the availability of competitive foods (foods from vending machines and other commercially prepared foods sold in school stores and at snack bars). Legislation passed by the U.S. Congress in 2004 mandated that school districts participating in the National School Lunch Program are required to have school wellness policies for nutrition education, physical activity opportunities, and other health-fostering activities.[29] Some districts have assembled Wellness Councils for each school district made up of members that include parents, teachers, administrators, and interested community members. Many registered dietitians volunteer to serve on these Councils. Chef volunteers can also help to advocate for and advise on the preparation of healthy, good-tasting foods.

Other organizations are also working to improve the nutritional and "taste" quality of foods in schools. Lists of approved products are available throughout the country. The Rhode Island Kids First organization, for example, developed product standards and has developed a list of 1,000 approved products in support of the Rhode Island State Wellness Policy Initiative. Individual states have also passed legislation concerning nutritional standards for the competitive foods offered. These apply to foods and beverages that are sold in schools but are not part of the school lunch program meals. Foods previously sold, that were high in sugar and processed carbohydrate content, have been eliminated. A study by the National Center for Education Statistics—Calories In, Calories Out has determined that 23% of public elementary schools offered such foods on school property and depended upon them to gain revenue for the schools.[30] Partnerships had been formed and product advertisements appeared throughout the entire school district on school buses and in sports stadiums. School administrators in cities around the country adopted such agreements to supplement school budgets, seemingly without regard for the nutritional significance of their decisions.[31]

Two newer initiatives that will positively impact the quality of foods available to schoolchildren include: *The Healthy, Hunger-Free Kids Act of 2010* and the *"Chefs Move to Schools"* program. *The Healthy, Hunger-Free Kids Act of 2010* mandates increased funding for school lunch meals, the elimination of unhealthy competitive foods in schools, the provision of water (at no cost to the student) at meals, and the improvement of the nutritional quality of foods in schools. Managers of school food programs will also be required to meet specific training standards.[32]

"Chefs Move to Schools," is being promoted by the First Lady, Michelle Obama. This USDA-run program partners chefs and culinary student volunteers with schools that would like to improve the quality of the foods offered to students.[33]

Food Behaviors

A child's appetite may vary dramatically from day to day. Offering snacks is a valuable way to meet nutrient needs since children benefit from eating more frequently than do adults. Parents should not confuse snacks with "treats." Snacks often consist of potato chips, soda, sweets and other empty-calorie foods.

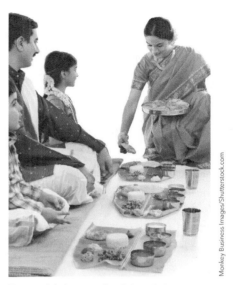

Even with busy schedules, it is valuable for parents to establish nutritionally sound food behaviors for the family at mealtimes.

These foods do not contain nutrients such as protein, iron, calcium, or fiber, which support growth, development, and health. Such foods should be "once in a while treats" rather than a regular part of the diet.

Parents are advised to respect a child's wish to vary food intake and to minimize the availability of competitive foods, rather than attempting to control the amount of food consumed. This approach avoids interference with natural satiety signals that can cause the child to develop the undesirable habit of overeating.[34] Attempts at controlling the intake of children, may lead to higher levels of body fat in children.[35]

During early childhood, parents have a "once in a lifetime" opportunity to strongly influence the type of food presented to the child and to shape food habits in a way that makes eating both nutritious and enjoyable. Respecting a child's food choices can improve the quality of home life by preventing power struggles and can have a positive effect on food experiences. Involving children in age-appropriate food preparation activities is another wise strategy to encourage children to try new foods and to develop healthy food attitudes and habits. As children move through childhood, they become more independent of parental influence and begin to separate psychologically, learning to strongly express personal desires and preferences.[36] Later, when the influences of friends and others outside the home are greater, food choices may consist mainly of fast food and snack choices, rather than of nutrient-rich, unprocessed foods.

Since current lifestyles often offer increased time limitations in the home—due to the busy schedules of both parents and children—less time is spent preparing food, and more food is consumed outside the home. This pattern can also interfere with the opportunity parents have to establish pleasurable and nutritionally sound food behaviors. A study of middle school children found that children who ate breakfast outside the home consumed more calories, fat, added sugars, and sugar-sweetened beverages than those who did not. In addition, fast food eaters ate fewer fruit, milk, and non-starchy vegetable servings.[37] With some knowledge of culinary nutrition, parents can provide healthy, delicious snacks and meals for children.

Health Concerns

There are several concerns related to the nutritional health of children. These include childhood obesity with the risk of early chronic disease, malnutrition due to lack of food or to poor food choices, low calcium and Vitamin D intake leading to inadequate mineralization of bones, and dental caries. All of these problems can damage children's physical and/or psychological health.

Childhood Obesity

Health professionals and government officials have recognized a growing problem of excessive weight gain during childhood that has resulted in a steadily increasing number of children who are overweight or obese (1 child in every 5).[38] This increase in weight is an alarming indicator that these children will experience the health problems that would have only affected parents and grandparents in past generations. Such health risks are related to the increased demands that excess weight places on a child's metabolism. For example, a greater amount of insulin is required to metabolize increased amounts of carbohydrate in high-calorie meals and snacks, and this in turn causes stress to the pancreas. High insulin levels can also change the biochemistry of the body and reduce controls for monitoring eating and for pursuing physical activity.[39]

Pediatricians, who care for the increasing number of overweight and obese children, are finding that these young people often have high blood pressure and high blood cholesterol levels as well as fatty livers. Some are even developing chronic diseases such as diabetes and cardiovascular disease, and are at risk for complications from these diseases for much longer periods than are adults who develop these medical problems later in life.[40]

Both parents and public health officials are attempting to identify and change the influences causing weight problems by using weight control management techniques. Medical and community organizations are now focusing on both the excessive caloric intakes and the low physical activity levels of overweight children. In addition to the physical results of high weight levels, overweight children often suffer psychological distress from social isolation and rejection by peers.

Children should not diet restrictively because they need energy to grow. Programs to assist children and parents in establishing good eating habits, and in finding enjoyable play activities that increase activity levels and replace long hours of television viewing, are important. Public service messages concerning behavioral changes should be directed towards parents because they purchase foods, set household schedules, monitor TV viewing and provide opportunities for physical activity. Weight control goals should include gradual weight gain and weight maintenance as growth occurs. Researchers have found that children are likely to be overweight if their parents are heavy and that their risk of having weight problems in adulthood doubles. A recent study indicates that children who consume high-sugar, low nutrient-density foods at a very young age have an increased risk for being overweight and obese. Young children, 2 1/2, 3 1/2, 4 1/2, and 5 years of age, who regularly consume sugar-sweetened beverages have 3 times the risk of being overweight at 4 1/2 years old as children who do not consume such beverages.[41]

Malnutrition

A child's ability to focus in school and to learn is decreased significantly if that child is hungry. Malnutrition related to a lack of key nutrients, such as iron, can reduce attention span and affect mood and behavior negatively. In addition to affecting healthy blood cell function, iron is needed in the normal activity of several substances that are required for a well-functioning brain and nervous system. Children with learning difficulties may be helped through a regular intake of adequate amounts of iron-rich foods or iron supplements. Early deprivation of iron in an infant may cause long-term childhood difficulties. Foods, such as lean meats, beans, whole-wheat bread with peanut butter, fortified breakfast cereals, and even canned spaghetti with meatballs can be rich sources of iron.

Hyperactivity

The medical condition **attention-deficit hyperactivity disorder (ADHD)** is often referred to as hyperactivity. This problem affects up to 10% of children and interferes with learning. A short attention span and several behavioral characteristics, such as restlessness and excessive activity, are associated with this condition. ADHD often leads to inappropriate behaviors that negatively affect relationships and adult interactions. According to recent studies, patients with ADHD have a more limited capacity in the various compartments of the brain. It is suggested that either factors affecting the development of the brain or genetics may be responsible for the condition and that the effects appear to be permanent.[42]

While parents, educators, and even some health professionals have linked ADHD to the consumption of particular foods, and special diets have been devised to treat the problem, there is no conclusive evidence to endorse diet as the sole approach to successful treatment for the majority of children with ADHD. One research study has shown improvements in ADHD symptoms with the use of a very restrictive diet, although not all experts agree with the results of the research.[43] Poor food choices, especially those high in sugar, caffeine, or certain additives, along with irregular eating schedules may leave a child hungry and fatigued and exaggerate the symptoms of ADHD. Simple strategies to organize the child's schedule and to provide a regular, balanced food intake may provide the best environment for improvement. Planning meals and snacks containing both carbohydrates and proteins and offering them on a consistent schedule may provide valuable support. Controlling television viewing and encouraging outside play may also help to establish a regular sleep pattern.

Autism Spectrum Disorder

Another condition for which a special diet is often suggested is autism spectrum disorder (ASD). Today, autism spectrum disorder is more frequently diagnosed. The condition is considered to be a spectrum disorder because the severity of symptoms ranges from mild, to moderate to severe. A popular, but unproven diet therapy among parents of children with autism is the gluten-free, casein-free diet. This diet excludes two dietary staple foods; wheat and milk, and any products made from these foods. The theory behind the diet is that some protein particles in these foods are not completely digested and they pass into the bloodstream, and then travel to the brain. Some individuals believe that long-term exposure to these protein fragments is thought to affect the maturing brain and to contribute to social awkwardness and behavioral issues that interfere with learning and relationships. The diet is restrictive and very difficult to follow, however, many parents consider it to be beneficial for their children. The role of the health professional should be a supportive one helping parents provide adequate calories and nutrients in spite of diet restrictions. Children with ASD may be poorly nourished even if they are not on a special diet because they can be very selective about the foods they will or will not eat; and they can be particularly choosy about food textures.[44, 45]

Dental Health

Avoiding high-sugar foods can improve dental health in children. The consumption of sweet, sticky foods encourages the growth of acid-producing bacteria that cause dental caries.[46] Frequent snacking can increase dental caries as well. Appropriate snacks such as fresh fruits, fresh and cooked vegetables, dairy products, and other protein foods promote good dental health and add nutrient density to children's diets. Crisp foods, such as popcorn, pretzels, toast, and foods high in fiber help to stimulate the production of saliva that helps to remove bacteria from the teeth. When sugar-starch containing foods such as cakes, cookies, and other soft, sticky foods are eaten, acid may be produced for more than an hour. Parents can help their children by regularly supervising their consumption of foods and by issuing a "tooth brushing reminder."[47]

Adolescence

The period of adolescence is a time of growth and development when an individual strives to create a new life, until reaching full maturity. Tremendous growth and other physical changes create a high need for nutrients. Social and psychological changes that are also taking place can make nutrient needs a low priority for these young adults. The growth spurt of adolescence is controlled by hormones and usually lasts about 2 1/2 years. Linear growth, the increase in height, occurs rapidly. Boys gain about 8 inches in height and about 45 pounds in weight, while girls grow about 6 inches and gain approximately 35 pounds. Individual teens may grow more or less in height and gain more or less weight depending upon factors such as the genetic pattern of the family, food intake, and their level of physical activity.

Energy Needs and Leading Nutrients

During adolescence, energy and nutrient needs are determined by body size and gender. Female hormones prepare girls for the possibility of future motherhood from the time menstruation begins. Female body fat increases and the shape of the body becomes more feminine. Boys gain more muscle due to the effect of male hormones. This change in body composition is reflected in significantly higher caloric intake needs. Between 11 and 18 years of age, adolescent girls need about 2,200 calories each day while teenage boys often require 2,500 to 3,000 calories. The lower energy need of teenage girls is due to a smaller body size and to the lesser number of calories needed to maintain body fat.

Due to a high growth rate during the teen years, all adolescents have special needs for iron and calcium. As a child's body grows, more iron is required to support the increased blood supply. This important nutrient is used to manufacture hemoglobin and additional blood cells as well as to increase myoglobin (a protein that carries and holds oxygen in muscle). When menstruation begins, girls also lose iron during their monthly cycle.

The need for calcium is critical in adolescence because that is when the highest rate of bone development occurs. The rate of absorption of calcium is at its peak because vitamin D is activated more efficiently than at any other time in the lifespan. Many adolescents, particularly girls, have been found to be deficient in vitamin D. If they do not consume foods rich in vitamin D, such as fortified milk or soy milk, they will need to take supplements so that their blood levels of vitamin D are sufficient to help promote calcium absorption from the diet. If teens do not take this opportunity to build bone, they may have low bone density levels and increase their risk of osteoporosis later in life. An extra serving of milk or other dairy product is recommended during adolescent years, increasing the daily servings to three. Table 10.12 illustrates the serving sizes and the number of servings for one meal based on the food pattern created by the United States Department of Agriculture for school lunch guidelines. This pattern also serves as a guide for planning two other meals and snacks to meet an individual's nutritional needs.

TABLE 10.12 Guide for Lunch Meal Plans for Teens	
School Lunch Patterns	
Food Group	High School (Grade)
	7–12
Meat or meat alternate	
1 serving:	
Lean meat, poultry, or fish	3 oz.
Cheese	3 oz.
Large egg(s)	1 ½
Cooked dry beans or peas	¾ cup
Peanut butter	6 tbsp
Vegetable and/or fruit	¾ cup
2 or more servings, both to total	10 per week
Bread or bread alternate	
Servings	1 cup
Milk	
1 serving of fluid milk	

Source: U.S. Department of Agriculture, 2000.

Food Behaviors

Teens want to eat what their friends enjoy, in addition to choosing foods with which they are familiar and that they enjoy. The appeal of the food at the moment is usually of greater interest to teens than the long-term effects of diet on health. Since teens are in the process of becoming more independent of parental influence, they may use food to assert a separate identity by eating what they choose. Parents are wise to create a family food experience that allows teens the freedom to make selections from a nutritionally sound and enjoyable assortment of foods. Research shows that family meals improve the nutritional quality of the diet even through the teen years. A food guide pyramid-based plan of popular foods, such as smoothies and wraps, can be valuable in helping teens eat well.

Medical Concerns

Obesity

As with children, the rate of overweight and obese teens is escalating and is raising concerns about the future health profiles of these young people. More than 20% of teens are overweight and at risk for type 2 diabetes, fatty liver, high blood pressure, and high blood cholesterol levels.[48] Being overweight can also cause social and psychological problems for teens at a time when they want and need to be accepted by their peers. Teen girls who attempt to lose weight are likely to restrict food intake and may begin a lifetime of dieting and discomfort with food. Boys attempting to reduce body weight are more apt to increase physical activity. Since discomfort with food and body image sets the stage for eating disorders that can damage the lives of teens and their family members, weight control initiatives for teens should emphasize fitness and health, rather than restrictive weight loss diets. Because of rising obesity rates, surgery is sometimes performed on obese adolescents so that their stomachs have a limited capacity to hold foods and are able to consume only small amounts of food. This is not an ideal solution and the teens must take multiple nutritional supplements for the long-term.

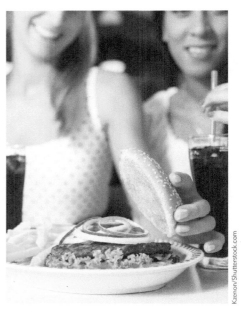

The appeal of the food at the moment is usually of greater interest to teens than the long-term effects of diet on health.

Acne

Acne, a serious problem for some teens, may be caused by a variety of factors including heredity and hormones. Although chocolate, fatty foods and colas are also suspected as acne-causing culprits, there are no definitive conclusions to support these claims. Medications that include vitamin A derivatives, such as Retin-A, are sometimes prescribed to aid this condition. Retin-A causes the skin to redden, to become tender, and then to peel to a healthier level of skin. Accutane is another medication that may be prescribed to inhibit the sebaceous glands (the glands that produce the skin's natural oil). Accutane may cause birth defects and young women must have a negative pregnancy test result before receiving a prescription for this drug.

Harmful Influences: Smoking, Alcohol, and Cocaine

Teens may use various forms of drugs that cause nutritional problems, as well as other consequences. Smoking, for example, has negative nutritional effects because it decreases hunger and reduces food intake. Lower intakes of fiber, vitamins A and C, folate, and beta-carotene have been found among smokers. This is especially significant in the case of inadequate vitamin C. Smokers need 90% more of this nutrient because they metabolize it at a high rate. A vitamin C deficiency in teens who smoke can also interfere with the vitamin E and the iron status because vitamin C is critical to the normal metabolism of these important nutrients. Low levels of vitamin A and beta-carotene, from an inadequate intake, may also increase the risk of lung cancer in smokers. Marijuana smoking may promote the consumption of foods that are high in sugar and salt, and low in valuable nutrients.

Alcohol provides calories, with no nutrients, and it interferes with the absorption and metabolism of several nutrients as it is rapidly absorbed and then detoxified in the liver. In addition, alcohol interferes with an enzyme that maintains blood sugar levels and can lead to low blood sugar levels, even in those without diabetes. Serious nutritional consequences are also related to cocaine abuse. The craving for this drug gradually overcomes natural hunger controls that lead to malnutrition.

Adult Stages

Adulthood

During **adulthood**, from age 20 until the end of life, sound nutritional choices remain critical for good health. Problems at this stage of life often result from past decisions that led to excess weight and related risk factors. Diets that provide a nutrient-dense variety of food choices are valuable in maintaining the body from early adulthood to old age (a period when the structure and the function of the body gradually changes and declines). In addition to a good diet, successful management of the progression of aging requires an ongoing commitment to regular physical activity.

Energy Needs and Leading Nutrients

Men continue to need more energy per kilogram during adulthood than do women, because of the larger amount of lean body mass in their bodies. However, the RDAs for energy for both men and women decrease for those aged 50 and older, because of a natural loss of muscle/lean body mass and an increase in body fat in people as they age. It is estimated that lean body mass is lost at a rate of approximately 2%–3% and that basal metabolic rate decreases by about 5% per decade, by middle adulthood. Yet, adults still need to meet nutrient needs that are similar to those of younger people who have higher calorie needs. Nutrient-dense food choices are more important than ever at this time. The national nutrition guidelines offer practical, easy-to-follow strategies that are valuable for those in middle and late adulthood.[49] A focus on appropriate serving sizes, such as those recommended in the USDA ChooseMyPlate food groups, is also important because portion sizes commonly served have increased significantly since the 1970s. Even the number of servings is reduced for recipes in a revised edition of the *Joy of Cooking* reflecting larger individual portion sizes.[50]

According to recent research, attention to the forms of carbohydrate and fat in the diet can be especially important for mid-life adults with decreasing caloric requirements and a need to control body weight. Carbohydrates that raise blood sugar at a moderate or slow rate are recommended to increase satiety and to delay the return of hunger, with the goal of reducing total calorie intake. These foods are also wise choices because many of them (whole-grain cereals, breads, fruits, and vegetables) are higher in fiber, low in saturated fat, known to be harmful to heart health.[51, 52] Moderate amounts of foods with "good fats" (those high in monounsaturated fat and omega-3 fatty acids) are recommended to replace saturated fat. Olives, olive oil, peanut butter, and nuts are foods that can be highlighted in heart-healthy menus to provide monounsaturated fat. "Oily fish," such as salmon, sardines, mackerel, and bluefish are sources of omega-3s, the "good fats," that also provide appetite control.[53]

Throughout adulthood, iron, calcium, and Vitamin D continue to be leading nutrients. Iron intake from food or from a supplement is especially important for women while they continue to menstruate. In older adults, iron deficiency is likely to occur if a poor diet is consumed or if a disease or physical problem interferes with the

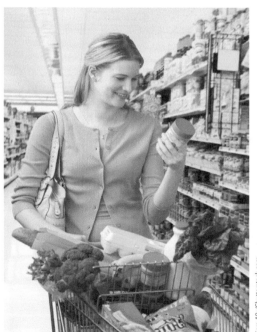

During adulthood, sound nutritional choices remain critical for good health.

body's use of iron. Calcium and Vitamin D are needed during early adulthood to continue building the maximum amount of bone possible since no additional calcium is added to bones after ages 30–35. In later years, calcium and vitamin D are recommended to prevent a rapid loss of bone.

How the Body Uses Nutrients

Adults who desire long-term weight control and the reduction of risk factors related to excess weight may benefit from carbohydrate foods that raise blood sugar more slowly, because they trigger a more gradual release of insulin. Glycemic index (GI) ratings have been assigned to foods according to the speed at which they raise the blood sugar level. Foods that increase blood sugar more slowly have moderate (56–70) or low (55 or less) ratings, while beans and phytochemical-rich whole grains, fruits, and vegetables, with lower caloric content and high nutrient density, have moderate GI levels. These foods do not raise blood sugar quickly, and the amount of insulin produced in response to the carbohydrate in them is also moderate, so the blood sugar level is decreased gradually. A decrease in blood sugar can increase satiety and delay the return of hunger, resulting in the consumption of fewer total calories, allowing for weight control.

High GI foods, however, can stimulate hunger because they raise blood sugar quickly and trigger a high insulin response that makes the blood sugar level fall quickly. This can be followed by a rapid return of the urge to eat and the likelihood that a greater number of calories will be consumed. These added calories are then efficiently stored as fat, because insulin also stimulates fat storage. The higher blood sugar and insulin levels triggered by high GI foods can also lead to overwork for the pancreas, poor blood sugar control, and an excessive deposit of fat in the arteries, which are risk factors for both diabetes and heart disease.[54]

Several factors in food can increase or decrease the glycemic index. These factors include: the cooking and processing methods, the physical form of the food, and the amounts of starch, soluble fiber, and sugar they contain. Cooking and processing changes the form of starch in foods such as popcorn, rice cakes, and corn flakes. This makes the food molecules more accessible to enzymes and leads to a more rapid rise in blood sugar levels (a higher GI). In addition to the glycemic index number, the amount of carbohydrates in the total serving is a factor in determining choices that will prevent rapid increases in blood sugar. Although carrots have a high glycemic index, for example, it is unlikely that a person would consume a large enough portion of carrots to cause blood sugar to surge to a high level.

Culinary nutrition professionals can provide recipes that include ingredients consisting of the more desirable carbohydrates that do not result in a rapid insulin response. Table 10.13 provides a "shopping list" for moderate and low GI foods to consider when planning menu items for those in middle adulthood.

In addition to careful decisions about the quality of carbohydrates in the diet, it is wise to choose fats that help to lower the risk of heart disease. Foods high in monounsaturated fat can lower bad cholesterol (LDLs) and raise good

TABLE 10.13 Examples of Foods with Moderate and Low Glycemic Index	
Moderate Glycemic Index (55–70)	Low Glycemic Index (55 or Less)
Quick oats	Old fashioned oats
Pita bread	All Bran™
Basmati rice	Grapenuts™
Bran Buds™	Special K™
Life cereal™	Apples
Rye bread	Pears
Raisins	Bananas
Pizza	Citrus fruits
Multi-Bran Chex™	Peaches
Gnocchi pasta	Plums
Mango	Legumes
Papaya	Most pasta
Fresh pineapple	Converted rice

Moderate Glycemic Index (55–70)	Low Glycemic Index (55 or Less)
Light microwave popcorn	Sweet potatoes or yams
Arborio risotto rice	Pearl barley
Whole-wheat bread	100% Stoneground wheat bread
Bean soups	Milk and yogurts

Source: Adapted from Brand-Miller, J., Foster-Powell, K., Wolverton, TMS. *The Glucose Revolution.* 1999. Marlowe and Company, NY.

cholesterol (HDLs). Omega-3 fatty acids are also important to heart health in adulthood, since this type of fat seems to reduce inflammation in the arteries and is said to decrease the tendency of blood to form clots. Recent studies have also found that sudden death from coronary heart disease is reduced in subjects consuming this type of fat on a regular basis.[55]

Attention to iron-rich foods continues to be important in adulthood for several reasons. Young women with regular menstrual periods have to balance monthly iron losses due to menstruation with a regular consumption of high-iron foods. Young adult women using oral contraceptives do not have such losses because iron is conserved when monthly periods are suppressed. At mid-life, iron deficiency is not a major concern after menopause (the end of the menstrual cycle), so the RDA for iron is lower for women 51 and older.

Older adults may have medical conditions that interfere with iron absorption. The functioning of the gastro-intestinal tract is less efficient in older individuals and iron absorption is decreased because less stomach acid is produced. A reduction in acid levels also puts older adults at risk for vitamin B_{12} deficiency. Even if they consume sources of animal products, older adults may require B_{12} injections.

Calcium is especially important in early adulthood, up until about age 30, to achieve peak bone mass. Even though the rate of increase in bone density is lower during the 20s than it is during adolescence, bone mass continues to increase until a maximum density is reached at about age 30. Sometime between the age of 30 and 40, a loss of bone density begins and this process continues throughout life. In later years, calcium's role is to help decrease the rate of bone loss as hormone levels change; particularly in women. Screening guidelines by the U.S. Preventive Services Task Force for osteoporosis recommend that women age 65 or older, age 60–64 who have been identified with risks such as low body weight, and women who do not use estrogen replacement therapy after menopause, undergo bone density testing.[56]

Another factor related to bone density during mid to late adulthood is the decreased ability of the skin to activate vitamin D. This negative influence on bone density prevents the body from absorbing calcium well. The RDA for vitamin D for those over 50 years of age has been increased to levels twice that of younger individuals. For those over 70, the recommendation for vitamin D is tripled. In a 3-year study, supplementation with 500 milligrams of calcium and 700 IUs of vitamin D resulted in less bone loss and fewer bone fractures.[57]

Diets high in protein and sodium accelerate bone loss by interfering with the absorption of calcium and by increasing the loss of this important mineral. Drug use can also increase calcium loss. Smoking, for example, can decrease bone density by 5%–10% below normal levels even before menopause, which is the time of greatest bone loss in women.

A diet rich in the phytochemicals found in plant foods can be especially valuable in maintaining good health in middle adulthood. By this stage of the lifespan, the cells of the body may have been damaged by the accumulation of substances called free radicals (unstable atoms or molecules that have 1 or more missing electrons). Antioxidants protect cell tissue and provide the needed electrons for free radicals to stop their damaging effects. These effects can interfere with the function of important organ systems and lead to serious diseases, such as type 2 diabetes, heart disease, and various cancers. Vitamins A, C, and E-containing foods, and many components of plant foods, have beneficial antioxidant effects on the body. Antioxidant supplements don't have the same health benefits as foods containing antioxidants.[58]

Food Behaviors

Social contact in adulthood continues to be as important an influence on dietary choices as it is during the other stages of the lifespan. Busy young adults may have limited time and money available for planning and purchasing food for a healthy diet. This can lead to an inadequate intake of nutrients that may set the stage for the chronic diseases in later years. Many young adults have grown up in homes where there was little food preparation. These young people may benefit from guidance at every step including how to prepare a grocery list, how to outfit the kitchen, how to choose recipes, and ultimately learning cooking techniques for preparing food. Culinary professionals can be key allies for good health by providing young people with tips on eating well in ways that are both economical and less time consuming.

At mid-life, economic success may make restaurant eating and food-oriented social events major recreational activities. Dining out frequently can contribute to excess weight gain and even obesity. Related increases in high blood pressure, cholesterol, and blood sugar may lead to health complications. Individuals at this stage of the lifespan will benefit from the skill of culinary experts who develop restaurant and event menus that include delicious and nutritionally rich choices. Menus based on the Mediterranean Diet can be "lifesavers." The monounsaturated fat, high fruit and vegetable intake, and low level of processed carbohydrates in such a plan can help to reduce high blood cholesterol, high blood sugar, and high blood pressure.

Lifestyle and Obesity

It is estimated that 50% of deaths in adulthood are related to lifestyle choices that include poor dietary habits, a lack of regular exercise, smoking, and the use of alcohol or other drugs. Diets high in fat and calories increase the risk for serious chronic diseases that are often diagnosed during middle adulthood. Risk factors for chronic disease reflect an individual's lifestyle, family history, and health status. Many lifestyle risk factors can be improved, even at mid-life, with a health-conscious diet. Excessive calories, high saturated fat and sodium intake and low fiber levels in the diet are all associated with atherosclerosis, hypertension, and type 2 diabetes. Adults must understand that a combination of several risk factors results in a greater total risk.

A healthy body weight is an important factor in health maintenance. Health professionals are showing great concern about the current levels of overweight and obese Americans, which is reported to be more than 60%. Death rates in adults are higher among those carrying extra weight, especially those with central obesity. This form of obesity increases the risks of cardiovascular disease, type 2 diabetes, and cancer. Central obesity is more common in men than in women and in smokers than in non-smokers.[59] Excess weight also increases pressure on the joints causing *osteoarthritis* (a disease with painful joint swelling). Achieving "ideal" body weight is desirable but just weight loss of 5%–10% of body weight can result in significant improvements in blood glucose, blood pressure and HDL. cholesterol.

Physical Activity

To counteract the effects of the aging process on body composition, and to avoid obesity, adults are advised to exercise. Exercise can minimize the loss of muscle, increase lean body mass, and raise caloric output. A commitment to regular aerobic activity and strength training cannot totally reverse the natural body composition changes caused by aging, but it can minimize the loss of lean body mass and help to limit weight gain. An aerobic exercise plan appropriate to an individual's fitness level can assist in burning body fat by changing the hormone balance in the body so that fat is broken down more easily. Exercise has been found to be valuable in preventing, as well as in controlling, type 2 diabetes and heart disease.[60] In a recent study, increased physical activity in daily living was found to help maintain weight control even in sedentary women.[61]

Older Adults

Regular physical activity has been identified as the most powerful influence on the ability of older adults to move about easily in later years.[62] The risk of falling and the chance of injury from falls are also reduced in more active older adults who have greater muscle strength. Weight training has been found to counteract the natural loss of bone in some individuals who exercise 2 or 3 days per week.[63, 64] Until recently, strength training was considered the only option for combating the effects of aging on muscle. However, new research shows that provision for adequate protein in the diet of older adults also helps build muscle. It is thought that the RDA for protein might need to be increased for older adults.[65]

Many older adults consume inadequate amounts of protein and other nutrients. Some older adults fall into dietary habits of convenience that some experts call "The Tea and Toast Syndrome." Many older adults live on their own, don't feel like preparing meals, and gradually narrow their foods down to those that are the most simple to prepare at the expense of vital nutrients and health. Older adults frequently have lost their teeth, and may have poorly fitting dentures that make it difficult for them to chew. These limitations further limit food selection.

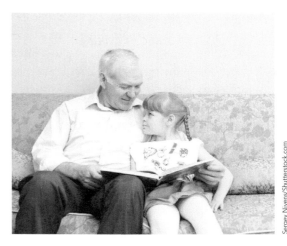

Contacts with children and grandchildren can be critical for seniors in maintaining a healthy diet and eating pattern.

During old age, nutrient-related changes can affect nutritional health in important ways. These changes, as seen in Table 10.14, are due to physical limitations that affect how the older body uses nutrients in food. The loss of muscle

TABLE 10.14 Nutrient-related Changes in Aging

Nutrient	Nutrient Changes in Aging	Related Issues
Water	Lack of thirst and decreased total body water make dehydration likely	Mild dehydration is a common cause of confusion. Difficulty obtaining water or getting to the bathroom adds to the problem.
Energy	Needs decrease	Physical activity moderates need for fewer calories.
Fiber	Likelihood of constipation increases with low intakes and changes in GI tract.	Inadequate water intakes and lack of physical activity, along with some medications, compound the problem.
Protein	Needs stay the same.	Low-fat, high-fiber legumes and grains can meet both protein and other nutrient needs
Vitamin A	Absorption increases	RDA may be high.
Vitamin D	Increased likelihood of inadequate intake; skin synthesis declines.	Daily limited sunlight exposure may be of benefit. DRI increased after age 70.
Vitamin B_{12}	Poor absorption due to decreased stomach acid	Injections of B_{12} are often necessary
Iron	In women, status improves after menopause; deficiencies are linked to chronic blood losses and low stomach acid output.	Adequate stomach acid is required for absorption; antacid or other medicine use may aggravate iron deficiency; vitamin C and meat increase absorption.
Zinc	Intakes may be low and absorption reduced; but needs may also decrease.	Medications interfere with absorption; deficiency may depress appetite and sense of taste.
Calcium	Intakes may be low; osteoporosis common.	Intake of other beverages commonly limits milk intake; calcium and vitamin D substitutes are needed.

function in the intestines, for example, may lead to discomfort from constipation and cause a lower rate of nutrient absorption as well as a limited interest in eating. Smoking and alcohol intake decreases the levels of some of the water-soluble vitamins. Smoking, for example, increases a need for vitamin C by 90%, while alcohol decreases folate levels which can increase the risk of colon cancer and heart disease.

At this stage, social contact is also likely to be sharply decreased due to the death of spouses, relatives, and friends. Older people who eat alone for the first time often lose interest in eating and increase their chances of malnutrition. Contacts with children and grandchildren can be helpful for seniors in maintaining a healthy diet and eating pattern.

Culinary Corner

The Bonus of Culinary Nutrition: Eating Well at Any Age

The ability to help individuals from pre-pregnancy to old age, to plan diets for the best possible nutritional intake, is a challenge. Valuable food assistance is provided by government agencies for targeted groups within the lifespan to make adequate energy and nutrients available. Pregnant and breastfeeding women and children up through age 5 are eligible for the **WIC program**, the Special Supplemental Food Program for Women, Infants, and Children (WIC). This U.S. government program provides education, nutrient-rich foods, and infant formula to clients through food vouchers. School feeding programs offer breakfast, lunch and after-school meals and snacks for children meeting low income requirements. Government funding assists older people at low-income levels by supporting group meals in community settings and by providing them access to Electronic Benefit Transfer (EBT) Cards. The Supplemental Nutrition Assistance Program or **SNAP** has replaced the Food Stamps Program and issues EBT cards that are similar to debit EBT cards that are that can be used to purchase foods. In recent years, both SNAP and WIC participants have been able to "purchase" foods from farmers' markets to encourage the intake of fruits and vegetables. Older adults may also be eligible for home-delivered meals through **Meals on Wheels** partnerships between the government and local agencies. The Administration on Aging (AOA), which is part of the U.S. Department of Health and Human Services, oversees both the Meals on Wheels Program and The **Congregate Dining Program.** The Meals on Wheels Program provides one home-delivered meal per day to income-eligible older adults. This program offers these adults an opportunity for social contact as well as the chance to have at least one nutritional meal each day. Volunteers deliver the meals directly to the older adults. Congregate dining programs are another alternative. These programs are funded by the AOA and sponsored by local agencies such as senior centers, where older adults can come and dine together in a social setting. Government programs are designed to provide food assistance to citizens who need it at every stage of the lifespan.

Nutrition is the science that establishes appropriate nutrient standards for humans at each life-stage. Culinary professionals who understand nutritional needs help both individuals and special groups to eat well by planning recipes and menus that are nutrient-dense and delicious. In a recent article, the Food Educators Network International supported the importance of education for culinary students in both nutrition and health. It concludes that an educational program that includes these goals will better prepare students for the restaurant industry and the changing environment. Innovative recipes with fewer calories and more healthful fats, or recipes with alternative foods for those who shouldn't consume wheat products or who are allergic to certain foods, are now expected by patrons.[66] They expect foods that accommodate their dietary needs and are tasty.[67] The health of the nation can be improved as more people enjoy eating healthfully.

References

1   L. M. De-Regil, A. C. Fernández-Gaxiola, T. Dowswell, J. P. Peña-Rosas, Micronutrients Unit, Department of Nutrition for Health and Development, World Health Organization, Geneva, "Effects and Safety of Periconceptional Folate Supplementation for Preventing Birth Defects," *Cochrane Database Cochrane Database Syst Rev.* 6 (2010): CD007950.

2   J. C. King, "Physiology of Pregnancy and Nutrient Metabolism," *American Journal of Clinical Nutrition* 71 (2000): 1218S–1225S.

3   L. M. De-Regil, A. C. Fernández-Gaxiola, T. Dowswell, J. P. Peña-Rosas, Micronutrients Unit, Department of Nutrition for Health and Development, World Health Organization, Geneva, "Effects and Safety of Periconceptional Folate Supplementation for Preventing Birth Defects," *Cochrane Database Cochrane Database Syst Rev.* 6 (2010): CD007950.

4   B. M. Zaadstra, J. C. Seidell, P. A. Van Noord, et al., "Fat and Female Fecundity: Prospective Study of Effect of Body Fat Distribution on Conception Rates," *British Medical Journal* 306 (1993): 484–487.

5   *Institute of Medicine*, "Nutrition During Pregnancy: Reexamining the Guidelines, Consensus Report: Weight Gain During Pregnancy," May 28, 2009. http://www.iom.edu/Activities/Women/PregWeightGain.aspx

6   L. M. De-Regil, A. C. Fernández-Gaxiola, T. Dowswell, J. P. Peña-Rosas, Micronutrients Unit, Department of Nutrition for Health and Development, World Health Organization, Geneva, "Effects and Safety of Periconceptional Folate Supplementation for Preventing Birth Defects," *Cochrane Database Cochrane Database Syst Review* 6 (2010): CD007950.

7   Position of the American Dietetic Association, "Nutrition and Lifestyle for a Healthy Pregnancy Outcome," *Journal of the American Dietetic Association* 102 (2002): 1479–1490.

8   U.S. Department of Agriculture, Food Safety and Inspection Service. "Fact Sheet: Protecting Your Baby and Yourself From Listeriosis," www.fsis.usda.gov. Last modified January 12, 2011.

9   E. Oken, J. S. Radesky, R. O. Wright, et al., "Maternal Fish Intake During Pregnancy, Blood Mercury Levels, and Child Cognition at Age 3 years in a US Cohort," *American Journal of Epidemiology* 167 (2008): 1171–1181.

10   E. Stokstad, "Salmon Survey Stokes Debate About Farmed Fish" *Science* 303 (2004): 154–155.

11   Centers for Disease Control, http://www.cdc.gov/parasites/toxoplasmosis/gen_info/pregnant.html "Toxoplasmosis and Pregnancy," Updated November 2, 2010.

12   E. L. Mortensen, K. F. Michaelsen, S. A. Sanders, et al., "The Association Between Duration of Breastfeeding and Adult Intelligence," *Journal of the American Medical Association* 287 (2002): 2365–2371.

13   F. R. Greer, S. Sicherer, A. W. Burks and The Committee on Nutrition and Section of Allergy and Immunology, "Effects of Early Nutritional Interventions on the Development of Atopic Disease in Infants and Children: The Role of Maternal Dietary Restriction, Breastfeeding, Timing of Introduction of Complementary Foods, and Hydrolyzed Formulas," *Pediatrics* 121 (2008): 183–191.

14   F. R. Hauck, J. M. Thompson, et al., "Breastfeeding and Reduced Risk of Sudden Infant Death syndrome: a Meta-Analysis," *Pediatrics* 128(2011):103-10.

15   American Academy of Pediatrics, "Starting Solid Foods," http://www.healthychildren.org/english/ages-stages/baby/feeding-nutrition/pages/Switching-To-Solid-Foods, Updated 11/10).

16   S. J. Fomon, "Feeding Normal Infants: Rationale for Recommendations," *Journal of The American Dietetic Association* 101 (2001): 1002–1005.

17   American Academy of Pediatrics, "Policy Re-affirmation: "The Use and Misuse of Fruit Juice in Pediatrics," *Pediatrics* 107 (2007): 1210–1213.

18   Federal Register, Department of Agriculture, Food and Nutrition Service, Special Supplemental Nutrition Program for Women, Infants and Children (WIC): Revisions in the Food Packages; Proposed Rule, August 7, 2006.

19   C. L. Wagner, F.R. Greer, "AAP Policy Statement: Section on Breastfeeding and Committee on Nutrition. Prevention of Rickets and Vitamin D Deficiency in Infants, Children and Adolescents," *Pediatrics* 122 (2008): 1142–1152.

20   J. D. Skinner, B. R. Carruth, B. Bounds, P. J. Ziegler, "Children's Food Preferences: A Longitudinal Analysis," *Journal of the American Dietetic Association* 102 (2002): 1638–1647.

21   F. R. Greer, S. Sicherer, A. W. Burks and The Committee on Nutrition and Section of Allergy and Immunology, "Effects of Early Nutritional Interventions on the Development of Atopic Disease in Infants and Children: The Role of Maternal Dietary Restriction, Breastfeeding, Timing of Introduction of Complementary Foods, and Hydrolyzed Formulas," *Pediatrics* 121 (2008): 183–91.

22   American Academy of Pediatrics, "Fetal Alcohol Syndrome and Alcohol-Related Neurodevelopmental Disorders," *Pediatrics* 106 (2000): 358–360.

23   L. T. Singer, R. Arendt, S. Minnes, et al., "Cognitive and Motor Outcomes of Cocaine-Exposed Infants," *Journal of the American Medical Association* 287 (2002): 1952–1959.

24   "Cocaine May Damage Developing Fetuses, Causing Lifelong Learning Disabilities (Brief Article)," *Pain & Central Nervous System Week* (March 25, 2002): 10.

25   C. R. Bauer, S. Shankaran, H. S. Bada, et al., "The Maternal Lifestyle Study: Drug Exposure During Pregnancy and Short-term Pregnancy Outcomes," *Journal of Obstetrics and Gynecology Research* 186 (2002): 3487–3489.

26   C. Belew, "Herbs and the Childbearing Woman. Guidelines for Midwives," *Journal of Nurse and Midwifery* 44 (1999): 231–252.

27   ChooseMyPlate.gov http://www.choosemyplate.gov/preschoolers/meal-and-snack-patterns-ideas.html May 3, 2013.

28   http://teamnutrition.usda.gov/healthierUS/index. Accessed May 3, 2013.

29   V. Yeager, "Local Wellness Policies: Securing a Healthy Tomorrow for Today's Youth," *Today's Dietitian* 7 (2006): 44–50.

30   B. Parsad and L. Lewis, *Calories In, Calories Out: Food and Exercise in Public Elementary Schools,* NCES 2006-057, Washington, DC: U.S. Department of Education, National Center for Education Statistics, 2005.

31   J. Wiecha et al., "School Vending Machine Use and Fast-Food Restaurant Use Are Associated with Sugar-Sweetened Beverage Intake in Youth," *Journal of the American Dietetic Association* 106 (2006): 1624–1630.

32   The Healthy, Hunger-Free Kids Act of 2010, United States Department of Agriculture. www.fns.usda.gov/cnd/governance/legislation/CNR_2010. Updated May 31, 2011.

33   R. Lustig et al., "Childhood Obesity: Behavioral Aberration or Biochemical Drive? Reinterpreting the First Law of Thermodynamics," *Nature Clinical Practice Endocrinology and Metabolism* 2 (2006): 447–458.

34   L. Dubois, A. Farmer, M. Girard, and K. Peterson, "Regular Sugar-Sweetened Beverage Consumption Between Meals Increases Risk of Overweight Among Preschool-Aged children," *Journal of the American Dietetic Association* 107 (2007): 924–935.

35   E. Satter, *Child of Mine: Feeding with Love and Good Sense,* Bull Publishing Company, Boulder, CO.: 2000.

36   D. Spruijt-Metz, C. H. Lindquist, L. L. Birch, et al., "Relationship between Mothers' Child-Feeding Practices and Children's Adiposity," *American Journal of Clinical Nutrition* 75 (2002): 581–586.

37   M. Nestle and M. F. Jacobson, "Halting the Obesity Epidemic: A Public Policy Approach." *Public Health Reports* 115 (2000): 12–24.

38   R. Sinha, G. Fisch, B. Teague, et al., "Prevalence of Impaired Glucose Tolerance Among Children and Adolescents with Marked Obesity," *New England Journal of Medicine* 346 (2002): 802–810.

39   D. S. Freedman, W. H. Dietz, S. R. Srinivasan, and G. S. Berenson, "The Relation of Overweight to Cardiovascular Risk Factors Among Children and Adolescents: The Bogalusa Heart Study," *Pediatrics* 103 (1999): 1175–1181.

40   G. Wang, and W. H. Dietz, "Economic Burden of Obesity in Youths Aged 6–17 Years: 1979–1999," *Pediatrics* 105 (2002): e81.

41   M. D. Castellanos, P. P. Lee, W. Sharp, et al., "Developmental Trajectories of Brain Volume Abnormalities in Children and Adolescents with Attention-Deficit/Hyperactivity Disorder," *Journal of the American Medical Association* 288 (2002): 1740–1748.

42   L. M. Pelsser, K. Frankena, J. Toorman, et. al. "Effects of A Restricted Elimination Diet on the Behaviour of Children with Attention-Deficit Hyperactivity Disorder (INCA study): A Randomized Controlled Trial," *The Lancet* (2011): 494–503.

43   S. Hyman, Original Research Presentation: "Dietary Treatment of Young Children with Autism: Behavioral Effects of the Gluten Free and Casein Free Diet," The International Meeting for Autism Research Philadelphia, May 22, 2010.

44   K. B. Nelson, J. K. Grether, L. A. Croen, et al., "Neuropeptides and Neurotrophins in Neonatal Blood of Children with Autism or Mental Retardation," *Ann Neurol* 49 (2001): 597–606.

45   M. P. Faine, and D. Oberg, "Survey of Dental Nutrition Knowledge of WIC Nutritionists and Public Health Dental Hygienists," *Journal of the American Dietetic Association* 95 (1995): 190–195.

46   M. P. Faine, and D. Oberg, "Survey of Dental Nutrition Knowledge of WIC Nutritionists and Public Health Dental Hygienists," *Journal of the American Dietetic Association* 95 (1995): 190–195.

47   R. P. Troiano and K. M. Flegal, "Overweight Children and Adolescents. Description, Epidem-iology, and Demograph-ics," *Pediatrics* 101 (1998): 497–504.

48   Dietary Guidelines for Americans, 2010. United States Department of Agriculture, Center for Nutrition and Policy Promotion, January 2011. http://www.cnpp.usda.gov/DGAs2010-PolicyDocument.htm

49   L. R. Young and M. Nestle, "The Contribution of Expanding Portion Size to the US Obesity Epidemic," *American Journal of Public Health* 92 (2002): 246–249.

50 J. Brand-Miller, K. Foster-Powell, and T. M. S. Wolverton, *The Glucose Revolution*, New York: Marlowe and Company, 1999.

51 K. McManus, L. Antinoro, and F. M. Sacks, "A Randomized Controlled Trial of a Moderate-Fat, Low-Energy Diet-Compared with a Low-Fat, Low-Energy Diet for Weight Loss in Overweight Adults," *International Journal of Obesity* 25 (2001): 1503–1511.

52 F. B. Hu, L. Bronner, W. C. Willett, et al., "Fish and Omega-3 Fatty Acid Intake and Risk of Coronary Heart Disease in Women," *Journal of the American Medical Association* 287 (2002): 1815–1821.

53 D. S. Ludwig, "The Glycemic Index: Physiological Mechanisms Relating to Obesity, Diabetes, and Cardiovascular Disease," *Journal of the American Medical Association* 287 (2002): 2414–2423.

54 C. M. Albert, H. Campos, M. J. Stampfer, et al., "Blood Levels of Long-Chain n-3 Fatty Acids and the Risk of Sudden Death," *New England Journal of Medicine* 346 (2002): 1113–1118.

55 U.S. Preventive Services Task Force, *Screening Guidelines for Osteoporosis in Postmenopausal Women: Recommendations and Rationale* 137 (2002): 526–528.

56 B. Dawson-Hughes, S. S. Harris, E. A. Krall, and G. E. Dallal, "Effect of Calcium and Vitamin D Supplementation on Bone Density in Men and Women 65 Years of Age or Older," *New England Journal of Medicine* 337(10), (1997): 671–675.

57 P. Knekt, J. Kumpulainen, R. Jarvinen, et al., "Flavonoid Intake and Risk of Chronic Diseases," *American Journal of Clinical Nutrition* 76 (2002): 560–568.

58 K. M. Flegal, M. D. Carroll, C. L. Ogden, and C. L. Johnson, "Prevalence and Trends in Obesity Among U.S. Adults, 1999–2000," *Journal of the American Medical Association* 288 (2002): 1723–1727.

59 J. L. Tuomilehto, J. G. Eriksson, et al., "Prevention of Type 2 Diabetes Mellitus by Changes in Lifestyle among Subjects with Impaired Glucose Tolerance," *New England Journal of Medicine* 344 (2001): 1343–1350.

60 R. L. Weinsier, G. R. Hunter, R. A. Desmond, et al., "Free-Living Activity Energy Expenditure in Women Successful and Unsuccessful at Maintaining a Normal Body Weight," *American Journal of Clinical Nutrition* 75 (2002): 499–504.

61 V. A. Hughes, W. R. Frontera, R. Roubenoff, W. R. Evans, and M. A. Fiatarone Singh, "Longitudinal Changes in Body Composition in Older Men and Women, Role of Body Weight Change and Physical Activity," *American Journal of Clinical Nutrition* 76 (2002): 473–479.

62 M. Nelson, M. A. Fiatarone, C. Morganti, et al., "Effects of High-Intensity Strength Training on Multiple Risk Factors for Osteoporotic Fractures," *Journal of the American Medical Association* 272 (1994): 1900–1914.

63 M. T. McGuire, R. R. Wing, M. L. Klem, et al., "Long-term Maintenance of Weight Loss: Do People Who Lose Weight Through Various Weight Loss Methods Use Different Behaviors to Maintain Weight?" *International Journal of Obesity* 22 (1998): 572–577.

64 T. B. Symons, T. L. Cocke, S. E. Schutzler et al., "Aging Does Not Impair the Anabolic Response to a Protein-rich Meal." *American Journal of Clinical Nutrition* 86 (2007): 451–456.

65 Welcoming Guests with Food Allergies to Restaurants, (2010). Food Allergy and Anaphylaxis Network. http://www.foodallergy.org/page/restaurants-guests-with-food-allergies

66 A. Jarman, "A Healthy Wholesome Education," *Chef Educator Today* 8 (2007): 18–20.

Put It into Practice

Define the Term

Review the section on Childhood/Health Concerns and explain the five most common conditions during this time period. Discuss the importance of nutrition and diet with relation to each of these conditions.

Myth vs. Fact

Determine if the following statement is a myth or fact and support your position with evidence from three research articles on the topic. *Statement: "All pregnant women crave pickles and ice cream."*

For each research article, summarize each component below.

A. Abstract
B. Methods
C. Results
D. Discussion
E. Conclusion

The Menu

Consumption of nutrient-dense foods should be encouraged throughout the life cycle. Particular nutrients are necessary during the high-growth segments of the lifespan (pregnancy, lactation, childhood, and adolescence). These nutrients are calcium, iron, vitamin A, and folate. Create a nutrient-dense dinner menus that include these four nutrients. Your menu must include an appetizer, an entrée, a vegetable, a starch, and a dessert. Highlight the foods that provide a good source of the nutrients.

Website Review

Navigate the U.S. Department of State's website on Global Hunger and Food Security though the following link: http://www.state.gov/s/globalfoodsecurity/index.htm In your opinion, how does this information impact the future of the food industry?

Navigate the "Food Day" website through the following link: http://www.foodday.org/. What is the actual date of "Food Day" and what is its purpose? What are the five "Food Day" principles? Click on the "Find a Community Coordinator" tab under the "Participate" tab. Is there a Community Coordinator in your state?

Build Your Career Toolbox

You are the Executive Chef/Dietitian for a large grocery market chain. You have been asked to develop educational materials and menus for consumers. Several grocery store customers are requesting specific shopping lists to accommodate their health concerns. Prepare a shopping list for a middle-aged couple who are overweight and have heart disease. Feature foods with moderate or low glycemic index ratings (see Table 10.13, Examples of Foods with Moderate and Low Glycemic Index) and include healthy fats.

Tina's Case Study

Tina is a 17-year old who is currently 5 months pregnant. Tina doesn't know much about nutrition and healthy foods, but she heard that she needs to eat foods high in calories since she is "eating for two." She met with her obstetrician who mentioned that she has been gaining the right amount of weight since becoming pregnant, which is important for both Tina and the baby.

She recently met with a WIC nutritionist who collected and analyzed a 24-hr recall, and provided recommendations for increasing calcium, iron, folate, and vitamin A. You are interning at WIC and have been asked to prepare a 1-day menu for Tina based on the nutritionist's assessment and recommendations.

Ht: 5'3"   Prepregnancy wt: 112 lbs   Prepregnancy BMI: 19.8 kg/m^2
Current wt: 123 lbs

Recommendations

Calorie needs: 2200–2400
Protein: 67–74 g
Calcium: 1300–1500 mg
Iron: 27–32 mg
Folate: 600–800 mcg
Vitamin A (RAE): 750–1000 mcg

Other recommendations: Avoid foods that are high-risk during pregnancy (undercooked meats/fish, sushi, deli meats, etc.); add omega-3 fatty acids

24-hr Recall

Breakfast: Glazed doughnut, medium iced coffee extra cream (3 oz), and sugar (8 tsp)

Lunch (at school): Chicken patty sandwich, potato wedges (2 pieces), 20-oz Gatorade, 2 tbsp ketchup

Dinner: 4-oz roasted chicken breast (no skin), 2/3 cup mashed potatoes, 1/2 cup steamed corn kernals w/2 tsp butter, 8-oz 1% milk

Snack: 1 cup vanilla ice cream

Preferences: She likes cereal, fruit, dairy products, and meats, and dislikes beans, spinach, and carrots.

Study Guide

Student Name _____ Date _____

Course Section _____ Chapter _____

TERMINOLOGY

Infancy_____	A. A growing baby's lifeline to the mother
WIC_____	B. The period from birth to one year
Adolescence_____	C. The second stage of pregnancy characterized by major organ formation
Occurs after the eighth week of pregnancy_____	D. A disease with painful joint swelling
Osteoarthritis_____	E. The period of growth in major organ systems that require specific nutrients
Critical period_____	F. Fetal development
Embryonic stage_____	G. A time of growth from puberty to full maturity
Placenta_____	H. A government program providing education wholesome foods, and infant formula to low income clients at no cost. Stands for Women, Infants and Children

Student Name _____   **Date** _____

Course Section _____   **Chapter** _____

LIFE STAGES AND LEADING NUTRIENTS WORKSHEET

Life Stage	Leading Nutrients	Nutritional Concerns
Pregnancy		
Breastfeeding (for mom)		

Life Stage	Leading Nutrients	Nutritional Concerns
Infancy		
Breastfeeding (for infant)		

Student Name _____   **Date** _____

Course Section _____   **Chapter** _____

Life Stage	Leading Nutrients	Nutritional Concerns
Childhood		
Adolescence		

Life Stage	Leading Nutrients	Nutritional Concerns
Young / Middle Adulthood		
Older Adults		

Student Name _____ Date _____

Course Section _____ Chapter _____

CASE STUDY DISCUSSION

Teen Pregnancy Case Study: Tina Eats School Lunch Daily

Review the section in Chapter 10 Adolescence, "Energy Needs and Leading Nutrients" and Table 10.12 "Guide for Lunch Meal plans for Teens". After reading the case study use the information to answer the following questions.

Using Tina's preferences from the case study, design a one day menu for breakfast, lunch, dinner and two snacks. The menu must include good sources of all four nutrients: Calcium, Iron, Vitamin A and Folate and meet the daily requirements for each food group for High School Grade levels.

Student Name _____ Date _____

Course Section _____ Chapter _____

PRACTICE TEST

Select the best answer.

1. The two leading nutrients throughout the lifespan are
   a. iron and protein
   b. iron and calcium
   c. fat and carbohydrates
   d. folic acid and vitamin C

2. The first stage of pregnancy is the
   a. critical
   b. embryo
   c. fetal
   d. zygote

3. During pregnancy, a normal weight woman should gain between
   a. 11-20 pounds
   b. 15-25 pounds
   c. 25-35 pounds
   d. 28-40 pounds

4. A food that may be high in mercury and should be avoided during both pregnancy and breastfeeding is
   a. feta cheese
   b. hotdogs
   c. raw milk
   d. swordfish

5. Cow's milk is **not** recommended for babies as their primary beverage until
   a. 3 months of age
   b. 6 months of age
   c. 9 months of age
   d. 12 months of age

Student Name _____   Date _____

Course Section _____   Chapter _____

TRUE OR FALSE

_____ Adolescence is a period of growth and development when an individual is able to create a new life until reaching full maturity.

_____ Older adults are at a greater risk for thiamine deficiencies.

_____ The highest rate of bone development occurs during adolescence.

_____ A diet high in phytochemicals is important to maintenance of health in the adult years.

_____ Breast milk contains probiotics.

List the 3 stages of pregnancy and discuss what is important about each one.

- _____
  _____
  _____

- _____
  _____
  _____

- _____
  _____
  _____

Explain the functions and target populations for the following programs:

- WIC_____

- SNAP_____

- **Meals on Wheels**_____

APPENDIX A

Sample Conversions and Calculations

Measurement Equivalents

Length

1 inch (in) = 2.54 centimeters (cm)
1 foot (ft) = 30.48 centimeters (cm)
1 meter (m) = 39.37 inches (in)

Temperature

Ice = 32°Fahrenheit (F) of 0°Celsius (C)
Body Temperature = 98.6°F or 37°C
Steam = 212°F or 100°C
To convert Fahrenheit (t_f) to Celsius (t_c):
$$T_c = \tfrac{5}{9}\,(t_f - 32)$$
To convert Celsius to Fahrenheit:
$$T_f = \tfrac{9}{5}\,(t_c + 32)$$

Volume

1 milliliter (ml) = ⅕ teaspoon (tsp) or 0.034 fluid ounce (fl oz)
1 teaspoon = 5 ml
1 tablespoon (tbs) = 3 tsp or 15 ml
1 fl oz = 2 tbs or 30 ml
1 cup (c) = 8 fl oz, 16 tbs, or 250 ml
1 quart (qt) = 32 fl oz, 4 c, or 0.95 liter (l)
1 l = 1.06 qt or 1000 ml
1 gallon (gal) = 16 c, 4 qt, 128 fl oz, or 3.79 l

Weight

1 microgram (μg or mcg) = ¹⁄₁₀₀₀ milligram (mg)
1 mg = ¹⁄₁₀₀₀ gram (g)
1 g = 1000 mg or ¹⁄₁₀₀₀ kilogram (kg)
1 kg = 1000 g or 2.2 pounds (lb)
1 lb = 16 ounce, weight (oz-wt) or 454 g
1 oz-wt = 28 g or ¹⁄₁₆ lb

Energy

1 kilocalorie (kcal)[a] = 4.2 kilojoules (kJ)
1 kJ = 0.24 kcal
1 g carbohydrate = 4 kcal or 17 kJ
1 g fat = 9 kcal or 37 kJ
1 g protein = 4 kcal or 17 kJ
1 g alcohol = 7 kcal or 29 kJ

Conversion Factors

Conversion factors are useful when it is necessary to change units which are known to be equivalent. The conversion factor uses both units in a fraction form. The fraction is equivalent to a value of one. Using the above measurement guide it is possible to convert fl oz to qt by setting up a conversion factor. This factor could be either

$$\frac{32\,\text{fl oz}}{1\,\text{qt}} \text{ or } \frac{1\,\text{qt}}{32\,\text{fl oz}}$$

[a]In this book and throughout the appendices, kilocalorie and calorie are often used interchangeably.

both of these fractions are equivalent to the same amount of fluid (or given an equivalent value of one).

Example

Convert 16 fl oz to qt.

1. Choose the conversion factor which has the units you need for your answer on the top.

$$\frac{1\,qt}{32\,fl\,oz}$$

2. Multiply the given amount by the conversion factor

$$16\,fl\,oz \times \frac{1\,qt}{32\,fl\,oz}$$

3. The result is 0.5 qt.

Additional Conversions or Equivalents

To convert International Units (IU) to

- mg vitamin D: divide by 40 or multiply by 0.025
- mg α-TE[b]: divide by 1.5

To convert grams (g) of Salt (NaCl) to milligrams (mg) of Sodium (Na)

- Grams (g) of salt (NaCL) ÷ 2.5 = grams of Sodium (Na)
- Grams (g) of Sodium (Na) × 1,000 = milligrams (mg) of Sodium
- Example: Amount of salt (NaCl): 5 g
  5g NaCl ÷ 2.5 = 2 g of Sodium (Na)
  2 g of Na × 1000 = 2000 mg of Na

To convert mcg of synthetic folate in supplements and enriched foods to Dietary Folate Equivalents (mcg DFE)

- mcg synthetic folate × 1.7 = mcg DFE

Vitamin A Equivalencies

- 1 RAE = 1 mcg retinal
  = 12 mcg beta-carotene
  = 24 mcg other vitamin A carotenoids
- 1 IU = 0.3 mcg retinal
  = 3.6 mcg beta-carotene
  = 7.2 mcg other vitamin A carotenoids

Percents

A percent compares one or more items to a standard number. This result is then multiplied by 100 in order to become a percent (per 100).

Example

Calculate the percent fat in a meal containing 25 g of fat and 900 kcal.

1. Convert g of fat to kcal of fat using a conversion factor.
   a. 1 g fat = 9 kcal so: 25 g fat × 9 kcal = 225 kcal fat

2. Divide kcal from fat from the kcal from the meal (the standard).
   a. 225 kcal fat / 900 kcal meal = 0.25

3. To turn into a percent, multiply by 100.
   a. 0.25 × 100 = 25 %

[b]Alpha-tocopherol equivalents (vitamin E)

APPENDIX B

Choose Your Foods Lists for Meal Planning

Healthy Eating, Physical Activity, and Your Weight

If you are at a healthy weight, you can maintain that weight by balancing the energy you take in from food and the energy you use for physical activity. You can lose weight by eating less and/or by increasing physical activity. If weight gain is desired, you can choose larger portions of a variety of nutrient rich foods; with an emphasis on selected fats as an excellent source of calories.

Planning Healthy Meals

Your Registered Dietitian/Nutritionist (RDN) will work with you to determine your calorie requirements. Based on your food preferences, your lifestyle and your calorie level, you and your RDN will be able to develop sample menus that will serve as an eating plan for you.

Your RDN will help you to adjust your eating plan when your lifestyle changes. For example, you can change your plan to fit your work, school, vacation, or travel or exercise schedule.

Measurement Abbreviations

Tbsp = tablespoon
tsp = teaspoon
oz = ounce
fl oz = fluid ounce
lb = pound

The Food Lists

The food lists group together foods that have about the same amount of carbohydrate, protein, fat, and calories. The term "choice" is used to describe a certain amount of food within a group of similar foods.

The following chart shows the approximate amount of nutrients in 1 choice from each list.

Food list	Carbohydrate (grams)	Protein (grams)	Fat (grams)	Calories
Carbohydrates				
Starch; breads; cereals; grains and pasta; starchy vegetables; crackers and snacks; and beans, peas, and lentils	15	3	1	80
Fruits	15	—	—	60
Milk and Milk Substitutes				
Fat-free, low-fat (1%)	12	8	0–2	100
Reduced-fat (2%)	12	8	5	120
Whole	12	8	8	160
Nonstarchy Vegetables	5	2	—	25
Sweets, Desserts, and Other Carbohydrates	15	varies	varies	varies
Proteins				
Lean	—	7	2	45
Medium-fat	—	7	5	75
High-fat	—	7	8	100
Plant-based	varies	7	varies	varies
Fats	—	—	5	45
Alcohol (1 alcohol equivalent)	varies	—	—	100

Other Features of *Choose Your Foods Meal Planning System*

- **Reading Food Labels:** Nutrition Facts panels on labels are a helpful nutrition guide.
- **Symbols:** The following symbols are used throughout this section to let you know which foods are good sources of fiber, which have extra fat, and which are high in sodium

  ✓ **A good source of fiber** = More than 3 grams of dietary fiber per choice.

  ! **Extra fat** = A food with extra fat.

  ‼ **Added fat** = A food with two extra fat choices or a food prepared with added fat.

  🧂 **High in sodium** = 480 milligrams or more of sodium per choice. (For foods listed as a main dish/meal on the **Combination Foods** and **Fast Foods** lists only, the symbol 🧂 represents more than 600 milligrams of sodium per choice.)

Foods that contain little carbohydrate and few calories are considered "free," when eaten in small amounts. See the **Free Foods** list.

Starch List

Breads, cereals, grains (including pasta and rice), starchy vegetables, crackers and snacks, and beans, peas, and lentils are starches. Examples of **1 starch choice** are :

- ½ cup of cooked cereal, grain, or starchy vegetable
- ⅓ cup of cooked rice or pasta

- 1 oz of a bread product, such as 1 slice of bread or ¼ of a large bagel
- ¾ to 1 oz of most snack foods (some snack foods may also have extra fat)

Nutrition Tips

- For information about a specific food, read the Nutrition Facts panel on its food label.
- Whole grains provide more vitamins, minerals and fiber.

> One starch choice has approximately 15 grams of carbohydrate, 3 grams of protein, 1 gram of fat, and 80 calories.

Bread

	Food	Serving size
	Bagel	¼ large bagel (1 oz)
!	Biscuit	1 biscuit (2½ inches across)
	Breads, loaf-type	
	white, whole-grain, French, Italian, pumpernickel, rye, sourdough, unfrosted raisin or cinnamon	1 slice (2 oz)
✓	reduced-calorie, light	2 slices (1 ½ oz)
	Breads, flat-type (flatbreads)	
	ciabatta	1 oz
	naan	3 ¼-inch square (1 oz)
	pita (6 inches across)	½ pita
✓	sandwich flat buns, whole-wheat	1 bun, including top and bottom (1 ½ oz)
!	taco shell	2 taco shells (each 5 inches across)
	tortilla, corn	1 small tortilla (6 inches across)
	tortilla, flour (white or whole-wheat)	1 small tortilla (6 inches across) or
	Cornbread	1¾-inch cube (1½ oz)
	English muffin	½ muffin
	Hot dog bun or hamburger bun	½ bun (¾ oz)
	Pancake	1 pancake (4 inches across ¼ inch thick)
	Roll, plain	1 small roll (1 oz)
!	Stuffing, bread	⅓ cup
	Waffle	1 waffle (4-inch square or 4 inches across)

Cereals

	Food	Serving Size
✓	Bran cereal (twigs, buds, or flakes)	½ cup
	Cooked cereals (oats, oatmeal)	½ cup
	Granola cereal	¼ cup

(continued)

Food	Serving Size
Grits, cooked	½ cup
Puffed cereal	1½ cups
Shredded wheat, plain	½ cup
Sugar-coated cereal	½ cup
Unsweetened, ready-to-eat cereal	¾ cup

One starch choice has approximately 15 grams of carbohydrate, 3 grams of protein, 1 gram of fat, and 80 calories.

Grains (Including Pasta and Rice)

Unless otherwise indicated, serving sizes listed are for cooked grains.

	Food	Serving Size
✓	Barley	⅓ cup
	Bran, dry	
✓	oat	¼ cup
✓	wheat	½ cup
✓	Bulgur	½ cup
	Couscous	⅓ cup
✓	Kasha	½ cup
	Millet	⅓ cup
	Pasta, white or whole-wheat (all shapes and sizes)	⅓ cup
	Polenta	⅓ cup
✓	Quinoa, all colors	⅓ cup
	Rice; white, brown, and other colors and types	⅓ cup
✓	Tabbouleh (tabouli), prepared	½ cup
	Wheat germ, dry	3 Tbsp
	Wild rice	½ cup

✓ Good source of fiber   ! Extra fat   🧂 High in sodium

Starch

Starchy Vegetables

All of the serving sizes for starchy vegetables on this list are for cooked vegetables.

	Food	Serving Size
	Breadfruit	¼ cup
	Cassava or dasheen	⅓ cup
	Corn	½ cup
	on cob	4- or 4½-inch piece (½ large cob)
✓	Hominy	¾ cup

✓	Mixed vegetables with corn or peas	1 cup
	Marinara, pasta, or spaghetti sauce	½ cup
✓	Parsnips	½ cup
✓	Peas, green	½ cup
	Plantain	⅓ cup
	Potato	
	baked with skin	¼ large potato (3 oz)
	boiled, all kinds	½ cup or ½ medium potato (3 oz)
!	mashed, with milk and fat	½ cup
	French-fried (oven-baked)*	1 cup (2 oz)
✓	Pumpkin puree, canned, no sugar added	¾ cup
✓	Squash, winter (acorn, butternut)	1 cup
✓	Succotash	½ cup
	Yam or sweet potato, plain	½ cup (3½ oz)

* Note: Restaurant-style French fries are on the **Fast Foods** list, page 54.

> One starch choice has approximately 15 grams of carbohydrate, 3 grams of protein, 1 gram of fat, and 80 calories.

Crackers and Snacks

Note: Some snacks are high in fat. Always check food labels.

	Food	Serving Size
	Crackers	
	animal	8 crackers
✓	crisp bread	2 to 5 pieces (¾ oz)
	graham, 2½-inch square	3 squares
	nut and rice	10 crackers
	oyster	20 crackers
!	round, butter-type	6 crackers
	saltine-type	6 crackers
!	sandwich-style, cheese or peanut butter filling	3 crackers
	whole-wheat baked	5 regular 1½-inch squares or 10 thinks (¾ oz)
	Granola or snack bar	1 bar (¾ oz)
	Matzoh, all shapes and sizes	¾ oz
	Melba toast	4 pieces (each about 2 by 4 inches)
	Popcorn	
✓	no fat added	3 cups
!!	with butter added	3 cups
	Pretzels	¾ oz

(*continued*)

	Food	Serving Size
	Rice cakes	2 cakes (4 inches across)
	Snack chips	
	baked (potato, pita)	about 8 chips (¾ oz)
!!	regular (tortilla, potato)	about 13 chips (1 oz)

! count as 1 starch choice + 1 fat choice (1 starch choice plus 5 grams of fat)
!! count as 1 starch choice + 2 fat choices (1 starch choice plus 10 grams of fat)
Note: For other snacks, see the **Sweets, Desserts,** and **Other Carbohydrates** list.

> **TIP** An open handful is equal to about 1 cup or 1 to 2 oz of snack food.

✓ Good source of fiber   ! Extra fat   High in sodium

Starch

Beans, Peas and Lentils

One choice counts on this list as 1 start choice + 1 lean protein choice.

	Food	Serving Size
✓	Baked beans, canned	⅓ cup
✓	Beans (black, garbanzo, kidney, lima, navy, pinto, white). Cooked or canned, drained and rinsed	½ cup
✓	Lentils (any color), cooked	½ cup
✓	Peas (black-eyed and split), cooked or canned, drained and rinsed	½ cup
✓	Refried beans, canned	½ cup

Note: Beans, lentils, and peas are also found on the **Protein** list, page 36.

✓ Good source of fiber   ! Extra fat   High in sodium

> **TIP** Canned beans, lentils, and peas can be high in sodium (salt). Draining and rinsing them reduces the sodium content by at least 40%.

Fruit List

Fresh, frozen, canned, and dried fruits and fruit juices are on this list. In general, **Examples of 1 fruit choice** are:

- ½ cup of canned or frozen fruit
- 1 small fresh fruit (¾ to 1 cup)
- ½ cup of unsweetened fruit juice
- 2 tablespoons of dried fruit

Nutrition Tips

- Fruit juices contain very little fiber. Choose fruits instead of juices whenever possible.

Selection Tips

- Serving sizes for canned fruits on the **Fruits** list are for the fruit and a small amount of juice (1 to 2 tablespoons).

Fruits

The weights listed include skin, core, seeds, and rind.

> One fruit choice has approximately 15 grams of carbohydrate, 0 grams of protein, 0 grams of fat, and 60 calories.

	Food	Serving Size
	Apple, unpeeled	1 small apple (4 oz)
	Apples, dried	4 rings
	Applesauce, unsweetened	½ cup
	Apricots	
	canned	½ cup
	dried	8 apricot halves
	fresh	4 apricots (5½ oz total)
	Banana	1 extra-small banana, about 4 inches long (4 oz)
✓	Blackberries	1 cup
	Blueberries	¾ cup
	Cantaloupe	1 cup diced
	Cherries	
	sweet, canned	½ cup
	sweet, fresh	12 cherries (3½ oz)
	Dates	3 small (deglet noor) dates or 1 large (medjool) date
	Dried fruits (blueberries, cherries, cranberries, mixed fruit, raisins)	2 Tbsp
	Figs	
	dried	3 small figs
✓	fresh	1½ large or 2 medium figs (3½ oz total)
	Fruit cocktail	½ cup
	Grapefruit	
	fresh	½ large grapefruit (5½ oz)
	sections, canned	¾ cup
	Grapes	17 small grapes (3 oz total)
✓	Guava	2 small guava (2½ oz total)

Food	Serving Size
Honeydew melon	1 cup diced
Kiwi	½ cup sliced
Loquat	¾ cup cubed
Mandarin oranges, canned	¾ cup

(continued)

	Food	Serving Size
	Mango	½ small mango (5½ oz) or ½ cup
	Nectarine	1 medium nectarine (5½ oz)
✓	Orange	1 medium orange (6½ oz)
	Papaya	½ papaya (8 oz) or 1 cup cubed
	Peaches	
	canned	½ cup
	fresh	1 medium peach (6 oz)
	Pears	
	canned	½ cup
	fresh	½ large pear (4 oz)
	Pineapple	
	canned	½ cup
	fresh	¾ cup
	Plantain, extra-ripe (black), raw	¼ plantain (2¼ oz)
	Plums	
	canned	½ cup
	dried (prunes)	3 prunes
	fresh	2 small plums (5 oz total)
	Pomegranate seeds (arils)	½ cup
✓	Raspberries	1 cup
✓	Strawberries	1¼ cup whole berries
	Tangerine	1 large tangerine (6 oz)
	Watermelon	1¼ cups diced

✓ Good source of fiber   ! Extra fat   🧂 High in sodium

Fruit Juice

	Food	Serving Size
	Apple juice/cider	½ cup
	Fruit juice blends, 100% juice	⅓ cup
	Grape juice	⅓ cup
	Grapefruit juice	½ cup
	Orange juice	½ cup
	Pineapple juice	½ cup
	Pomegranate juice	½ cup
	Prune juice	⅓ cup

Milk and Milk Substitutes

Different types of milk products, and milk substitutes are included on this list. However, certain types of milk and milk-like products are found on other lists:

- Cheeses are on the **Protein** list (rich in protein, minimal carbohydrate)
- Butter, cream, coffee creamers, and unsweetened nut milks are on the **Fats** list Many nut milks are very low in fat; your RDN can help you with individualized adjustments.
- Ice cream and frozen yogurt are on the **Sweets, Desserts, and Other Carbohydrates** list.

Nutrition Tips

- Milk and yogurt are good sources of calcium and protein.
- Greek yogurt contains more protein and less carbohydrate than other yogurts.

Selection Tip

- 1 cup equals 8 fluid oz or ½ pint.

One milk choice has 12 grams of carbohydrate and 8 grams of protein and:

- One fat-free (skim) or low-fat (1%) milk choice has 0–3 grams of fat and 100 calories per serving.
- One reduced-fat (2%) milk choice has 5 grams of fat and 120 calories per serving.
- One whole milk choice has 8 grams of fat and 160 calories per serving.

Milk and Yogurts

Food	Serving Size	Choices per Serving
Fat-free (skim) or low-fat (1%)		
milk, buttermilk, acidophilus milk, lactose-free milk	1 cup	1 fat-free milk
evaporated milk	½ cup	1 fat-free milk
yogurt, plain or Greek may be sweetened with an artificial sweetener	⅔ cup (6 oz)	1 fat-free milk
chocolate milk	1 cup	1 fat-free milk + 1 carbohydrate
Reduced-fat (2%)		
milk, acidophilus milk, kefir, lactose-free milk	1 cup	1 reduced-fat milk
yogurt, plain	⅔ cup (6 oz)	1 reduced-fat milk
Whole		
milk, buttermilk, goat's milk	1 cup	1 whole milk
evaporated milk	½ cup	1 whole milk
yogurt, plain	1 cup (8 oz)	1 whole milk
chocolate milk	1 cup	1 whole milk + 1 carbohydrate

Other Milk Foods and Milk Substitutes

Food	Serving Size	Choices per Serving
Eggnog		
fat-free	⅓ cup	1 carbohydrate
low-fat	⅓ cup	1 carbohydrate + ½ fat
whole milk	⅓ cup	1 carbohydrate + 1 fat
Rice drink		
plain, fat-free	1 cup	1 carbohydrate
flavored low-fat	1 cup	2 carbohydrates
Soy milk		
light or low-fat, plain	1 cup	½ carbohydrate + ½ fat
regular, plain	1 cup	½ carbohydrate + 1 fat
Yogurt with fruit, low-fat	2/3 cup (6 oz)	1 fat-free milk + 1 carbohydrate

Nonstarchy Vegetables List

- ½ cup of cooked vegetables or vegetable juice
- 1 cup of raw vegetables

Note: Salad greens (like arugula, chicory, endive, escarole, lettuce, radicchio, romaine, and watercress) are on the **Free Foods** list.

Nutrition Tips

- Try to choose a variety of vegetables and **eat at least 2 to 3 nonstarchy vegetable choice daily.**

One nonstarchy vegetable choice (½ cup-cooked or 1 cup raw) has approximately 5 grams of carbohydrate, 2 grams of protein, 0 grams of fat, and 25 calories.

Nonstarchy Vegetables

Amaranth leaves (Chinese spinach)			Hearts of palm
Artichoke		✓	Jicama
Artichoke hearts (no oil)			Kale
Asparogus			Kohlrabi
Baby corn			Leeks
Bamboo shoots			Mixed vegetables (without starchy vegetables, legumes, or pasta)
Bean sprouts (alfalfa, mung, soybean)			
Beans (green, wax, Italian, yard-long beans)			Mushrooms, all kinds, fresh
Beets			Okra
Broccoli			Onions

	Broccoli slaw, packaged, no dressing		Pea pods
✓	Brussels sprouts		Peppers (all varieties)
	Cabbage (green, red, bok choy, Chinese)		Radishes
✓	Carrots		Rutabaga
	Cauliflower	⑤	Sauerkraut, drained and rinsed
	Celery		Spinach
	Chayote		Squash, summer varieties (yellow, patty pan, crookneck, zucchini)
	Coleslaw, packaged, no dressing		
	Cucumber		Sugar snap peas
	Daikon		Swiss chard
	Eggplant		Tomatoe
	Fennel		Tomatoes, canned
	Gourds (bitter, bottle, luffa, bitter melon)	⑤	Tomato sauce (unsweetened)
	Green onions or scallions		Tomato/vegetable juice
	Greens (collard, dandelion, mustard, purslane, turnip)		Turnips
			Water chestnuts

Symbols: ✓ Good source of fiber   ! Extra fat   ⑤ High in sodium

Sweets Desserts, and Other Carbohydrate Lists

Some foods on this list have added sugars or fat.

Nutrition Tips

- Choose foods from this less often. They do not have as many vitamins or minerals or as much fiber as choices from other lists.

A choice in this list has approximately 15 grams of carbohydrate and about 70 calories. Many choices have more calories due to added fator more, depending on fat content.

Common Measurements

Dry	Liquid
3 tsp = 1 Tbsp	
4 oz = ½ cup	4 Tbsp = ¼ cup
8 oz = 1 cup	8 oz = 1 cup or ½ pint

Beverages, Soda, and Sports Drinks

Food	Serving Size	Choices per Serving
Cranberry juice cocktail	½ cup	1 carbohydrate
Fruit drink or lemonade	1 cup (8 oz)	2 carbohydrates

(continued)

Food	Serving Size	Choices per Serving
Hot chocolate, regular	1 envelope (2 Tbsp or ¾ oz added to 8 oz water)	1 carbohydrate
Soft drink (soda), regular	1 can (12 oz)	2½ carbohydrates
Sports drink fluid replacement type	1 cup (8 oz)	1 carbohydrate

> One carbohydrate choice has approximately 15 grams of carbohydrate and about 70 calories. One fat choice has 5 grams of fat and 45 calories.

Brownies, Cake, Cookies, Gelatine, pie and Pudding

Food	Serving Size	Cholees per Serving
Biscotti	1 oz	1 carbohydrate + 1 fat
Brownie, small unfrosted	1¼-inch square, ⅞-inch high (about 1 oz)	1 carbohydrate + 1 fat
Cake		
angel food, unfrosted	⅟₁ of cake (about 2 oz)	2 carbohydrates
frosted	2-inch square (about 2 oz)	2 carbohydrates + 1 fat
unfrosted	2-inch square (about 1 oz)	1 carbohydrate + 1 fat
Cookies		
100-calorie pack	1 oz	1 carbohydrate + 1 fat
chocolate chip cookies	2 cookies, 2¼ inches across	1 carbohydrate + 2 fats
gingersnaps	3 small cookies, 1½ inches across	1 carbohydrate
large cookie	2 cookie, 6 inches across (about 3 oz)	4 carbohydrates + 3 fats
sandwich cookies with crème filling	2 small cookies (about ⅔ oz)	1 carbohydrate + 1 fat
sugar-free cookies	1 large or 3 small cookies (¾ to 1 oz)	1 carbohydrate + 1 to 2 fats
vanilla wafer	5 cookies	1 carbohydrate + 1 fat
Cupcake, frosted	1 small cupcake (about 1¾ oz)	2 carbohydrates + 1 to 1½ fats
Flan	½ cup	2½ carbohydrates + 1 fat
Fruit cobbler	½ cup (3½ oz)	3 carbohydrates + 1 fat
Gelatin, regular	½ cup	1 carbohydrate
Pie		
commercially prepared fruit, 2 crusts	⅙ of 8-inch pie	3 carbohydrates + 2 fats
pumpkin or custard	⅛ of 8-inch pie	1½ carbohydrates + 1½ fats
Pudding		
regular (made with reduced-fat milk)	½ cup	2 carbohydrates
sugar-free or sugar- and fat-free (made with fat-free milk)	½ cup	1 carbohydrate

Candy, Spreads, Sweets, Sweeteners, Syrups, and Toppings

Food	Serving Size	Choice per Serving
Blended sweeteners (mixtures of artificial sweeteners and sugar)	1½ Tbsp	1 carbohydrate
Candy		
chocolate, dark or milk type	1 oz	1 carbohydrate + 2 fats
chocolate "kisses"	5 pieces	1 carbohydrate + 1 fat
hard	3 pieces	1 carbohydrate
Coffee creamer, nondairy type		
powdered, flavored	4 tsp	½ carbohydrate + ½ fat
liquid, flavored	2 Tbsp	1 carbohydrate
Fruit snacks, chewy (pureed fruit concentrate)	1 roll (¾ oz)	1 carbohydrate
Fruit spreads, 100% fruit	1½ Tbsp	1 carbohydrate
Honey	1 Tbsp	1 carbohydrate
Jam or jelly, regular	1 Tbsp	1 carbohydrate
Sugar	1 Tbsp	1 carbohydrate
Syrup		
chocolate	2 Tbsp	2 carbohydrates
light (pancake-type)	2 Tbsp	1 carbohydrate
regular (pancake-type)	1 Tbsp	1 carbohydrate

Condiments and Sauces

	Food	Serving Size	Choice per Serving
	Barbecue sauce	3 Tbsp	1 carbohydrate
	Cranberry sauce jellied	¼ cup	1½ carbohydrates
🧂	Curry sauce	1 oz	1 carbohydrate + 1 fat
🧂	Gravy, canned or bottled	½ cup	½ carbohydrate + ½ fat
	Hoisin sauce	1 Tbsp	½ carbohydrate
	Marinade	1 Tbsp	½ carbohydrate
	Plum sauce	1 Tbsp	½ carbohydrate
	Salad dressing, fat-free, cream-based	3 Tbsp	1 carbohydrate
	Sweet-and-sour sauce	3 Tbsp	1 carbohydrate

Note: You can also check the **Fats** list and **Free Foods** list for other condiments.

🧂 High in sodium

One carbohydrate choice has approximately 15 grams of carbohydrate and about 70 calories. One fat choice has 5 grams of fat and 45 calories.

Doughnuts, Muffins, Pastries, and Sweet Breads

Food	Serving Size	Choice per Serving
Banana nut bread	1-inch slice (2 oz)	2 carbohydrates + 1 fat
Doughnut		
cake, plain	1 medium doughnut (1½ oz)	1½ carbohydrates + 2 fats
hole	2 holes (1 oz)	1 carbohydrate + 1 fat
yeast-type, glazed	1 doughnut, 3¾ across (2 oz0	2 carbohydrates + 2 fats
Muffin		
regular	1 muffin (4 oz)	4 carbohydrates + 2½ fats
lower-fat	1 muffin (4 oz)	4 carbohydrates + ½ fat
Scone	1 scone (4 oz)	4 carbohydrates + 3 fats
Sweet roll or Danish	1 pastry (2½ oz)	2½ carbohydrates + 2 fats

Frozen Bars, Frozen Desserts, Frozen Yogurt, and Ice Cream

Food	Serving Size	Choice per Serving
Frozen pops	1	½ carbohydrate
Fruit juice bars, frozen, 100% juice	1 bar (3 oz)	1 carbohydrate
Ice cream		
fat-free	½ cup	1½ carbohydrates
light	½ cup	1 carbohydrate + 1 fat
no sugar-added	½ cup	1 carbohydrate + 1 fat
regular	½ cup	1 carbohydrate + 2 fats
Sherbet, sorbet	½ cup	2 carbohydrates
Yogurt, frozen		
fat-free	1/3 cup	1 carbohydrate
regular	½ cup	1 carbohydrate + 0 to 1 fat
Greek, lower-fat or fat-free	½ cup	1½ carbohydrates

✓ Good source of fiber   ! Extra fat   🧂 High in sodium

Protein List

Foods from this list are divided into four groups based on the amount of fat they contain. The following chart shows you what one protein choice includes.

	Carbohydrate (grams)	Protein (grams)	Fat (grams)	Calories
Lean protein	–	7	2	45
Medium-fat protein	–	7	5	75
High-fat protein	–	7	8	100
Plant-based protein	varies	7	varies	varies

Some meals may have more than 1 protein choice and the fat content may vary. For example, a breakfast sandwich may be made with 1 ounce of cheese and 1 egg. Since 1 ounce of cheese counts as 1 protein choice and 1 egg counts as 1 protein choice, this meal would contain 2 protein choices. The cheese is counted as a high-fat protein choice and the egg is a medium-fat protein choice. As another example, if you eat 3 ounces of cooked chicken at dinner, this protein would equal 3 protein choices because each ounce counts as 1 protein choice. Chicken without skin is a lean protein choice.

Portion Sizes

Portion size is an important part of meal planning. The **Protein** list is based on cooked weight (for example, 4 oz of raw meat is equal to 3 oz of cooked meat) after bone and fat have been removed. Try using the following comparisons to help estimate potion sizes.

- 1 oz cooked meat, poultry, or fish is about the size of a small matchbox.
- 3 oz cooked meat, poultry, or fish is about the size of a deck of playing cards.
- 2 tablespoons peanut butter is about the size of a golf ball.
- The palm of a woman's hand is about the size of 3 to 4 oz of cooked, boneless meat. The palm of a man's hand is about the size of 4 to 6 oz of cooked, boneless meat.
- 1 oz cheese is about the size of 4 dice.

> One lean protein choice has 0 grams of carbohydrate, approximately 7 grams of protein, 2 grams of fat, and 45 calories.

Lean Protein

	Food	Serving Size
	Beef: ground (90% or higher lean/10% or lower fat): select or choice grades trimmed of fat: roast (chuck, round, rump sirloin), steak (cubed, flank, porterhouse, T-bone), tenderloin	1 oz
s	Beef jerky	½ oz
	Cheeses with 3 grams of fat or less per oz	1 oz
	Curd-style cheeses: cottage-type (all kinds): ricotta (fat-free or light)	¼ cup (2 oz)
	Egg whites	2
	Fish	
	fresh or frozen, such as catfish, cod, flounder, haddock, halibut.	1 oz
	salmon, fresh or canned	1 oz
	sardines, canned	2 small sardines
	tuna, fresh or canned in water or oil and drained	1 oz
s	smoked: herring or salmon (lox)	1 oz
	Game: buffalo, ostrich, rabbit, venison	1 oz
s	Hot dog with 3 grams of fat or less per oz Note: May contain carbohydrate.	1 hot dog (1¾ oz)
	Lamb: chop, leg, or roast	1 oz
	Organ meats: heart, kidney, liver Note: May be high in cholesterol.	1 oz
	Oysters, fresh or frozen	6 medium oysters

(continued)

Food		Serving Size
	Pork, lean	
[s]	Canadian bacon	1 oz
[s]	ham	1 oz
	rib or loin chop/roast, tenderloin	1 oz
	Poultry, without skin: chicken, Cornish hen: domestic duck or goose (well-drained of fat): turkey: lean ground turkey or chicken	
[s]	Processed sandwich meats with 3 grams of fat or less per oz: chipped beef, thin-sliced deli meats, turkey ham, turkey pastrami	1 oz
[s]	Sausage with 3 grams of fat or less per oz	1 oz
	Shellfish: clams, crab, imitation shellfish, lobster, scallops, shrimp Veal: cutlet (no breading), loin chop, roast	1 oz

✓ Good source of fiber   ! Extra fat

[s] High in sodium (based on the sodium content of a typical 3-oz serving of meat, unless 1 oz or 2 oz is the normal serving size)

> One medium-fat protein choice has approximately 0 grams of carbohydrate, 7 grams of protein, 5 grams of fat, and 75 calories.

Medium-Fat Protein

	Food	Serving Size
	Beef trimmed of visible fat: ground beef (85% or lower lean/15% or higher fat), corned beef, meatloaf, prime cuts of beef (rib roast), short ribs, tongue	1 oz
	Cheeses with 4 to 7 grams of fat per oz: feta, mozzarella, pasteurized processed cheese spread, reduced-fat cheeses	1 oz
	Cheese, ricotta (regular or part-skim)	¼ cup (2 oz)
	Egg	1 egg
	Fish: any fried	1 oz
	Lamb: ground, rib roast	1 oz
	Pork: cutlet, ground shoulder roast	1 oz
	Poultry with skin: chicken, dove, pheasant, turkey, wild duck, or goose: fried chicken	1 oz
[s]	Sausage with 4 to 7 grams of fat per oz	1 oz

> One high-fat protein choice has approximately 0 grams of carbohydrate, 7 grams of protein, 8 grams of fat, and 100 calories.

High-Fat Protein

These foods are high in saturated fat, and calories. Try to eat 3 or fewer choices from this group per week.

Note: 1 oz is usually the serving size of meat, fish, poultry, or hard cheeses.

	Food	Sending Size
	Bacon, pork	2 slices (1 oz each before cooking)
[s]	Bacon, turkey	3 slices (½ oz each before cooking)

	Cheese, regular: American, blue-veined, brie, cheddar, hard goat, Monterey jack, Parmesan, queso, and Swiss	1 oz
!	Hot dog: beef, pork, or combination	1 hot dog (10 hot dogs per 1 lb-sized package)
	Hot dog: turkey or chicken	1 hot dog (10 hot dogs per 1 lb-sized package
	Pork: sausage, spareribs	1 oz
🧂	Processed sandwich meats with 8 grams of fat or more per oz: bologna, hard salami, pastrami	1 oz
🧂	Sausage with 8 grams fat or more per oz: bratwurst, chorizo, Italian, Knockwurst, Polish, smoked, summer	1 oz

✓ Good source of fiber   ! Extra fat

🧂 High in sodium (based on the sodium content of a typical 3-oz serving of meat, unless 1 oz or 2 oz is the normal serving size)

Note

- Beans, peas, and lentils are also found on the **Starch** list
- Nuts butters in smaller amounts are found on the **Fats** list.
- Conned beans, lentils, and peas can be high in sodium unless they're labeled *no-salt-added* or *low-sodium*. Draining and rinsing canned beans, peas, and lentils reduces sodium content by at least 40%.

Plant-Based Protein

Because carbohydrate content varies among plant-based protein foods, read food labels.

Many plant-based protein foods also contain carbohydrate and are counted as 1 or more **Starch** choices

	Food	Serving Size	Choices per Serving
	"Bacon" strips, soy-based	2 strips (½ oz)	1 loan protein
✓	Baked beans, canned	⅓ cup	1 starch + 1 lean protein
✓	Beans (black, garbanzo, kidney, lima, navy, pinto, white), cooked or canned, drained and rinsed	½ cup	1 starch + 1 lean protein
	"Beef" or "sausage" crumbles, meatless	1 oz	1 lean protein
	"Chicken" nuggets, soy-based	2 nuggets (1½ oz)	½ starch + 1 medium-fat protein
✓	Edamame, shelled	½ cup	½ starch + 1 lean protein
	Falafel (spiced chickpea and wheat parties)	3 patties (about 2 inches across)	1 starch + 1 high-fat protein
	Hot dog, meatless, soy-based	1 hot dog (1½ oz)	1 lean protein
✓	Hummus	⅓ cup	1 starch + 1 medium-fat protein
✓	Lentils, any color, cooked or canned, drained and rinsed	½ cup	1 starch + 1 lean protein
	Meatless burger, soy-based	3 oz	½ starch + 2 lean proteins

(continued)

	Food	Serving Size	Choices per Serving
✓	Meatless burger, vegetable and starch-based	1 patty (about 2½ oz)	½ starch + 1 lean protein
	Meatless deli slices	1 oz	1 lean protein
	Mycoprotein ("chicken" tenders or crumbles), meatless	2 oz	½ starch + 1 lean protein
	Nut spreads almond butter, cashew butter, peanut butter, soy nut butter	1 Tbsp	1 high-fat protein
✓	Peas (black-eyed and split peas), cooked or canned, drained and rinsed	½ cup	1 starch + 1 lean protein
🧂 ✓	Refried beans, canned	½ cup	1 starch + 1 lean protein
	"Sausage" breakfast-type patties, meatless	1 (1½ oz)	1 medium-fat protein
	Soy nuts, unsalted	¾ oz	½ starch + 1 medium-fat protein
	Tempeh, plan, unflavored	¼ cup (1½ oz)	1 medium-fat protein
	Tofu	½ cup (4 oz)	1 medium-fat protein
	Tofu, light	½ cup (4 oz)	1 lean protein

Fats List

Nutrition Tips

- In general, **1 fat choice** equals:
  - 1 teaspoon of oil or solid fat
  - 1 tablespoon of salad dressing

Nuts and seeds are good sources of unsaturated fats and have small amounts of fiber and protein.

One fat choice has approximately 5 grams of fat and 45 calories.

Good sources of omega-3 fatty acids include:

- Fish such as albacore tuna, halibut, herring, mackerel, salmon, sardines, and trout
- Flaxseeds and English walnuts and their oils, canola and soy oil.

Unsaturated Fats—Monounsaturated Fats

Food	Serving size
Avocado, medium	2 Tbsp (1 oz)
Nut butters (*trans* fat-free): almond butter, cashew butter, peanut butter (smooth or crunchy)	1½ tsp
Nuts	
almonds	6 nuts
Brazil	2 nuts

cashews	6 nuts
filberts (hazelnuts)	5 nuts
macadamia	3 nuts
mixed (50% peanuts)	6 nuts
peanuts	10 nuts
pecans	4 halves
pistachios	16 nuts
Oil: canola, olive peanut	1 tsp
Olives	
black (ripe)	8
green, stuffed	10 large
Spread, plant stanol ester-type	
light	1 Tbsp
regular	2 tsp

Unsaturated Fats—Polyunsaturated Fats

Food	Serving size
Margarine	
lower-fat spread (30 to 50% vegetable oil, *trans* fat-free)	1 Tbsp
stick, tub (*trans* fat-free), or squeeze (*trans* fat-free)	1 tsp
Mayonnaise	
reduced-fat	1 Tbsp
regular	1 tsp
Mayonnaise-style salad dressing	
reduced-fat	1 Tbsp
regular	2 tsp
Nuts	
pignolia (pine nuts)	1 Tbsp
walnuts, English	4 halves
Oil: corn, cottonseed, flaxseed, grapeseed, safflower soybean, sunflower.	1 tsp
Salad dressing	
reduced-fat (Note: May contain carbohydrate)	2 Tbsp
regular	1 Tbsp
Seeds	
flaxseed, ground	1½ Tbsp
pumpkin, sesame, sunflower	1 Tbsp
Tahini or sesame paste	2 tsp

Portion Tip

Your thumb is about the same size and volume as 1 tablespoon of salad dressing, mayonnaise, margarine, or oil. It is also about the same size as 1 ounce of cheese. A thumb tip is about the size of 1 teaspoon of margarine, mayonnaise, or other fats and oils.

> One fat choice has approximately 5 grams of fat and 45 calories.

Saturated Fats

Food	Serving size
Bacon, cooked, regular or turkey	1 slice
Butter	
reduced-fat	1 Tbsp
stick	1 tsp
whipped	2 tsp
Butter blends made with oil	
reduced-fat or light	1 Tbsp
regular	1½ tsp
Chitterlings, boiled	2 Tbsp (½ oz)
Coconut, sweetened, shredded	2 Tbsp
Coconut milk, canned, thick	
light	⅓ cup
regular	1½ Tbsp
Cream	
half-and-half	2 Tbsp
heavy	1 Tbsp
light	1½ Tbsp
whipped	2 Tbsp
Cream cheese	
reduced-fat	1½ Tbsp (¾ oz)
regular	1 Tbsp (½ oz)
Lard	1 tsp
Oil: coconut, palm, palm kernel	1 tsp
Salt park	¼ oz
Shortening, solid	1 tsp
Sour cream	
reduced-fat or light	3 Tbsp
regular	2 Tbsp

Fats

Similar Foods in Other Lists

- Bacon and nut butters, when used in smaller amounts, are counted as fat choices. When used in larger amounts, they are counted as high-fat protein choices (see the **Protein** list)
- Fat-free salad dressings are on the **Sweets, Desserts, and Other Carbohydrates** list.

Free Foods List

A "free" food is any food or drink choice that has less than 20 calories and 5 grams or less of carbohydrate per serving.

Selection Tips

- If a "free" food is listed with a serving size, limit yourself to 3 servings or fewer of that food per day, and spread the servings throughout the day.
- Food and drink choices listed here without a serving size can be used whenever you like.

Low-Carbohydrate Foods

Food	Serving size
Candy, hard (regular or sugar-free)	1 piece
Fruits	
Cranberries or rhubarb, sweetened with sugar substitute	½ cup
Gelatin dessert, sugar-free, any flavor	
Gum, sugar-free	
Jam or jelly, light or no-sugar-added	2 tsp
Salad greens (such as arugula, chicory, endive, escarole, leaf or loeberg lettuce, purslane, romaine, radicchio, spinach, watercress)	
Sugar substitutes (artificial sweeteners)	
Syrup, sugar-free	2 Tbsp
Vegetables: any **raw** nonstarchy vegetables (such as broccoli, cabbage, carrots, cucumber, tomato)	½ cup
Vegetables: any **cooked** nonstarchy vegetables (such as carrots, cauliflower, green beans)	¼ cup

Free Foods

Reduced-Fat or Fat-Free Foods

Food	Serving Size
Cream cheese, fat-free	1 Tbsp (½ oz)
Coffee creamers, non dairy	
liquid, flavored	1½ tsp
liquid, sugar-free, flavored	4 tsp
powdered, flavored	1 tsp
powdered, sugar-free, flavored	2 tsp
Margarine spread	
fat-free	1 Tbsp
reduced-fat	1 tsp

(continued)

Food	Serving Size
Mayonnaise	
fat-free	1 Tbsp
reduced-fat	1 tsp
Mayonnaise-style salad dressing	
fat-free	1 Tbsp
reduced-fat	2 tsp
Salad dressing	
fat-free	1 Tbsp
fat-free, Italian	2 Tbsp
Sour cream, fat-free or reduced fat	1 Tbsp
Whipped topping	
light or fat-free	1 Tbsp
regular	1 Tbsp

Condiments

	Food	Serving Size
	Barbecue sauce	2 tsp
	Catsup (ketchup)	1 Tbsp
	Chili sauce, sweet, tomato-type	2 tsp
	Horseradish	
	Hot pepper sauce	
	Lemon juice	
	Miso	1½ tsp
	Mustard	
	honey	1 Tbsp
	brown, Dijon, horseradish-flavored, wasabi-flavored or yellow	
	Parmesan cheese, grated	1 Tbsp
	Pickle relish (dill or sweet)	1 Tbsp
	Pickles	
🧂	dill	1½ medium pickles
	sweet, bread and butter	2 slices
	sweet, gherkin	¾ oz
	Pimento	
	Salsa	¼ cup
🧂	Soy sauce, light or regular	1 Tbsp
	Sweet-and-sour sauce	2 tsp

Taco sauce	1 Tbsp
Vinegar	
Worcestershire sauce	
Yogurt, any type	2 Tbsp

! Extra fat   (s) High in sodium

Free Foods
Free Snack Suggestions

When you are hungry between meals, try to choose whole foods as snacks instead of highly processed options. The foods listed below are examples of nutritious free-food snacks:

- ½ choice from the **Nonstarchy Vegetables** list on pages 384–385: for example, ½ cup raw broccoli, carrots, cucumber, or tomato
- ⅓ choice from the **Fruits** list on page 380; for example. ¼ cup blueberries or blackberries, ⅓ cup melon, 6 grapes, or 2 tsp dried fruits
- ¼ choice from **Starch** list on pages 376–378; for example, 2 animal crackers, 1½ saltine-type crackers, ¾ cup no-fat-added popcorn, or ½ regular-sized rice or popcorn cake
- ½ choice from the nuts and seeds portion of the **Fats** list on pages 392–394; for example, 8 pistachios, 3 almonds, 4 black olives, or 1½ tsp sunflower seeds
- ½ choice from the **Lean Protein** list on pages 388–392; for example. ½ oz slice of fat-free cheese or ½ oz of lean cooked meat

Drinks/Mixes

(s)
- Bouillon, broth, consommé
- Bouillon or broth, low-sodium
- Carbonated or mineral water
- Club soda
- Cocoa powder, unsweetened (1 Tbsp)
- Coffee, unsweetened or with sugar substitute
- Diet soft drinks, sugar-free
- Drink mixes (powder or liquid drops), sugar-free
- Tea, unsweetened or with sugar substitute
- Tonic water, sugar-free
- Water
- Water, flavored, sugar-free

Seasonings

- Flavoring extracts (for example, vanilla, peppermint)
- Garlic, fresh or powder
- Herbs, fresh or dried
- Kelp
- Nonstick cooking spray
- Spices
- Wine, used in cooking

Combination Foods

Many of the foods you eat, such as casseroles and frozen entrees, are mixed together. These "combination" foods do not fit into any one choice list. This list of some typical "combination" food choices will help you fit these foods into your eating plan. Ask your RDN about the nutrient information for other combination foods you would like to eat, including your own recipes.

Entrees

	Food	Serving Size	Choices per Serving
🧂	Casserole-type entrees (tuna noodle, lasagna, spaghetti with meatballs, chili with beans, macaroni and cheese)	1 cup (8 oz)	2 starches + 2 medium-fat proteins
🧂	Stews (beef/other meats and vegetables)	1 cup (8 oz)	1 starches + 1 medium-fat proteins + 0 to 3 fats

Frozen Meals/Entrees

	Food	Serving Size	Choices per Serving
🧂 ✓	Burrito (beef and bean)	1 burrito (5 oz)	3 starches + 1 lean protein + 2 fats
	Dinner-type healthy meal (includes dessert and is usually less than 400 calories)	about 9–12 oz	2 to 3 starches + 1 to 2 lean proteins + 1 fat
	"Healthy"-type entrée (usually less than 300 calories)	about 7–10 oz	2 starches + 2 lean proteins
	Pizza		
🧂	cheese/vegetarian, thin crust	¼ of a 12-inch pizza (4½ –5oz)	2 starches + 2 medium-fat proteins
🧂	meat topping, thin crust	¼ of a 12-inch pizza (5oz)	2 starches + 2 medium-fat proteins + 1½ fats
🧂	cheese/vegetarian or meat topping, rising crust	⅙ of 12-inch pizza (4 oz)	2½ starches + 2 medium-fat proteins
🧂	Pocket sandwich	1 sandwich (4½ oz)	3 starches + 1 lean protein + 1 to 2 fats
🧂	Pot pie	1 pot pie (7 oz)	3 starches + 1 medium-fat protein + 3 fats

✓ Good source of fiber 　　　! Extra fat 　　　🧂 High in sodium

Combination of Foods

Salads (Deli-Style)

	Food	Serving Size	Choices per Serving
	Coleslaw	½ cup	1 starch + 1½ fats
	Macaroni/pasta salad	½ cup	2 starches + 3 fats
🧂	Potato salad	½ cup	1½ to 2 starches + 1 to 2 fats
	Tuna salad or chicken salad	½ cup (3½ oz)	½ starch + 2 lean proteins + 1 fat

Soups

	Food	Serving Size	Choices per Serving
✓ 🧂	Bean, lentil, or split pea soup	1 cup (8 oz)	1½ starches + 1 lean protein
🧂	Chowder (made with milk)	1 cup (8 oz)	1 starch + 1 lean protein + 1½ fats
🧂	Cream soup (reconstituted with water)	1 cup (8 oz)	1 starch + 1 fat
🧂	Miso soup	1 cup (8 oz)	½ starch + 1 lean protein
🧂	Ramen noodle soup	1 cup (8 oz)	2 starches + 2 fats
	Rice soup/porridge (congee)	1 cup (8 oz)	1 starch
🧂	Tomatoe soup (made with water) borscht	1 cup (8 oz)	1 starch
🧂	Vegetable beef, chicken noodle, or other broth-type soup (including "healthy" -type soups, such as those lower in sodium and/or fat	1 cup (8 oz)	1 starch + 1 lean protein

✓ Good source of fiber   ! Extra fat   🧂 High in sodium

Fast Foods

You can get specific nutrition information for almost every fast food or restaurant chain.

Main Dishes/Entrees

	Food	Serving Size	Choices per Serving
	Chicken		
🧂	breast, breaded and fried *	1 (about 7 oz)	1 starch + 6 medium-fat proteins
	breast, meat only**	1	4 lean proteins
	drumstick, breaded and fried*	1 (about 2½ oz)	½ starch + 2 medium-fat proteins
	drumstick, meat only**	1	1 lean protein + ½ fat
🧂	nuggets or tenders	6 (about 3½ oz)	1 starch + 2 medium-fat proteins + 1 fat
🧂	thigh, breaded and fried*	1 (about 5 oz)	1 starch + 3 medium-fat proteins + 2 fats
	thigh, meat only**	1	2 lean proteins + ½ fat
	wing, breaded and fried*	1 wing (about 2 oz)	½ starch + 2 medium-fat proteins
	wing, meat only **	1 wing	1 lean protein
🧂 ✓	Main dish salad (grilled chicken-type, no dressing or croutons)	1 salad (about 11½ oz)	1 starch + 4 lean proteins
	Pizza		
🧂	cheese, pepperoni, or sausage, regular or thick crust	⅛ of a 14-inch pizza (about 4 oz)	2½ starches + 1 high-fat protein + 1 fat
🧂	cheese, pepperoni, or sausage, thin crust	⅛ of a 14-inch pizza (about 2¾ oz)	1½ starches + 1 high-fat protein + 1 fats
🧂	cheese, meat, and vegetable, regular crust	⅛ of a 14-inch pizza (about 5 oz)	2½ starches + 2 high-fat proteins

* Definition and weight refer to food **with** bone, skin, and breading.
** Definition **refers** to above food **without** bone, skin, and breading.
✓ Good source of fiber   ! Extra fat   🧂 High in sodium

Fast Foods

Asian

	Food	Serving Size	Choices per Serving
🧂	Beef/chicken/shrimp with vegetables in sauce	1 (about 6 oz)	1 starch + 2 lean proteins + 1 fat
	Egg roll, meat	1 egg roll (about 3 oz)	1½ starches + 1 lean protein + 1½ fats
	Fried rice, meatless	1 cup	2½ starches + 2 fats
	Fortune cookie	1 cookie	½ starch
🧂	Hot-and-sour soup	1 cup	½ starch + ½ fat
🧂	Meat with sweet sauce	1 cup (about 6 oz)	3½ starches + 3 medium-fat proteins + 3 fats
🧂	Noodles and vegetables in sauce (chow mein, lo mein)	1 cup	2 starches + 2 fats

Mexican

	Food	Serving Size	Choices per Serving
🧂 ✓	Burrito with beans and cheese	1 small burrito (about 6 oz)	3½ starches + 1 medium-fat protein + 1 fat
🧂	Nachos with cheese	1 small order (about 8 nachos)	2½ starches + 1 high-fat protein + 2 fats
🧂	Quesadilla, cheese only	1 small order (about 5 oz)	2½ starches + 3 high-fat proteins
	Taco, crisp, with meat and cheese	1 small taco (about 3 oz)	1 starch + 1 medium-fat protein + ½ fat
🧂 ✓	Taco salad with chicken and tortilla bowl	1 salad (1 lb, including tortilla bowl)	2½ starches + 4 medium-fat proteins + 3 fats
🧂	Tostada with beans and cheese	1 small tostada (about 5 oz)	2 starches + 1 high-fat protein

Sandwiches

	Food	Serving Size	Choices per Serving
	Breakfast Sandwiches		
🧂	Breakfast burrito with sausage egg, cheese	1 burrito (about 4 oz)	1½ starches + 2 high -fat proteins
🧂	Egg, cheese, meat on an English muffin	1 sandwich	2 starches + 3 medium-fat proteins + ½ fat
🧂	Egg, cheese, meat on a biscuit	1 sandwich	2 starches + 3 medium-fat proteins + 2 fats
🧂	Sausage biscuit sandwich	1 sandwich	2 starches + 1 high-fat protein + 4 fats
	Chicken Sandwiches		
🧂	grilled with bun, lettuce, tomatoes, spread	1 sandwich (about 7½ oz)	3 starches + 4 lean proteins

🧂	crispy, with bun, lettuce, tomatoes, spread	1 sandwich (about 6 oz)	3 starches + 2 lean proteins + 3½ fats
	Fish sandwich with tartar sauce and cheese	1 sandwich (5 oz)	2½ starches + 2 medium-fat proteins + 1½ fats
	Hamburger		
	regular with bun and condiments (catsup, mustard, onion, pickle)	1 burger (about 3½ oz)	2 starches + 1 medium-fat protein + 1 fat
🧂	4 oz meat with cheese, bun, and condiments (catsup, mustard, onion, pickle)	1 burger (about 8½ oz)	3 starches + 4 medium-fat protein + 2½ fast
🧂	Hot dog with bun, plain	1 hot dog (about 3½ oz)	1½ starches + 1 high-fat protein + 2 fats

Submarine sandwich
(no cheese or sauce)

🧂	less than 6 grams fat	1 6-inch sub	3 starches + 2 lean proteins
🧂	regular	1 6-inch sub	3 starches + 2 lean proteins + 1 fat
🧂	Wrap, grilled chicken, vegetables, cheese, and spread	1 small wrap (about 4 to 5 oz)	2 starches + 2 lean proteins + 1½ fats

✓ Good source of fiber   ! Extra fat   🧂High in sodium

Fast Foods
Sides/Appetizers

	Food	Serving Size	Choices per Serving
🧂 !	French fries	1 small order (about 3½ oz)	2½ starches + 2 fats
		1 medium order (about 5 oz)	3½ starches + 3 fats
		1 larger order (about 6 oz)	4½ starches + 4 fats
!	Hash browns	1 cup/medium order (about 5 oz)	3 starches + 6 fats
!	Onion rings	1 serving (8 to 9 rings about 4 oz).	3½ starches + 4 fats
	Salad, side (no dressing croutons or cheese)	1 small salad	1 nonstarchy vegetable

Beverages and Desserts

Food	Serving Size	Choices per Serving
Coffee, latte (fat-free milk)	1 small order (about 12 oz)	1 fat-free milk
Coffee, mocha (fat-free milk, no whipped cream)	1 small order (about 12 oz)	1 fat-free milk + 1 starch
Milkshake, any flavour	1 small shake (about 12 oz)	5½ starches + 3 fats
	1 medium shake (about 16 oz)	7 starches + 4 fats
	1 large shake (about 22 oz)	10 starches + 5 fats
Soft-serve ice cream cone	1 small	2 starches + ½ fat

APPENDIX C

Dietary Reference Intake Tables

Dietary Reference Intakes (DRIs): Estimated Average Requirements
Food and Nutrition Board, Institute of Medicine, National Academies

Life Stage Group	Calcium (mg/d)	CHO (g/d)	Protein (g/kg/d)	Vit A (µg/d)[a]	Vit C (mg/d)	Vit D (µg/d)	Vit E (mg/d)[b]	Thiamin (mg/d)	Ribo-flavin (mg/d)	Niacin (mg/d)[c]
Infants										
0 to 6 mo										
6 to 12 mo			1.0							
Children										
1–3 y	500	100	0.87	210	13	10	5	0.4	0.4	5
4–8 y	800	100	0.76	275	22	10	6	0.5	0.5	6
Males										
9–13 y	1,100	100	0.76	445	39	10	9	0.7	0.8	9
14–18 y	1,100	100	0.73	630	63	10	12	1.0	1.1	12
19–30 y	800	100	0.66	625	75	10	12	1.0	1.1	12
31–50 y	800	100	0.66	625	75	10	12	1.0	1.1	12
51–70 y	800	100	0.66	625	75	10	12	1.0	1.1	12
>70 y	1,000	100	0.66	625	75	10	12	1.0	1.1	12
Females										
9–13 y	1,100	100	0.76	420	39	10	9	0.7	0.8	9
14–18 y	1,100	100	0.71	485	56	10	12	0.9	0.9	11
19–30 y	800	100	0.66	500	60	10	12	0.9	0.9	11
31–50 y	800	100	0.66	500	60	10	12	0.9	0.9	11
51–70 y	1,000	100	0.66	500	60	10	12	0.9	0.9	11
>70 y	1,000	100	0.66	500	60	10	12	0.9	0.9	11
Pregnancy										
14–18 y	1,000	135	0.88	530	66	10	12	1.2	1.2	14
19–30 y	800	135	0.88	550	70	10	12	1.2	1.2	14
31–50 y	800	135	0.88	550	70	10	12	1.2	1.2	14
Lactation										
14–18 y	1,000	160	1.05	885	96	10	16	1.2	1.3	13
19–30 y	800	160	1.05	900	100	10	16	1.2	1.3	13
31–50 y	800	160	1.05	900	100	10	16	1.2	1.3	13

Note: An Estimated Average Requirement (EAR) is the average daily nutrient intake level estimated to meet the requirements of half of the healthy individuals in a group. EARs have not been established for vitamin K, pantothenic acid, biotin, choline, chromium, fluoride, manganese, or other nutrients not yet evaluated via the DRI process.

[a] As retinol activity equivalents (RAEs). 1 RAE = 1 µg retinol, 12 µg β-carotene, 24 mg α-carotene, or 24 mg β-cryptoxanthin. The RAE for dietary provitamin A carotenoids is two-fold greater than retinol equivalents (RE), whereas the RAE for preformed vitamin A is the same as RE.

[b] As α-tocopherol. α-Tocopherol includes *RRR*-α-tocopherol, the only form of α-tocopherol that occurs naturally in foods, and the *2R*-stereoisomeric forms of α-tocopherol (*RRR*-, *RSR*-, *RRS*-, and *RSS*-α-tocopherol) that occur in fortified foods and supplements. It does not include the *2S*-stereoisomeric forms of a-tocopherol (*SRR*-, *SSR*-, *SRS*-, and *SSS*-α-tocopherol), also found in fortified foods and supplements.

[c] As niacin equivalents (NE). 1 mg of niacin = 60 mg of tryptophan.

[d] As dietary folate equivalents (DFE). 1 DFE = 1 µg food folate = 0.6 µg of folic acid from fortified food or as a supplement consumed with food = 0.5 µg of a supplement taken on an empty stomach.

Vit B$_6$ (mg/d)	Folate (µg/d)^d	Vit B$_{12}$ (µg/d)	Copper (µg/d)	Iodine (µg/d)	Iron (mg/d)	Magnesium (mg/d)	Molybdenum (µg/d)	Phosphorus (mg/d)	Selenium (µg/d)	Zinc (mg/d)
					6.9					2.5
0.4	120	0.7	260	65	3.0	65	13	380	17	2.5
0.5	160	1.0	340	65	4.1	110	17	405	23	4.0
0.8	250	1.5	540	73	5.9	200	26	1,055	35	7.0
1.1	330	2.0	685	95	7.7	340	33	1,055	45	8.5
1.1	320	2.0	700	95	6	330	34	580	45	9.4
1.1	320	2.0	700	95	6	350	34	580	45	9.4
1.4	320	2.0	700	95	6	350	34	580	45	9.4
1.4	320	2.0	700	95	6	350	34	580	45	9.4
0.8	250	1.5	540	73	5.7	200	26	1,055	35	7.0
1.0	330	2.0	685	95	7.9	300	33	1,055	45	7.3
1.1	320	2.0	700	95	8.1	255	34	580	45	6.8
1.1	320	2.0	700	95	8.1	265	34	580	45	6.8
1.3	320	2.0	700	95	5	265	34	580	45	6.8
1.3	320	2.0	700	95	5	265	34	580	45	6.8
1.6	520	2.2	785	160	23	335	40	1,055	49	10.5
1.6	520	2.2	800	160	22	290	40	580	49	9.5
1.6	520	2.2	800	160	22	300	40	580	49	9.5
1.7	450	2.4	985	209	7	300	35	1,055	59	10.9
1.7	450	2.4	1,000	209	6.5	255	36	580	59	10.4
1.7	450	2.4	1,000	209	6.5	265	36	580	59	10.4

Sources: *Dietary Reference Intakes for Calcium, Phosphorous, Magnesium, Vitamin D, and Fluoride* (1997); *Dietary Reference Intakes for Thiamin, Riboflavin, Niacin, Vitamin B$_6$, Folate, Vitamin B$_{12}$, Pantothenic Acid, Biotin, and Choline* (1998); *Dietary Reference Intakes for Vitamin C, Vitamin E, Selenium, and Carotenoids* (2000); *Dietary Reference Intakes for Vitamin A, Vitamin K, Arsenic, Boron, Chromium, Copper, Iodine, Iron, Manganese, Molybdenum, Nickel, Silicon, Vanadium, and Zinc* (2001); *Dietary Reference Intakes for Energy, Carbohydrate, Fiber, Fat, Fatty Acids, Cholesterol, Protein, and Amino Acids* (2002/2005); and *Dietary Reference Intakes for Calcium and Vitamin D* (2011). These reports may be accessed via www.nap.edu.

Dietary Reference Intakes (DRIs): Recommended Dietary Allowances and Adequate Intakes, Vitamins Food and Nutrition Board, Institute of Medicine, National Academies

Life Stage Group	Vitamin A (µg/d)[a]	Vitamin C (mg/d)	Vitamin D (µg/d)[b,c]	Vitamin E (mg/d)[d]	Vitamin K (µg/d)	Thiamin (mg/d)	Riboflavin (mg/d)
Infants							
0 to 6 mo	400*	40*	10	4*	2.0*	0.2*	0.3*
6 to 12 mo	500*	50*	10	5*	2.5*	0.3*	0.4*
Children							
1–3 y	**300**	**15**	**15**	**6**	30*	**0.5**	**0.5**
4–8 y	**400**	**25**	**15**	**7**	55*	**0.6**	**0.6**
Males							
9–13 y	**600**	**45**	**15**	**11**	60*	**0.9**	**0.9**
14–18 y	**900**	**75**	**15**	**15**	75*	**1.2**	**1.3**
19–30 y	**900**	**90**	**15**	**15**	120*	**1.2**	**1.3**
31–50 y	**900**	**90**	**15**	**15**	120*	**1.2**	**1.3**
51–70 y	**900**	**90**	**15**	**15**	120*	**1.2**	**1.3**
>70 y	**900**	**90**	**20**	**15**	120*	**1.2**	**1.3**
Females							
9–13 y	**600**	**45**	**15**	**11**	60*	**0.9**	**0.9**
14–18 y	**700**	**65**	**15**	**15**	75*	**1.0**	**1.0**
19–30 y	**700**	**75**	**15**	**15**	90*	**1.1**	**1.1**
31–50 y	**700**	**75**	**15**	**15**	90*	**1.1**	**1.1**
51–70 y	**700**	**75**	**15**	**15**	90*	**1.1**	**1.1**
>70 y	**700**	**75**	**20**	**15**	90*	**1.1**	**1.1**
Pregnancy							
14–18 y	**750**	**80**	**15**	**15**	75*	**1.4**	**1.4**
19–30 y	**770**	**85**	**15**	**15**	90*	**1.4**	**1.4**
31–50 y	**770**	**85**	**15**	**15**	90*	**1.4**	**1.4**
Lactation							
14–18 y	**1,200**	**115**	**15**	**19**	75*	**1.4**	**1.6**
19–30 y	**1,300**	**120**	**15**	**19**	90*	**1.4**	**1.6**
31–50 y	**1,300**	**120**	**15**	**19**	90*	**1.4**	**1.6**

Note: This table (taken from the DRI reports, see www.nap.edu) presents Recommended Dietary Allowances (RDAs) in **bold type** and Adequate Intakes (AIs) in ordinary type followed by an asterisk (*). An RDA is the average daily dietary intake level; sufficient to meet the nutrient requirements of nearly all (97–98 percent) healthy individuals in a group. It is calculated from an Estimated Average Requirement (EAR). If sufficient scientific evidence is not available to establish an EAR, and thus calculate an RDA, an AI is usually developed. For healthy breastfed infants, an AI is the mean intake. The AI for other life stage and gender groups is believed to cover the needs of all healthy individuals in the groups, but lack of data or uncertainty in the data prevent being able to specify with confidence the percentage of individuals covered by this intake.

[a]As retinol activity equivalents (RAEs). 1 RAE = 1 mg retinol, 12 mg β-carotene, 24 mg α-carotene, or 24 mg α-cryptoxanthin. The RAE for dietary provitamin A carotenoids is two-fold greater than retinol equivalents (RE), whereas the RAE for preformed vitamin A is the same as RE.

[b]As cholecalciferol. 1 µg cholecalciferol = 40 IU vitamin D.

[c]Under the assumption of minimal sunlight.

[d]As α-tocopherol. α-Tocopherol includes *RRR*-α-tocopherol, the only form of α-tocopherol that occurs naturally in foods, and the *2R*-stereoisomeric forms of α-tocopherol (*RRR*-, *RSR*-, *RRS*-, and *RSS*-α -tocopherol) that occur in fortified foods and supplements. It does not include the *2S*-stereoisomeric forms of α-tocopherol (*SRR*-, *SSR*-, *SRS*-, and *SSS*-α-tocopherol), also found in fortified foods and supplements.

[e]As niacin equivalents (NE). 1 mg of niacin = 60 mg of tryptophan; 0–6 months = preformed niacin (not NE).

Niacin (mg/d)[e]	Vitamin B$_6$ (mg/d)	Folate (µg/d)[f]	Vitamin B$_{12}$ (µg/d)	Pantothenic Acid (mg/d)	Biotin (µg/d)	Choline (mg/d)[g]
2*	0.1*	65*	0.4*	1.7*	5*	125*
4*	0.3*	80*	0.5*	1.8*	6*	150*
6	0.5	150	0.9	2*	8*	200*
8	0.6	200	1.2	3*	12*	250*
12	1.0	300	1.8	4*	20*	375*
16	1.3	400	2.4	5*	25*	550*
16	1.3	400	2.4	5*	30*	550*
16	1.3	400	2.4	5*	30*	550*
16	1.7	400	2.4[h]	5*	30*	550*
16	1.7	400	2.4[h]	5*	30*	550*
12	1.0	300	1.8	4*	20*	375*
14	1.2	400[i]	2.4	5*	25*	400*
14	1.3	400[i]	2.4	5*	30*	425*
14	1.3	400[i]	2.4	5*	30*	425*
14	1.5	400	2.4[h]	5*	30*	425*
14	1.5	400	2.4[h]	5*	30*	425*
18	1.9	600[j]	2.6	6*	30*	450*
18	1.9	600[j]	2.6	6*	30*	450*
18	1.9	600[j]	2.6	6*	30*	450*
17	2.0	500	2.8	7*	35*	550*
17	2.0	500	2.8	7*	35*	550*
17	2.0	500	2.8	7*	35*	550*

[f]As dietary folate equivalents (DFE). 1 DFE = 1 µg food folate = 0.6 µg of folic acid from fortified food or as a supplement consumed with food = 0.5 µg of a supplement taken on an empty stomach.

[g]Although AIs have been set for choline, there are few data to assess whether a dietary supply of choline is needed at all stages of the life cycle, and it may be that the choline requirement can be met by endogenous synthesis at some of these stages.

[h]Because 10 to 30 percent of older people may malabsorb food-bound B$_{12}$, it is advisable for those older than 50 years to meet their RDA mainly by consuming foods fortified with B$_{12}$ or a supplement containing B$_{12}$.

[i]In view of evidence linking folate intake with neural tube defects in the fetus, it is recommended that all women capable of becoming pregnant consume 400 µg from supplements or fortified foods in addition to intake of food folate from a varied diet.

[j]It is assumed that women will continue consuming 400 µg from supplements or fortified food until their pregnancy is confirmed and they enter prenatal care, which ordinarily occurs after the end of the periconceptional period—the critical time for formation of the neural tube.

Sources: Dietary Reference Intakes for Calcium, Phosphorous, Magnesium, Vitamin D, and Fluoride (1997); Dietary Reference Intakes for Thiamin, Riboflavin, Niacin, Vitamin B$_6$, Folate, Vitamin B$_{12}$, Pantothenic Acid, Biotin, and Choline (1998); Dietary Reference Intakes for Vitamin C, Vitamin E, Selenium, and Carotenoids (2000); Dietary Reference Intakes for Vitamin A, Vitamin K, Arsenic, Boron, Chromium, Copper, Iodine, Iron, Manganese, Molybdenum, Nickel, Silicon, Vanadium, and Zinc (2001); Dietary Reference Intakes for Water, Potassium, Sodium, Chloride, and Sulfate (2005); and Dietary Reference Intakes for Calcium and Vitamin D (2011). These reports may be accessed via www.nap.edu.

Dietary Reference Intakes (DRIs): Recommended Dietary Allowances and Adequate Intakes, Elements Food and Nutrition Board, Institute of Medicine, National Academies

Life Stage Group	Calcium (mg/d)	Chromium (µg/d)	Copper (µg/d)	Fluoride (mg/d)	Iodine (µg/d)	Iron (mg/d)	Magnesium (mg/d)	Manganese (mg/d)
Infants								
0 to 6 mo	200*	0.2*	200*	0.01*	110*	0.27*	30*	0.003*
6 to 12 mo	260*	5.5*	220*	0.5*	130*	**11**	75*	0.6*
Children								
1–3 y	**700**	11*	**340**	0.7*	**90**	**7**	**80**	1.2*
4–8 y	**1,000**	15*	**440**	1*	**90**	**10**	**130**	1.5*
Males								
9–13 y	**1,300**	25*	**700**	2*	**120**	**8**	**240**	1.9*
14–18 y	**1,300**	35*	**890**	3*	**150**	**11**	**410**	2.2*
19–30 y	**1,000**	35*	**900**	4*	**150**	**8**	**400**	2.3*
31–50 y	**1,000**	35*	**900**	4*	**150**	**8**	**420**	2.3*
51–70 y	**1,000**	30*	**900**	4*	**150**	**8**	**420**	2.3*
>70 y	**1,200**	30*	**900**	4*	**150**	**8**	**420**	2.3*
Females								
9–13 y	**1,300**	21*	**700**	2*	**120**	**8**	**240**	1.6*
14–18 y	**1,300**	24*	**890**	3*	**150**	**15**	**360**	1.6*
19–30 y	**1,000**	25*	**900**	3*	**150**	**18**	**310**	1.8*
31–50 y	**1,000**	25*	**900**	3*	**150**	**18**	**320**	1.8*
51–70 y	**1,200**	20*	**900**	3*	**150**	**8**	**320**	1.8*
>70 y	**1,200**	20*	**900**	3*	**150**	**8**	**320**	1.8*
Pregnancy								
14–18 y	**1,300**	29*	**1,000**	3*	**220**	**27**	**400**	2.0*
19–30 y	**1,000**	30*	**1,000**	3*	**220**	**27**	**350**	2.0*
31–50 y	**1,000**	30*	**1,000**	3*	**220**	**27**	**360**	2.0*
Lactation								
14–18 y	**1,300**	44*	**1,300**	3*	**290**	**10**	**360**	2.6*
19–30 y	**1,000**	45*	**1,300**	3*	**290**	**9**	**310**	2.6*
31–50 y	**1,000**	45*	**1,300**	3*	**290**	**9**	**320**	2.6*

Note: This table (taken from the DRI reports, see www.nap.edu) presents Recommended Dietary Allowances (RDAs) in **bold type** and Adequate Intakes (AIs) in ordinary type followed by an asterisk (*). An RDA is the average daily dietary intake level; sufficient to meet the nutrient requirements of nearly all (97–98 percent) healthy individuals in a group. It is calculated from an Estimated Average Requirement (EAR). If sufficient scientific evidence is not available to establish an EAR, and thus calculate an RDA, an AI is usually developed. For healthy breastfed infants, an AI is the mean intake. The AI for other life stage and gender groups is believed to cover the needs of all healthy individuals in the groups, but lack of data or uncertainty in the data prevent being able to specify with confidence the percentage of individuals covered by this intake.

Molybdenum (µg/d)	Phosphorus (mg/d)	Selenium (µg/d)	Zinc (mg/d)	Potassium (g/d)	Sodium (g/d)	Chloride (g/d)
2*	100*	15*	2*	0.4*	0.12*	0.18*
3*	275*	20*	3	0.7*	0.37*	0.57*
17	460	20	3	3.0*	1.0*	1.5*
22	500	30	5	3.8*	1.2*	1.9*
34	1,250	40	8	4.5*	1.5*	2.3*
43	1,250	55	11	4.7*	1.5*	2.3*
45	700	55	11	4.7*	1.5*	2.3*
45	700	55	11	4.7*	1.5*	2.3*
45	700	55	11	4.7*	1.3*	2.0*
45	700	55	11	4.7*	1.2*	1.8*
34	1,250	40	8	4.5*	1.5*	2.3*
43	1,250	55	9	4.7*	1.5*	2.3*
45	700	55	8	4.7*	1.5*	2.3*
45	700	55	8	4.7*	1.5*	2.3*
45	700	55	8	4.7*	1.3*	2.0*
45	700	55	8	4.7*	1.2*	1.8*
50	1,250	60	12	4.7*	1.5*	2.3*
50	700	60	11	4.7*	1.5*	2.3*
50	700	60	11	4.7*	1.5*	2.3*
50	1,250	70	13	5.1*	1.5*	2.3*
50	700	70	12	5.1*	1.5*	2.3*
50	700	70	12	5.1*	1.5*	2.3*

Sources: Dietary Reference Intakes for Calcium, Phosphorous, Magnesium, Vitamin D, and Fluoride (1997); Dietary Reference Intakes for Thiamin, Riboflavin, Niacin, Vitamin B₆, Folate, Vitamin B₁₂, Pantothenic Acid, Biotin, and Choline (1998); Dietary Reference Intakes for Vitamin C, Vitamin E, Selenium, and Carotenoids (2000); and Dietary Reference Intakes for Vitamin A, Vitamin K, Arsenic, Boron, Chromium, Copper, Iodine, Iron, Manganese, Molybdenum, Nickel, Silicon, Vanadium, and Zinc (2001); Dietary Reference Intakes for Water, Potassium, Sodium, Chloride, and Sulfate (2005); and Dietary Reference Intakes for Calcium and Vitamin D (2011). These reports may be accessed via www.nap.edu.

Dietary Reference Intakes (DRIs): Recommended Dietary Allowances and Adequate Intakes, Total Water and Macronutrients Food and Nutrition Board, Institute of Medicine, National Academies

Life Stage Group	Total Water[a] (L/d)	Carbohydrate (g/d)	Total Fiber (g/d)	Fat (g/d)	Linoleic Acid (g/d)	α-Linolenic Acid (g/d)	Protein[b] (g/d)
Infants							
0 to 6 mo	0.7*	60*	ND	31*	4.4*	0.5*	9.1*
6 to 12 mo	0.8*	95*	ND	30*	4.6*	0.5*	**11.0**
Children							
1–3 y	1.3*	**130**	19*	ND[c]	7*	0.7*	**13**
4–8 y	1.7*	**130**	25*	ND	10*	0.9*	**19**
Males							
9–13 y	2.4*	**130**	31*	ND	12*	1.2*	**34**
14–18 y	3.3*	**130**	38*	ND	16*	1.6*	**52**
19–30 y	3.7*	**130**	38*	ND	17*	1.6*	**56**
31–50 y	3.7*	**130**	38*	ND	17*	1.6*	**56**
51–70 y	3.7*	**130**	30*	ND	14*	1.6*	**56**
>70 y	3.7*	**130**	30*	ND	14*	1.6*	**56**
Females							
9–13 y	2.1*	**130**	26*	ND	10*	1.0*	**34**
14–18 y	2.3*	**130**	26*	ND	11*	1.1*	**46**
19–30 y	2.7*	**130**	25*	ND	12*	1.1*	**46**
31–50 y	2.7*	**130**	25*	ND	12*	1.1*	**46**
51–70 y	2.7*	**130**	21*	ND	11*	1.1*	**46**
>70 y	2.7*	**130**	21*	ND	11*	1.1*	**46**
Pregnancy							
14–18 y	3.0*	**175**	28*	ND	13*	1.4*	**71**
19–30 y	3.0*	**175**	28*	ND	13*	1.4*	**71**
31–50 y	3.0*	**175**	28*	ND	13*	1.4*	**71**
Lactation							
14–18	3.8*	**210**	29*	ND	13*	1.3*	**71**
19–30 y	3.8*	**210**	29*	ND	13*	1.3*	**71**
31–50 y	3.8*	**210**	29*	ND	13*	1.3*	**71**

Note: This table (take from the DRI reports, see www.nap.edu) presents Recommended Dietary Allowances (RDA) in **bold type** and Adequate Intakes (AI) in ordinary type followed by an asterisk (*). An RDA is the average daily dietary intake level; sufficient to meet the nutrient requirements of nearly all (97–98 percent) healthy individuals in a group. It is calculated from an Estimated Average Requirement (EAR). If sufficient scientific evidence is not available to establish an EAR, and thus calculate an RDA, an AI is usually developed. For healthy breastfed infants, an AI is the mean intake. The AI for other life stage and gender groups is believed to cover the needs of all healthy individuals in the groups, but lack of data or uncertainty in the data prevent being able to specify with confidence the percentage of individuals covered by this intake.

[a]*Total* water includes all water contained in food, beverages, and drinking water.
[b]Based on g protein per kg of body weight for the reference body weight, e.g., for adults 0.8 g/kg body weight for the reference body weight.
[c]Not determined.
Source: Dietary Reference Intakes for Energy, Carbohydrate, Fiber, Fat, Fatty Acids, Cholesterol, Protein, and Amino Acids (2002/2005) and *Dietary Reference Intakes for Water, Potassium, Sodium, Chloride, and Sulfate* (2005). The report may be accessed via www.nap.edu.

Dietary Reference Intakes (DRIs): Acceptable Macronutrient Distribution Ranges
Food and Nutrition Board, Institute of Medicine, National Academies

Macronutrient	Range (percent of energy)		
	Children, 1–3 y	Children, 4–18 y	Adults
Fat	30–40	25–35	20–35
n-6 polyunsaturated fatty acids[a] (linoleic acid)	5–10	5–10	5–10
n-3 polyunsaturated fatty acids[a] (α-linolenic acid)	0.6–1.2	0.6–1.2	0.6–1.2
Carbohydrate	45–65	45–65	45–65
Protein	5–20	10–30	10–35

[a]Approximately 10 percent of the total can come from longer-chain n-3 or n-6 fatty acids.

Source: Dietary Reference Intakes for Energy, Carbohydrate, Fiber, Fat, Fatty Acids, Cholesterol, Protein, and Amino Acids (2002/2005). The report may be accessed via www.nap.edu.

Dietary Reference Intakes (DRIs): Acceptable Macronutrient Distribution Ranges
Food and Nutrition Board, Institute of Medicine, National Academies

Macronutrient	Recommendation
Dietary cholesterol	As low as possible while consuming a nutritionally adequate diet
Trans fatty Acids	As low as possible while consuming a nutritionally adequate diet
Saturated fatty acids	As low as possible while consuming a nutritionally adequate diet
Added sugars[a]	Limit to no more than 25 % of total energy

[a]Not a recommended intake. A daily intake of added sugars that individuals should aim for to achieve a healthful diet was not set.

Source: Dietary Reference Intakes for Energy, Carbohydrate, Fiber, Fat, Fatty Acids, Cholesterol, Protein, and Amino Acids (2002/2005). The report may be accessed via www.nap.edu.

Dietary Reference Intakes (DRIs): Tolerable Upper Intake Levels, Vitamins
Food and Nutrition Board, Institute of Medicine, National Academies

Life Stage Group	Vitamin A (µg/d)[a]	Vitamin C (mg/d)	Vitamin D (µg/d)	Vitamin E (mg/d)[b,c]	Vitamin K	Thiamin	Riboflavin
Infants							
0 to 6 mo	600	ND[e]	25	ND	ND	ND	ND
6 to 12 mo	600	ND	38	ND	ND	ND	ND
Children							
1–3 y	600	400	63	200	ND	ND	ND
4–8 y	900	650	75	300	ND	ND	ND
Males							
9–13 y	1,700	1,200	100	600	ND	ND	ND
14–18 y	2,800	1,800	100	800	ND	ND	ND
19–30 y	3,000	2,000	100	1,000	ND	ND	ND
31–50 y	3,000	2,000	100	1,000	ND	ND	ND
51–70 y	3,000	2,000	100	1,000	ND	ND	ND
>70 y	3,000	2,000	100	1,000	ND	ND	ND
Females							
9–13 y	1,700	1,200	100	600	ND	ND	ND
14–18 y	2,800	1,800	100	800	ND	ND	ND
19–30 y	3,000	2,000	100	1,000	ND	ND	ND
31–50 y	3,000	2,000	100	1,000	ND	ND	ND
51–70 y	3,000	2,000	100	1,000	ND	ND	ND
>70 y	3,000	2,000	100	1,000	ND	ND	ND
Pregnancy							
14–18 y	2,800	1,800	100	800	ND	ND	ND
19–30 y	3,000	2,000	100	1,000	ND	ND	ND
31–50 y	3,000	2,000	100	1,000	ND	ND	ND
Lactation							
14–18 y	2,800	1,800	100	800	ND	ND	ND
19–30 y	3,000	2,000	100	1,000	ND	ND	ND
31–50 y	3,000	2,000	100	1,000	ND	ND	ND

Note: Tolerable Upper Intake Level (UL) is the highest level of daily nutrient intake that is likely to pose no risk of adverse health effects to almost all individuals in the general population. Unless otherwise specified, the UL represents total intake from food, water, and supplements. Due to a lack of suitable data, ULs could not be established for vitamin K, thiamin, riboflavin, vitamin B_{12}, pantothenic acid, biotin, and carotenoids. In the absence of a UL, extra caution may be warranted in consuming levels above recommended intakes. Members of the general population should be advised not to routinely exceed the UL. The UL is not meant to apply to individuals who are treated with the nutrient under medical supervision or to individuals with predisposing conditions that modify their sensitivity to the nutrient.
[a]As preformed vitamin A only.
[b]As α-tocopherol; applies to any form of supplemental α-tocopherol.

Niacin (mg/d)[c]	Vitamin B$_6$ (mg/d)	Folate (µg/d)[c]	Vitamin B$_{12}$	Pantothenic Acid	Biotin	Choline (g/d)	Carotenoids[d]
ND	ND	ND	ND	ND	ND	ND	ND
ND	ND	ND	ND	ND	ND	ND	ND
10	30	300	ND	ND	ND	1.0	ND
15	40	400	ND	ND	ND	1.0	ND
20	60	600	ND	ND	ND	2.0	ND
30	80	800	ND	ND	ND	3.0	ND
35	100	1,000	ND	ND	ND	3.5	ND
35	100	1,000	ND	ND	ND	3.5	ND
35	100	1,000	ND	ND	ND	3.5	ND
35	100	1,000	ND	ND	ND	3.5	ND
20	60	600	ND	ND	ND	2.0	ND
30	80	800	ND	ND	ND	3.0	ND
35	100	1,000	ND	ND	ND	3.5	ND
35	100	1,000	ND	ND	ND	3.5	ND
35	100	1,000	ND	ND	ND	3.5	ND
35	100	1,000	ND	ND	ND	3.5	ND
30	80	800	ND	ND	ND	3.0	ND
35	100	1,000	ND	ND	ND	3.5	ND
35	100	1,000	ND	ND	ND	3.5	ND
30	80	800	ND	ND	ND	3.0	ND
35	100	1,000	ND	ND	ND	3.5	ND
35	100	1,000	ND	ND	ND	3.5	ND

[c] The ULs for vitamin E, niacin, and folate apply to synthetic forms obtained from supplements, fortified foods, or a combination of the two.
[d] β-Carotene supplements are advised only to serve as a provitamin A source for individuals at risk of vitamin A deficiency.
[e] ND = Not determinable due to lack of data of adverse effects in this age group and concern with regard to lack of ability to handle excess amounts. Source of intake should be from food only to prevent high levels of intake.
Sources: Dietary Reference Intakes for Calcium, Phosphorous, Magnesium, Vitamin D, and Fluoride (1997); Dietary Reference Intakes for Thiamin, Riboflavin, Niacin, Vitamin B$_6$, Folate, Vitamin B$_{12}$, Pantothenic Acid, Biotin, and Choline (1998); Dietary Reference Intakes for Vitamin C, Vitamine E, Selenium, and Carotenoids (2000); Dietary Reference Intakes for Vitamin A, Vitamin K, Arsenic, Boron, Chromium, Copper, Iodine, Iron, Manganese, Molybdenum, Nickel, Silicon, Vanadium, and Zinc (2001); and Dietary Reference Intakes for Calcium and Vitamin D (2011). These reports may be accessed via www.nap.edu.

Dietary Reference Intakes (DRIs): Tolerable Upper Intake Levels, Elements
Food and Nutrition Board, Institute of Medicine, National Academies

Life Stage Group	Arsenic[a]	Boron (mg/d)	Calcium (mg/d)	Chromium	Copper (µg/d)	Fluoride (mg/d)	Iodine (µg/d)	Iron mg/d)	Magnesium (mg/d)[b]
Infants									
0 to 6 mo	ND[e]	ND	1,000	ND	ND	0.7	ND	40	ND
6 to 12 mo	ND	ND	1,500	ND	ND	0.9	ND	40	ND
Children									
1–3 y	ND	3	2,500	ND	1,000	1.3	200	40	65
4–8 y	ND	6	2,500	ND	3,000	2.2	300	40	110
Males									
9–13 y	ND	11	3,000	ND	5,000	10	600	40	350
14–18 y	ND	17	3,000	ND	8,000	10	900	45	350
19–30 y	ND	20	2,500	ND	10,000	10	1,100	45	350
31–50 y	ND	20	2,500	ND	10,000	10	1,100	45	350
51–70 y	ND	20	2,000	ND	10,000	10	1,100	45	350
>70 y	ND	20	2,000	ND	10,000	10	1,100	45	350
Females									
9–13 y	ND	11	3,000	ND	5,000	10	600	40	350
14–18 y	ND	17	3,000	ND	8,000	10	900	45	350
19–30 y	ND	20	2,500	ND	10,000	10	1,100	45	350
31–50 y	ND	20	2,500	ND	10,000	10	1,100	45	350
51–70 y	ND	20	2,000	ND	10,000	10	1,100	45	350
>70 y	ND	20	2,000	ND	10,000	10	1,100	45	350
Pregnancy									
14–18 y	ND	17	3,000	ND	8,000	10	900	45	350
19–30 y	ND	20	2,500	ND	10,000	10	1,100	45	350
31–50 y	ND	20	2,500	ND	10,000	10	1,100	45	350
Lactation									
14–18 y	ND	17	3,000	ND	8,000	10	900	45	350
19–30 y	ND	20	2,500	ND	10,000	10	1,100	45	350
31–50 y	ND	20	2,500	ND	10,000	10	1,100	45	350

Note: A Tolerable Upper Intake Level (UL) is the highest level of daily nutrient intake that is likely to pose no risk of adverse health effects to almost all individuals in the general population. Unless otherwise specified, the UL represents total intake from food, water, and supplements. Due to a lack of suitable data, ULs could not be established for vitamin K, thiamin, riboflavin, vitamin B₁₂, pantothenic acid, biotin, and carotenoids. In the absence of a UL, extra caution may be warranted in consuming levels above recommended intakes. Members of the general population should be advised not to routinely exceed the UL. The UL is not meant to apply to individuals who are treated with the nutrient under medical supervision or to individuals with predisposing conditions that modify their sensitivity to the nutrient.
[a]Although the UL was not determined for arsenic, there is no justification for adding arsenic to food or supplements.
[b]The ULs for magnesium represent intake from a pharmacological agent only and do not include intake from food and water.
[c]Although silicon has not been shown to cause adverse effects in humans, there is no justification for adding silicon to supplements.

Manganese (mg/d)	Molybdenum (μg/d)	Nickel (mg/d)	Phosphorus (g/d)	Selenium (μg/d)	Silicon[c]	Vanadium (mg/d)[d]	Zinc (mg/d)	Sodium (g/d)	Chloride (g/d)
ND	ND	ND	ND	45	ND	ND	4	ND	ND
ND	ND	ND	ND	60	ND	ND	5	ND	ND
2	300	0.2	3	90	ND	ND	7	1.5	2.3
3	600	0.3	3	150	ND	ND	12	1.9	2.9
6	1,100	0.6	4	280	ND	ND	23	2.2	3.4
9	1,700	1.0	4	400	ND	ND	34	2.3	3.6
11	2,000	1.0	4	400	ND	1.8	40	2.3	3.6
11	2,000	1.0	4	400	ND	1.8	40	2.3	3.6
11	2,000	1.0	4	400	ND	1.8	40	2.3	3.6
11	2,000	1.0	3	400	ND	1.8	40	2.3	3.6
6	1,100	0.6	4	280	ND	ND	23	2.2	3.4
9	1,700	1.0	4	400	ND	ND	34	2.3	3.6
11	2,000	1.0	4	400	ND	1.8	40	2.3	3.6
11	2,000	1.0	4	400	ND	1.8	40	2.3	3.6
11	2,000	1.0	4	400	ND	1.8	40	2.3	3.6
11	2,000	1.0	3	400	ND	1.8	40	2.3	3.6
9	1,700	1.0	3.5	400	ND	ND	34	2.3	3.6
11	2,000	1.0	3.5	400	ND	ND	40	2.3	3.6
11	2,000	1.0	3.5	400	ND	ND	40	2.3	3.6
9	1,700	1.0	4	400	ND	ND	34	2.3	3.6
11	2,000	1.0	4	400	ND	ND	40	2.3	3.6
11	2,000	1.0	4	400	ND	ND	40	2.3	3.6

[d]Although vanadium in food has not been shown to cause adverse effects in humans, there is no justification for adding vanadium to food and vanadium supplements should be used with caution. The UL is based on adverse effects in laboratory animals and this data could be used to set a UL for adults but not children and adolescents.

[e]ND = Not determinable due to lack of data of adverse effects in this age group and concern with regard to lack of ability to handle excess amounts. Source of intake should be from food only to prevent high levels of intake.

Sources: Dietary Reference Intakes for Calcium, Phosphorous, Magnesium, Vitamin D, and Fluoride (1997); Dietary Reference Intakes for Thiamin, Riboflavin, Niacin, Vitamin B₆, Folate, Vitamin B₁₂ Pantothenic Acid, Biotin, and Choline (1998); Dietary Reference Intakes for Vitamin C, Vitamin E, Selenium, and Carotenoids (2000); Dietary Reference Intakes for Vitamin A, Vitamin K, Arsenic, Boron, Chromium, Copper, Iodine, Iron, Manganese, Molybdenum, Nickel, Silicon, Vanadium, and Zinc (2001); Dietary Reference Intakes for Water, Potassium, Sodium, Chloride, and Sulfate (2005); and Dietary Reference Intakes for Calcium and Vitamin D (2011). These reports may be accessed via www.nap.edu.

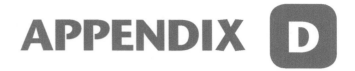

APPENDIX D

Anthropometric Measures

Height & Weight Table For Women*			
Height Feet Inches	Small Frame	Medium Frame	Large Frame
4' 10"	102–111	109–121	118–131
4' 11"	103–113	111–123	120–134
5' 0"	104–115	113–126	122–137
5' 1"	106–118	115–129	125–140
5' 2"	108–121	118–132	128–143
5' 3"	111–124	121–135	131–147
5' 4"	114–127	124–138	134–151
5' 5"	117–130	127–141	137–155
5' 6"	120–133	130–144	140–159
5' 7"	123–136	133–147	143–163
5' 8"	126–139	136–150	146–167
5' 9"	129–142	139–153	149–170
5' 10"	132–145	142–156	152–173
5' 11"	135–148	145–159	155–176
6' 0"	138–151	148–162	158–179

Weights at ages 25–59 based on lowest mortality. Weight in pounds according to frame (in indoor clothing weighing 3 lbs.; shoes with 1" heels)

*Note: This information is not intended to be a substitute for professional medical advice and should not be regarded as an endorsement or approval of any product or service.

Source: From http://www.metlife2000.org by Metropolitan Life Insurance Company. Copyright © 1996, 1999 by Metropolitan Life Insurance Company.

Weight Categories as an Indicator of Nutrition Status

>120	Obese
110–120	Overweight
90–109	Adequate
80–89	Mildly undernourished
70–79	Moderately undernourished
<70	Severely undernourished

Height & Weight Table For Men*

Height Feet Inches	Small Frame	Medium Frame	Large Frame
5' 2"	128–134	131–141	138–150
5' 3"	130–136	133–143	140–153
5' 4"	132–138	135–145	142–156
5' 5"	134–140	137–148	144–160
5' 6"	136–142	139–151	146–164
5' 7"	138–145	142–154	149–168
5' 8"	140–148	145–157	152–172
5' 9"	142–151	148–160	155–176
5' 10"	144–154	151–163	158–180
5' 11"	146–157	154–166	161–184
6' 0"	149–160	157–170	164–188
6' 1"	152–164	160–174	168–192
6' 2"	155–168	164–178	172–197
6' 3"	158–172	167–182	176–202
6' 4"	162–176	171–187	181–207

Weights at ages 25–59 based on lowest mortality. Weight in pounds according to frame (in indoor clothing weighing 5 lbs.; shoes with 1" heels)
*Note: This information is not intended to be a substitute for professional medical advice and should not be regarded as an endorsement or approval of any product or service.
Source: From http://www.metlife2000.org by Metropolitan Life Insurance Company. Copyright © 1996, 1999 by Metropolitan Life Insurance Company.

Weight Categories as an Indicator of Nutrition Status

>120	Obese
110–120	Overweight
90–109	Adequate
80–89	Mildly undernourished
70–79	Moderately undernourished
<70	Severely undernourished

Body Mass Index Table for Adults

	Normal						Overweight					Obese										Extreme Obesity															
BMI	19	20	21	22	23	24	25	26	27	28	29	30	31	32	33	34	35	36	37	38	39	40	41	42	43	44	45	46	47	48	49	50	51	52	53	54
Height (inches)																		Body Weight (pounds)																		
58	91	96	100	105	110	115	119	124	129	134	138	143	148	153	158	162	167	172	177	181	186	191	196	201	205	210	215	220	224	229	234	239	244	248	253	258
59	94	99	104	109	114	119	124	128	133	138	143	148	153	158	163	168	173	178	183	188	193	198	203	208	212	217	222	227	232	237	242	247	252	257	262	267
60	97	102	107	112	118	123	128	133	138	143	148	153	158	163	168	174	179	184	189	194	199	204	209	215	220	225	230	235	240	245	250	255	261	266	271	276
61	100	106	111	116	122	127	132	137	143	148	153	158	164	169	174	180	185	190	195	201	206	211	217	222	227	232	238	243	248	254	259	264	269	275	280	285
62	104	109	115	120	126	131	136	142	147	153	158	164	169	175	180	186	191	196	202	207	213	218	224	229	235	240	246	251	256	262	267	273	278	284	289	295
63	107	113	118	124	130	135	141	146	152	158	163	169	175	180	186	191	197	203	208	214	220	225	231	237	242	248	254	259	265	270	278	282	287	293	299	304
64	110	116	122	128	134	140	145	151	157	163	169	174	180	186	192	197	204	209	215	221	227	232	238	244	250	256	262	267	273	279	285	291	296	302	308	314
65	114	120	126	132	138	144	150	156	162	168	174	180	186	192	198	204	210	216	222	228	234	240	246	252	258	264	270	276	282	288	294	300	306	312	318	324
66	118	124	130	136	142	148	155	161	167	173	179	186	192	198	204	210	216	223	229	235	241	247	253	260	266	272	278	284	291	297	303	309	315	322	328	334
67	121	127	134	140	146	153	159	166	172	178	185	191	198	204	211	217	223	230	236	242	249	255	261	268	274	280	287	293	299	306	312	319	325	331	338	344
68	125	131	138	144	151	158	164	171	177	184	190	197	203	210	216	223	230	236	243	249	256	262	269	276	282	289	295	302	308	315	322	328	335	341	348	354
69	128	135	142	149	155	162	169	176	182	189	196	203	209	216	223	230	236	243	250	257	263	270	277	284	291	297	304	311	318	324	331	338	345	351	358	365
70	132	139	146	153	160	167	174	181	188	195	202	209	216	222	229	236	243	250	257	264	271	278	285	292	299	306	313	320	327	334	341	348	355	362	369	376
71	136	143	150	157	165	172	179	186	193	200	208	215	222	229	236	243	250	257	265	272	279	286	293	301	308	315	322	329	338	343	351	358	365	372	379	386
72	140	147	154	162	169	177	184	191	199	206	213	221	228	235	242	250	258	265	272	279	287	294	302	309	316	324	331	338	346	353	361	368	375	383	390	397
73	144	151	159	166	174	182	189	197	204	212	219	227	235	242	250	257	265	272	280	288	295	302	310	318	325	333	340	348	355	363	371	378	386	393	401	408
74	148	155	163	171	179	186	194	202	210	218	225	233	241	249	256	264	272	280	287	295	303	311	319	326	334	342	350	358	365	373	381	389	396	404	412	420
75	152	160	168	176	184	192	200	208	216	224	232	240	248	256	264	272	279	287	295	303	311	319	327	335	343	351	359	367	375	383	391	399	407	415	423	431
76	156	164	172	180	189	197	205	213	221	230	238	246	254	263	271	279	287	295	304	312	320	328	336	344	353	361	369	377	385	394	402	410	418	426	435	443

Source: Adapted from Clinical Guidelines on the Identification, Evaluation, and Treatment of Overweight and Obesity in Adults: The Evidence Report.
Note: BMI Categories for Adults:
  - Underweight = <18.5
  - Normal weight = 18.5–24.9
  - Overweight = 25–29.9
  - Class 1 Obesity 30–34.9
  - Class 2 Obesity 35–39.9
  - Class 3 Obesity >BMI of 40 or greater

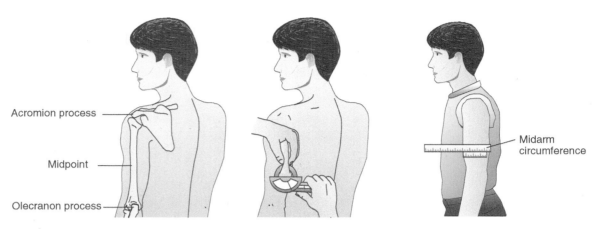

Acromion process

Midpoint

Olecranon process

Midarm circumference

The Triceps fatfold measurement together with the midarm circumference measurement can be used to calculate the midarm muscle circumference, a measure of lean body mass. The percentile standards are on Appendix page 313.

A. Find the midpoint of the arm:

1. Ask the subject to bend his or her arm at the elbow and lay the hand across the stomach. (If he or she is right-handed, measure the left arm, and vice versa.)

2. Feel the shoulder to locate the acromion process. It helps to slide your fingers along the clavicle to find the acromion process. The olecranon process is the tip of the elbow.

3. Place a measuring tape from the acromion process to the tip of the elbow. Divide this measurement by 2, and mark the midpoint of the arm with a pen.

B. Measure the fatfold:

1. Ask the subject to let his or her arm hang loosely to the side.

2. Grasp the fold of skin and subcutaneous fat between the thumb and forefinger slightly above the midpoint mark. Gently pull the skin away from the underlying muscle. (This step takes a lot of practice. If you want to be sure you don't have muscle as well as fat, ask the subject to contract and relax the muscle. You should be able to feel if you are pinching muscle.)

1. Place the calipers over the fatfold at the midpoint mark, and read the measurement to the nearest 1.0 millimeter in two to three seconds. (If using plastic calipers, align pressure lines, and read the measurement to the nearest 1.0 millimeter in two to three seconds.)

4. Repeat steps 2 and 3 twice more. Add the three readings, and then divide by 3 to find the average.

5. Ask the subject to let his or her arm hang loosely to the side. Place the measuring tape horizontally around the arm at the midpoint mark. This measurement is the midarm circumference. Use the following equation to calculate the midarm muscle circumference: Midarm muscle circumference (cm) = midarm circumference (cm) − [0.314[a] × triceps fatfold (mm)].

[a]This factor converts the fatfold measurement to a circumference measurement and millimeters to centimeters.

Triceps Fatfold Percentiles (Millimeters)

Age	Male					Female				
	5TH	25TH	50TH	75TH	95TH	5TH	25TH	50TH	75TH	95TH
1–1.9	6	8	10	12	16	6	8	10	12	16
2–2.9	6	8	10	12	15	7	9	10	12	16
3–3.9	6	8	10	11	15	7	9	11	12	15
4–4.9	6	8	9	11	14	6	8	10	12	16
5–5.9	6	8	9	11	15	6	8	10	12	18
6–6.9	5	7	8	10	16	6	8	10	12	16
7–7.9	5	7	9	12	17	6	9	11	13	18
8–8.9	5	7	8	10	16	8	9	12	15	24
9–9.9	6	7	10	13	18	7	10	13	16	22
10–10.9	6	8	10	14	21	7	10	12	17	27
11–11.9	6	8	11	16	24	8	10	13	18	28
12–12.9	6	8	11	14	28	8	11	14	18	27
13–13.9	5	7	10	14	26	9	12	15	21	30
14–14.9	4	7	9	14	24	8	13	16	21	28
15–15.9	4	6	8	11	24	10	12	17	21	32
16–16.9	4	6	8	12	22	10	15	18	22	31
17–17.9	5	6	8	12	19	10	13	19	24	37
18–18.9	4	6	9	13	24	10	15	18	22	30
19–24.9	4	7	10	15	22	10	14	18	24	34
25–34.9	5	8	12	16	24	12	16	21	27	37
35–44.9	5	8	12	16	23	12	18	23	29	38
45–54.9	6	8	12	15	25	12	20	25	30	40
55–64.9	5	8	11	14	22	12	20	25	31	38
65–74.9	4	8	11	15	22	12	18	24	29	36

Note: If measurements fall between the percentiles shown here, the percentile can be estimated from the information in this table. For example, a measurement of 7 millimeters for a 27-year-old male would be about the 20th percentile.
Source: Adapted from A. R. Frisancho, New norms of upper limb fat and muscle areas for assessment of nutritional status. *American Journal of Clinical Nutrition* 34 (1981). 2540–2545.

Midarm Muscle Circumference Percentiles (Centimeters)

Age	Male					Female				
	5TH	25TH	50TH	75TH	95TH	5TH	25TH	50TH	75TH	95TH
1–1.9	11.0	11.9	12.7	13.5	14.7	10.5	11.7	12.4	13.9	14.3
2–2.9	11.1	12.2	13.0	14.0	15.0	11.1	11.9	12.6	13.3	14.7
3–3.9	11.7	13.1	13.7	14.3	15.3	11.3	12.4	13.2	14.0	15.2
4–4.9	12.3	13.3	14.1	14.8	15.9	11.5	12.8	13.6	14.4	15.7
5–5.9	12.8	14.0	14.7	15.4	16.9	12.5	13.4	14.2	15.1	16.5
6–6.9	13.1	14.2	15.1	16.1	17.7	13.0	13.8	14.5	15.4	17.1
7–7.9	13.7	15.1	16.0	16.8	19.0	12.9	14.2	15.1	16.0	17.6
8–8.9	14.0	15.4	16.2	17.0	18.7	13.8	15.1	16.0	17.1	19.4
9–9.9	15.1	16.1	17.0	18.3	20.2	14.7	15.8	16.7	18.0	19.8
10–10.9	15.6	16.6	18.0	19.1	22.1	14.8	15.9	17.0	18.0	19.7
11–11.9	15.9	17.3	18.3	19.5	23.0	15.0	17.1	18.1	19.6	22.3
12–12.9	16.7	18.2	19.5	21.0	24.1	16.2	18.0	19.1	20.1	22.0
13–13.9	17.2	19.6	21.1	22.6	24.5	16.9	18.3	19.8	21.1	24.0
14–14.9	18.9	21.2	22.3	24.0	26.4	17.4	19.0	20.1	21.6	24.7
15–15.9	19.9	21.8	23.7	25.4	27.2	17.5	18.9	20.2	21.5	24.4
16–16.9	21.3	23.4	24.9	26.9	29.6	17.0	19.0	20.2	21.6	24.9
17–17.9	22.4	24.5	25.8	27.3	31.2	17.5	19.4	20.5	22.1	25.7
18–18.9	22.6	25.2	26.4	28.3	32.4	17.4	19.1	20.2	21.5	24.5
19–24.9	23.8	25.7	27.3	28.9	32.1	17.9	19.5	20.7	22.1	24.9
25–34.9	24.3	26.4	27.9	29.8	32.6	18.3	19.9	21.2	22.8	26.4
35–44.9	24.7	26.9	28.6	30.2	32.7	18.6	20.5	21.8	23.6	27.2
45–54.9	23.9	26.5	28.1	30.0	32.6	18.7	20.6	22.0	23.8	27.4
55–64.9	23.6	26.0	27.8	29.5	32.0	18.7	20.9	22.5	24.4	28.0
65–74.9	22.3	25.1	26.8	28.4	30.6	18.5	20.8	22.5	24.4	27.9

Source: Adapted from A. R. Frisancho, New norms of upper limb fat and muscle areas for assessment of nutritional status, *American Journal of Clinical Nutrition* 34 (1981): 2540–2545.

CDC Growth Charts: United States

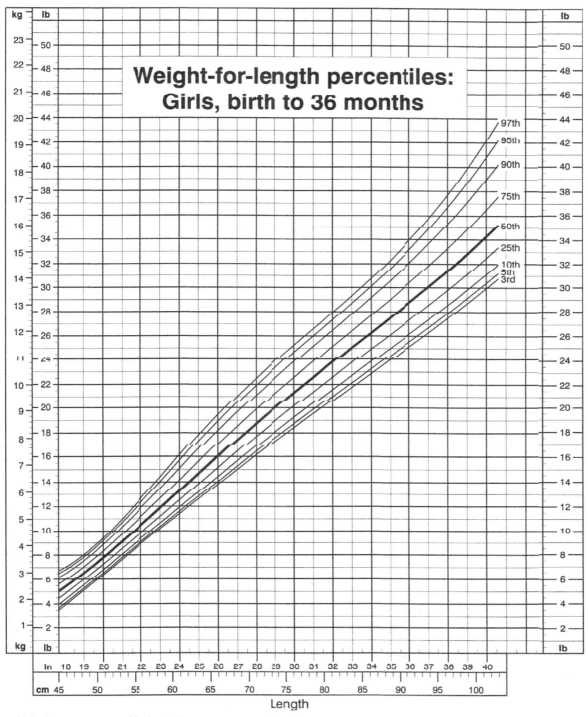

**Weight-for-length percentiles:
Girls, birth to 36 months**

Length

Published May 30, 2000 (modified 6/8/00).
Source: Developed by the National Center for Health Statistics In collaboration with the National Center for Chronic Disease Prevention and Health Promotion (2000).

CDC Growth Charts: United States

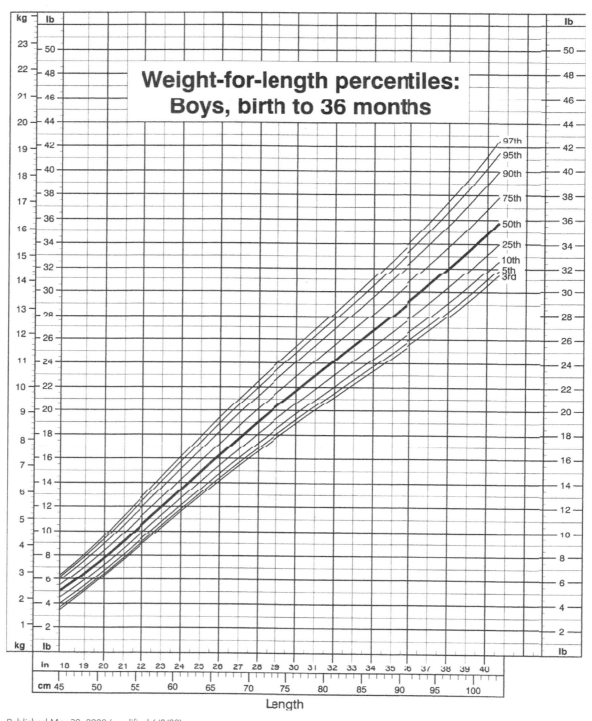

Weight-for-length percentiles:
Boys, birth to 36 months

Length

Published May 30, 2000 (modified 6/8/00).
Source: Developed by the National Center for Health Statistics in collaboration with the National Center for Chronic Disease Prevention and Health Promotion (2000).

CDC Growth Charts: United States

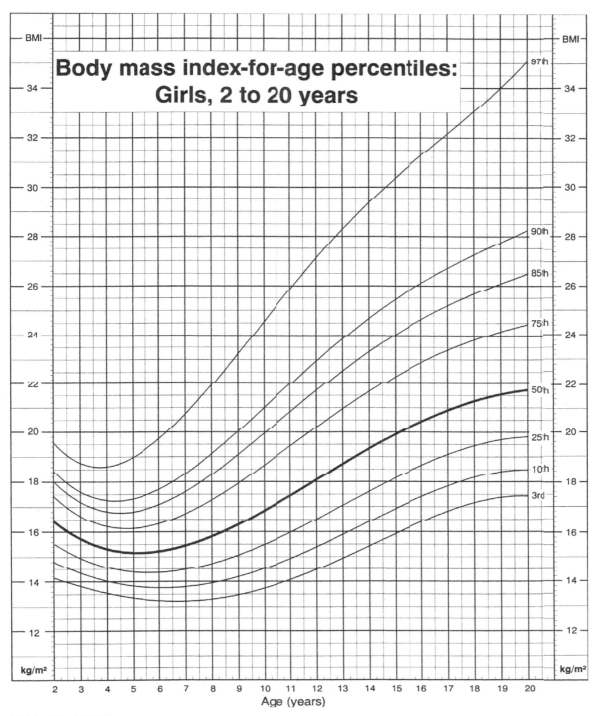

Body mass index-for-age percentiles: Girls, 2 to 20 years

Published May 30, 2000.
Source: Developed by the National Center for Health Statistics in collaboration with the National Center for Chronic Disease Prevention and Health Promotion (2000).
Note: BMI Categories for ages 2–20:
- Underweight (≤ 15 percentile)
- Overweight (≥ 85 percentile)
- Obese (≥ 95 percentile)

CDC Growth Charts: United States

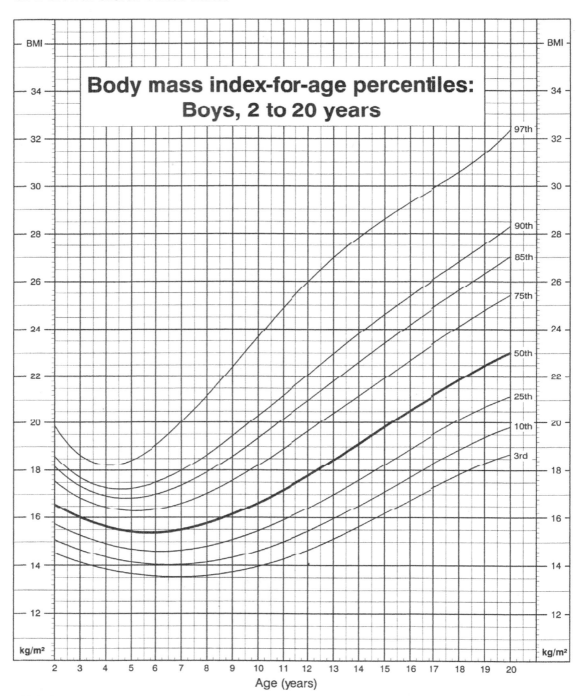

Published May 30, 2000.
Source: Developed by the National Center for Health Statistics in collaboration with the National Center for Chronic Disease Prevention and Health Promotion (2000).
Note: BMI Categories for ages 2–20:
- Underweight (≤ 15 percentile)
- Overweight (≥ 85 percentile)
- Obese (≥ 95 percentile)

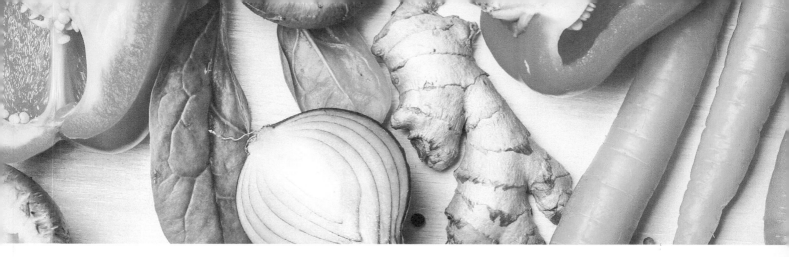

Culinary Nutrition Glossary

AAP The Association of the American Academy of Pediatrics.

Absorption The transport of nutrients through the wall of the intestines.

Accutane A brand of isotretinoin that may be prescribed to treat acne. It works by inhibiting the glands that produce the skin's natural oil (the sebaceous glands).

Active transport The movement of molecules across a cellular membrane from a lower to a higher concentration, which requires the use of energy.

Adequate Intake Nutrient intake goals for healthy individuals that are derived from the Estimated Average Requirements. They are set when insufficient scientific data is available to establish the RDA value.

ADHD Attention deficit hyperactivity disorder.

Adipose tissue The storage center for fats in the body.

Adolescence The period between puberty and adulthood in human development, which extends over the teen years and ends when the age of maturity is reached.

Adulthood The time in your life when physical growth has stopped and full development is reached.

Aerobic activity An activity that requires the presence of oxygen.

Alcohol A nonessential nutrient that yields 7 calories per gram and contains the intoxicating ingredient ethanol or ethyl alcohol.

Alpha-lactalbumin A protein found in breast milk.

Amenorrhea the absence of the menstrual cycle.

Academy of Nutrition and Dietetics (AND) The national association responsible for approving undergraduate, graduate, and post graduate programs in the field of nutrition.

Amino acids The building blocks of protein.

Amylopectin The part of a starch molecule that is made up of a branched chain of glucose molecules.

Amylose Part of a starch molecule made up of a linear chain of glucose molecules.

Anabolism The synthesis of complex substances from simpler ones.

Anaerobic activity An activity that does not require the presence of oxygen.

Ancillary organs Organs that assist in the digestive process. These include the liver, gall bladder, and the pancreas.

Anorexia nervosa (AN) The eating disorder is characterized by the refusal to maintain a minimally normal body weight in the context of age, sex development trajectory, and physical health. Self-starvation is imposed, and a distorted perception of body weight and shape occurs.

Anthropometry The use of body measures in studying body composition and development.

Antibody The part of the body's immune system that helps to destroy or inactivate foreign substances.

Anticoagulant A substance that prevents the clotting of blood.

Antioxidant A substance acting as a scavenger of free oxygen, such as vitamin E, which can reduce the activity of ROS.

Anus The opening at the end of the gastrointestinal tract where waste products are excreted.

Appetite A desire for food or drink.

Atherosclerosis A disease where there is clogging, narrowing, and hardening of the body's large arteries and medium-sized blood vessels.

ATP Adenosine triphosphate is a compound that can be created through catabolism, which captures energy in its bonds for future use.

Autism spectrum disorder A spectrum of psychological conditions characterized by widespread abnormalities of social interactions and communication as well as restricted interests and repetitive behavior.

Autoimmune A process of creating antibodies within one's self, as in the disease rheumatoid arthritis.

Bariatric surgery A surgical method for weight loss which involves reducing the stomach size and bypassing a significant part of the small intestine.

Basal metabolic rate (BMR) The minimum amount of energy needed to sustain life, measured in humans by the heat given off per unit time, and expressed as the calories released per kilogram of body weight per hour.

Behavior modification The adjustment of unwanted behavior by means of biofeedback or conditioning.

Bicarbonate A substance produced by the pancreas and secreted into the upper small intestine to neutralize acid chyme.

Bile A yellow, green liquid made by the liver and stored in the gallbladder. It is used to emulsify fat for digestion.

Binge-drinking The consumption in excess of 4 to 5 drinks consecutively.

Binge Eating Disorder (BED) An eating disorder characterized by an uncontrollable and excessive intake of food that often occurs following stressful events.

Bioavailability How well a nutrient can be absorbed and used by the body.

Biochemical Analysis in Nutrition Assessment The use of body tissues or fluids (blood and/or urine) to determine nutritional status.

Bioelectrical impedance A technique used to estimate body composition based on the difference in electrical conductive properties of various tissues. Lean tissue and fluids conduct a mild current whereas fat tissue does not.

Biological need to eat An internal signal in the body to consume food to continue functioning.

Body composition Used to describe the percentages of fat, bone, and muscle in human bodies.

Body mass index (BMI) A mathematical formula used to assess body composition, which uses both a person's height and weight. BMI equals a person's weight in kilograms divided by height in meters squared. (BMI=kg/m^2)

Bolus A semi-solid mixture that is formed after food is chewed and mixed with saliva.

Breastfeeding Feeding a baby mother's breast milk.

Bulimia Nervosa (BN) A condition that involves recurring episodes of binge eating that are combined with a morbid fear of becoming fat. The binging is typically followed by self-induced vomiting or other compensatory behavior.

Calorie A measurement of heat energy.

Carbohydrate One of the six essential nutrients whose primary function is to provide energy to the body.

Carbohydrate loading A diet used by athletes that first depletes the body's glycogen stores by routine training exercise and a low-carbohydrate diet. A high-carbohydrate diet is then consumed to improve glycogen storage and to increase athletic endurance.

Carcinogenesis The development of a cancer.

Cardiac sphincter A ring of smooth muscle fibers at the junction of the esophagus and stomach, also known as the lower esophageal sphincter.

Carotenoids A plant pigment referred to as provitamin A.

Catabolism The metabolic breakdown of complex molecules into simpler ones, usually resulting in the release of energy.

Celiac Disease a disorder of the gastrointestinal tract characterized by inflammation and injury of the mucosal lining of the small intestine.

Central obesity A large amount of visceral fat located in the abdominal area.

Chemical digestion Occurs throughout the digestive system due to powerful chemical secretions such as enzymes that breakdown food.

Childhood The time between the first and eleventh birthday when a steady, slow, physical, and mental development take place.

Cholecalciferol A form of vitamin D found in animal products.

Cholecystokinin A hormone produced in the upper small intestine that sends a message to the gall bladder to release bile into the small intestine.

ChooseMyPlate A guide developed by the USDA in 2011 to help to educate individuals in making appropriate food choices.

Choose Your Foods: Food Lists for Diabetes A system designed by the American Diabetes Association and the Academy of Nutrition and Dietetics to assist in meal planning for individuals with diabetes.

Choroid Part of the vascular tunic responsible for absorbing and retaining light in the eye.

Chylomicrons The form of lipoprotein that carries triglycerides to body cells.

Chyme The thick semi-fluid mass of partly digested food that is passed from the stomach into the duodenum.

Cilia Olfactory hairs contained in the mucous membranes of the olfactory epithelium.

Ciliary Body A muscle found in the vascular tunic that is involved in the focusing of images.

Circulatory syste The bloodstream that is attached to the intestinal tract by a variety of blood vessels.

Clinical Methods of Nutrition Assessment The use of historical information and physical examination to determine nutritional status.

Coenzyme A molecule that binds to an enzyme so that the enzyme can do its metabolic work in the body.

Competitive foods Low nutrient-density foods which typically interfere with the selections from the National School Lunch or Breakfast programs.

Complementary foods Foods other than breast milk or infant formula (liquids, semisolids, and solids) introduced to an infant to provide nutrients.

Complementary protein Two food sources that complement each other with their amino acid profile so that all essential amino acids are present.

Complete protein A food that contains all the essential amino acids.

Complex carbohydrates A type of carbohydrate containing many glucose units.

Congregate dining program A program funded by the Administration on Aging whereby seniors can come and dine together in a social setting.

Constipation A condition of the bowels where the feces become dry and hardened and defecation is difficult.

Coupled reactions Pairs of chemical reactions that occur when energy is released from the breakdown of a compound (catabolism) and used to form another compound (anabolism).

Cretinism A condition during pregnancy when an iodine deficiency in the diet may cause irreversible mental and physical retardation of the fetus.

Critical period Periods of growth in major organ systems that require specific amounts of nutrients.

Cystic fibrosis A chronic disease of the exocrine glands, characterized by production of viscous mucous. The excess mucous obstructs the pancreatic ducts and bronchi, leading to infection and fibrosis.

Deamination A process which occurs in the liver where nitrogen is removed from an amino acid.

Deficiency An inadequate level of nutrients in the body with potential negative health effects.

Dehydration Excessive water loss in comparison to the amount of water consumed.

Denature To change the structural configuration of a protein.

Dental carries Tooth decay.

Dextrose A simple carbohydrate made of glucose molecules.

Diabetes A chronic disease of abnormal carbohydrate metabolism characterized by elevated blood glucose levels.

Diaphragm A muscle that separates the chest (thoracic) cavity from the abdomen located at the end of the esophagus

Diet The sum of all the foods and fluids consumed.

Dietary Approaches to Stop Hypertension (DASH) The lifestyle approach to prevent and manage hypertension that focuses on a diet rich in fruits, vegetables, nuts, low-fat dairy foods, and reduced saturated and total fats.

Dietary Goals A set of goals designed for healthy individuals to reflect the percentage of calories that should be consumed from each of the three major nutrients.

Dietary Guidelines A set of guidelines developed by the USDA to convert nutrients into general recommendations about foods that should be consumed and/or avoided.

Dietary Methods of Nutrition Assessment Involves the use of food intake records and a nutritional analysis of these intakes.

Dietary Reference Intakes A set of dietary standards determined jointly by American and Canadian scientists to replace the RDA and the RNI.

Dietary standards A set of guidelines designed to meet the nutrient needs of the majority of healthy persons.

Dietetic Technician Registered (DTR) An individual who completes an Associate's degree from a college or university accredited by the Academy of Nutrition and Dietetics and who participates in a supervised practice experience under an approved Dietetic Technician Program.

Digestion The process by which food is broken down and converted into substances that can be absorbed and assimilated by the body.

Disaccharide A simple sugar consisting of two sugar molecules.

Diuretic A substance or drug that increases urinary output.

Diverticular Disease An inflammation of diverticuli in the mucosal wall of the intestinal tract.

Diverticuli The development of small pouches along the intestinal tract.

Docosahexaenoic acid A very long chain omega-3 fatty acid that is important in the developing fetus and infant for brain development. It is also important in retina health and cognitive improvement.

Eating disorders Disorders that are classified as disturbances in eating behavior that jeopardize physical and psychological health.

Edema The retention of fluid in the body

Eicosapentaenoic acid A very long chain omega-3 fatty acid associated with a decrease in platelet aggregation, promoting vasodilation, inhibition of the inflammatory response, and a decreased risk of a second heart attack.

Electrolyte A substance containing free ions that make the substance electrically conductive.

Electron Transport Chain The last stage of energy production occurring in the mitochondria.

Embryonic stage The earliest stage of development that lasts through the first eight weeks of pregnancy.

Empty-calorie foods Foods that have a high level of calories and a limited amount of nutrients.

Emulsifier A compound that is partly soluble in water and partly soluble in oil.

Energy The capacity to do work.

Energy yielding-nutrients Compounds found in carbohydrates, proteins, and fats that provide the body with energy to remain active.

Enzyme Proteins produced by living organisms that function as biological catalysts to speed up chemical reactions.

Epidemiology The branch of medicine or research design that deals with the incidence and prevalence of disease in large populations.

Epiglottis The thin elastic structure that closes over the larynx, blocking the entrance to the lungs via the trachea. It prevents food or fluid from entering the trachea.

Ergocalciferol A form of vitamin D found in plant products.

Esophagus The muscular tube where food passes from the pharynx to the stomach.

Essential amino acid Amino acids that must be supplied through diet because the body cannot make them in sufficient quantities.

Essential fatty acids Fatty acids that must be supplied by diet because the body cannot make them in sufficient quantities.

Essential nutrients Nutrients that must be supplied by the diet to provide the body with energy for growth, maintenance, and repair.

Estimated Average Requirement A set of nutrient requirements used in nutrition research and policy making that serve as the basis upon which RDA values are set.

Esophagitis An inflammation of the esophagus.

Ergogenic aid A substance that claims to improve athletic performance.

Extracellular The fluid found outside of the cell.

Extrusion reflex An involuntary movement of the tongue when food is placed in an infant's mouth with a spoon.

Facilitated diffusion A simple diffusion process in which a "helper molecule," or specific carrier transports molecules over the cell membrane.

Fasting hypoglycemia A condition associated with an abnormally low fasting blood glucose level.

Fat-soluble vitamins A category of vitamins that includes vitamins A, D, E, and K.

Fatfold Measurement A measurement taken at different areas on the surface of the body to determine body fat percentage.

Female Athlete Triad An eating disorder that includes a combination of three conditions: disordered eating, amenorrhea, and osteoporosis.

Fetal Alcohol Syndrome A syndrome found in infants of women with high alcohol intake that causes permanent mental retardation and a variety of physical abnormalities.

Fetal Stage The period of week 9 until the end of a normal pregnancy (about 40 weeks)

Fiber A form of polysaccharide that is non-digestible by humans.

Fibrous Tunic The outer protective layer of the eye that contains the sclera and cornea.

Flavor Adaptation A situation that occurs when taste buds adjust or become dulled because similar flavors are consistently consumed.

Fluorohydroxyapatite A compound made of fluoride, calcium and phosphorus which makes teeth more resistant to damage from acids and bacteria.

Fluorosis A discoloration of the teeth resulting from high intakes of fluoride.

Food Allergy An immune system response to a food that the body mistakenly believes is harmful.

Food Composition Tables A set of nutrient tables that provide numerical data on a variety of nutrients found in foods.

Food Guide Pyramid A guide developed by the USDA designed to help individuals make good food choices.

Food intolerance The development of gastrointestinal symptoms such as bloating and diarrhea, which are stimulated by substances in foods.

Food sensitivities See food intolerances

Free radicals Substances that are formed during metabolic processes that damage biological marcromolecules such as DNA, carbohydrates, and proteins. Also known as a reactive oxygen species (ROS).

Fructose The monosaccharide found in fruits.

Galactose The monosaccharide used in the formation of the milk sugar, lactose.

Gallbladder A small, pear-shaped muscular sac located under the right lobe of the liver, in which bile is stored until needed by the body for fat digestion.

Gallstones A crystalline substance formed within the gallbladder typically made up of cholesterol, bilirubin, and calcium salts.

Gastric juice The watery, acidic digestive fluid secreted by various glands in the mucous membrane of the stomach. It consists mainly of hydrochloric acid, pepsin, rennin, and mucin.

Gastric lipase An enzyme in the stomach that aids in the digestion of milk fat.

Gestational diabetes A medical condition in women who exhibit abnormal blood sugar levels at around the twentieth week of pregnancy.

Gastrointestinal tract (GI tract) A long mucous-secreting, muscular hollow tube that extends from the mouth to the anus and functions in digestion and elimination. Its main components are the mouth, esophagus, stomach, small intestine, and large intestine.

Glucagon A hormone produced by the pancreas that stimulates the liver to breakdown glycogen into glucose.

Gluconeogenesis The synthesis of glucose from a non-carbohydrate source such as protein.

Glucose A monosaccharide found in blood.

Glutamate An amino acid present in a variety of protein-rich foods, which is particularly abundant in aged cheese.

Glycemic Index (GI) A measurement used to evaluate the rise in blood sugar level evoked from a 50 gram dose of a carbohydrate.

Glycemic Load (GL) The product of the foods glycemic index and its total available carbohydrate content: GL = [GI X carbohydrate (g)]/100.

Glycogen A form of polysaccharide that is stored in the liver and muscles of the body.

Glycolysis The first process in energy production where a glucose molecule is converted to two pyruvate molecules.

Goiter An enlargement of the thyroid caused by iodine deficiency.

Gram The metric unit used to measure weight.

Gustatory Cells The taste cells located in the taste buds.

Hamwi method A mathematical equation used to determine an individual's Ideal Body Weight (IBW) for height.

Healthy People 2020 A plan developed by the U.S. Department of Health and Human Services to establish healthy objectives for the nation.

Heartburn A burning sensation, that is usually centered in the middle of the chest, caused by acid reflux from stomach fluids that enter the lower end of the esophagus. The medical term for the condition is gastroesophageal reflux disease (GERD).

Heimlich maneuver A technique to dislodge the food from the trachea of a choking person.

Heme The form of iron found in meats, poultry, and fish.

Hemochromatosis A condition which occurs when too much iron builds up in the body.

Hemoglobin The compound that carries oxygen in the blood.

Hemorrhoids An itching or painful mass of dilated veins located in swollen anal tissue.

Hidden fats Fats in foods that are not readily seen.

Homeostasis A balance of bodily functions.

Homocysteine A sulfur containing amino acid found primarily in animal products.

Hormone A chemical messenger that is secreted by one area of the body and travels through the blood to a different destination. At its final destination a "chemical message" is given to this second site to complete a task.

Hunger The physiological need to consume food.

Hydrogenation A process that adds hydrogen to unsaturated fats to make them more saturated, consequently more stable and solid in nature.

Hydrophilic The property of having a strong affinity for water. A tendency to dissolve in, mix with, or be wetted by water.

Hyperglycemia A condition of elevated blood glucose levels.

Hyperkalemia A high level of potassium in the blood.

Hypertension A condition of elevated blood pressure.

Hypoglycemia Low blood glucose levels.

Hypokalemia A low level of potassium in the blood.

Hypothyroidism A condition in which the thyroid gland does not make enough thyroid hormone.

Ideal body weight An anthropometric measure used to determine acceptable weight for height ranges.

Ileocecal valve A muscular structure at the junction of the small intestine and large intestine.

Incomplete protein A food that is lacking one or more of the essential amino acids.

Infancy The early stage of growth or development, between birth and the first birthday.

Innate An inherent or intrinsic characteristic that is possessed from birth.

Inorganic A compound that does not contain the element carbon.

Insoluble fiber A polysaccharide that is insoluble in water that promotes bowel regularity and reduces the risk of diverticular disease.

Insulin A hormone produced by the pancreas that signals the body's cells to take up glucose.

Intestine The portion of the gastrointestinal tract extending from the stomach to the anus, and consisting of two segments, the small intestine and the large intestine.

Intracellular The fluid found inside of the cell.

Iris A circular shaped muscle that surrounds the pupil, and is part of the vascular tunic.

Iron-deficiency anemia A form of anemia caused by a lack of iron in the diet or excessive iron loss due to chronic bleeding.

Isoflavone One of the phytoestrogens found in soy protein.

Keratinization A condition caused by Vitamin A deficiency, whereby the skin becomes dry and scaly.

Ketone A substance formed when fat is used as an energy source.

Ketosis A buildup of ketones in the blood caused when fat is improperly broken down for energy.

Krebs Cycle Also known as the Citric Acid Cycle. The third stage of energy production occurring in the mitochondria.

Kwashiorkor A deficiency of high-quality protein that occurs despite the intake of adequate calories, which can result in retarded growth.

Lactose A disaccharide made up of glucose and galactose that is found in dairy products.

Large intestine The portion of the intestine that extends from the ileum to the anus, and includes the cecum, colon, and rectum.

Learned Preference A taste that is developed over time. Often referred to as acquired taste.

Licensure of Dietitians/Nutritionists A state-to-state requirement for dietitians to protect the consumer from fraudulent professionals and/or practices.

Limiting amino acid An essential amino acid that is at its lowest concentration in relation to the body's needs.

Lipid peroxidation The oxidation of polyunsaturated fatty acids.

Lipoprotein A molecule made up of protein and lipid used in the transportation of fats.

Liver A large, reddish-brown, organ located in the upper right quadrant of the abdominal cavity that produces bile and is active in the formation of certain blood proteins and in the metabolism of carbohydrates, fats, and proteins.

Lymphatic system The system to which fat molecules and fat soluble vitamins are absorbed from the digestive tract.

Macronutrient A nutrient found in large quantities in the body.

Major minerals Essential nutrients found in the body in amounts greater than 5 grams.

Malabsorption The body's inability to absorb one or more nutrients.

Malnutrition Poor nutrition resulting from a dietary intake of one or more nutrients that is either above or below the amount required to meet the body's needs.

Maltose A disaccharide made up of two glucose units.

Marasmus A severe deficiency of protein and calories in the diet, often characterized by a wasted skeletal appearance.

Mastication The process by which food is crushed and ground by teeth, i.e., chewing.

Maximum heart rate The age-related number of beats per minute of the heart when working at its maximum. It is usually estimated at 220 minus one's age.

Meals on wheels A partnership between the government and local agencies to provide older adults with home-delivered meals.

Mechanical digestion The process that occurs when food is chewed to be broken down into smaller units.

Mediterranean Food Pyramid A food guide pyramid plan similar in nature to the USDA Food Guide Pyramid that reflects the food intake of individuals in Spain, Portugal, Southern France, Syria, and Israel.

Menaquinone A form of vitamin K synthesized by bacteria and found in animal products.

Menopause The period characterized by the permanent cessation of menstruation, which usually occurs between the ages of 45 and 55.

Menstruation The monthly discharge of blood and mucosal tissue from the uterus, which occurs from puberty to menopause in non-pregnant women.

Metabolic equivalents (METS) A physiological concept expressing the energy cost of physical activities as multiples of basal metabolic rate (BMR) and is defined as the ratio of metabolic rate (and therefore the rate of energy consumption) during a specific physical activity to a reference rate of metabolic rate at rest.

Metabolic Syndrome A combination of medical disorders that increase the risk of developing cardiovascular disease and diabetes

Metabolism The many chemical processes that occur in a living cell and are required for the maintenance of life.

Metabolomics The interaction between nutrition and metabolic pathways in the body.

Micronutrient A nutrient needed in very small quantities in the body.

Microparticulated A process used to prepare protein for use as a fat replacer.

Mineral An inorganic element that is essential to the functioning of the human body, which must be obtained from foods.

Monosaccharide A simple sugar containing one sugar unit.

Monounsaturated A fatty acid chain with only one point of unsaturation, i.e., one double bond.

Morning sickness Nausea occurring in the early part of the day, often seen during the first months of pregnancy.

Mouth An opening in the body through which food is taken in.

Mouthfeel A term used to describe the texture of food in the mouth.

Mucus The viscous substance that is secreted by cells and glands of the mucous membranes as a protective lubricant coating.

Mutual supplementation The concept of combining two complementary proteins sources to make a complete protein.

Myoglobin The oxygen transporting protein of muscle.

Neuromuscular Having to do with both nerves and muscles.

Neurotransmitter A chemical messenger that transmits a signal from nerve cells to other parts of the body.

Nitrogen balance The measure of protein intake in the diet contrasted with that which is used and excreted by the body.

Non-energy yielding nutrients Nutrients that assist in the energy production process but do not supply energy themselves.

Nonnutrient Compounds other than the six essential nutrients found in foods. These include compounds found in herbs and spices.

Nonessential amino acids Amino acids that can be synthesized by the body.

Nonessential fatty acids Fatty acids that the body is able to make.

Nonheme The form of iron found in vegetables, fruits, and grains.

Nonnutritive sweetener A sweetener that provides no energy or nutritive value to the body.

Non-taster An individual with a low number of taste buds.

Nutrient Substances or compounds that make up foods.

Nutrient dense Foods containing a high level of nutrients and a lower number of calories.

Nutrigenomic The interaction between nutrition and a person's genome.

Nutrition A science that studies the substances in food and their interactions in the body.

Nutrition Facts Panel A portion of the Food Label where manufacturers provide required nutritional information on certain nutrients that are in the product.

Nutritional assessment The technique of evaluating an individual's or a population's nutritional status by using comprehensive approaches such as anthropometrics, biochemical analysis, clinical methods, and dietary approaches.

Nutritional status A person's health, as influenced by both the intake and utilization of nutrients.

Nutritive sweetener A sweetener that has the ability to provide the body with energy.

Obesity High body weight caused by an excessive accumulation of fat.

Objective evaluation of food A type of food testing involving the use of various instruments.

Olfactory The part of the body having to do with the nose.

Oligosaccharides A carbohydrate source containing a small number (typically two to ten) of component sugars.

Omega-3 fatty acids The type of fatty acids found in fatty fish, that are associated with a reduced frequency of coronary heart disease

Omega-6 fatty acids The type of fatty acids found in high quantities in vegetable oils such as corn and sunflower. These are associated with an increased risk of heart attacks, strokes, and various inflammatory conditions.

Organic Nutrients that contain the element carbon.

Osteoarthritis A disease with painful joint swelling.

Osteomalacia The condition of adult rickets caused by a deficiency of vitamin D. Bones become weak and may fracture in the weight-bearing bones such as the hips and spine.

Osteoporosis A decrease in bone mass and bone density.

Overfatness Obesity with a BMI over 30.

Overhydration Intake of water above what the kidney can handle.

Overnutrition Malnutrition resulting from an excess intake of one or more nutrients.

Overweight Weight above that considered normal for height

Oxidation The process that occurs when a substance combines with oxygen.

Pancreas A long, irregularly shaped gland located behind the stomach that secretes pancreatic juice into the duodenum, and insulin and glucagon into the bloodstream.

Papillae Small, pink bumps located on the tongues surface where the taste buds can be found.

Parathyroid hormone A hormone involved with the regulation of blood calcium levels.

Peripheral Neuropathy A problem with the nerves that carry information to and from the brain and spinal cord to the rest of the body—can produce pain, a loss of sensation, and an inability to control muscles.

Peristalsis The wavelike muscular contractions of the gastrointestinal tract that is responsible for moving ingested material.

Phenylketonuria A genetic disease in which an individual cannot convert the essential amino acid phenylalanine into the nonessential amino acid tyrosine.

Phospholipid A compound similar to a triglyceride that has a phosphorus molecule rather than one of the fatty acids attached to the glycerol chain.

Phylloquinone The plant form of vitamin K.

Physical activity The activity of exerting muscles in various ways to keep fit.

Phytochemical A nonnutrient compound in plant-derived foods that displays weak biological activity in the body.

Placenta The organ formed in the lining of the uterus connecting the uterine mucous membrane with the membranes of the fetus. The placenta provides nourishment for the fetus and eliminates its waste products.

Polysaccharide A sugar made up of many glucose molecules.

Polyunsaturated A fatty acid chain with more than one point of unsaturation, i.e., two or more double bonds.

Portal system A system of blood vessels that begins and ends in capillaries. Water soluble nutrients (water, water-soluble vitamins, amino acids, and simple sugars) enter the blood via the portal system and then enter the portal vein to the liver.

Postprandial hypoglycemia Abnormally low blood glucose levels after the consumption of a meal.

Prebiotics Substances such as inulin and lactulose, which provide a food source to the probiotic.

Pregnancy The time from conception to birth when a woman carries a developing fetus in her uterus.

Probiotic Bacteria-producing foods, such as milk and yogurt, which may favorably alter the microflora composition of the gut.

Protein sparing The use of carbohydrates rather than protein for the body's energy needs.

Proteomics The interaction between nutrition and the protein encoding genes.

Prothrombin A protein in plasma involved in blood coagulation.

Psychological reason for food selection An external stimulus contributing to food selection.

Puberty The age at which a person is first capable of the sexual reproduction of an offspring: commonly presumed to be around 14 years in the male and 12 years in the female.

Pyloric sphincter A ring of smooth muscle fibers found at the junction of the stomach and the duodenum.

Rancidity The deterioration of fat caused by the presence of oxygen or high heat.

Reactive oxygen species (ROS) Formed through an oxidation reaction, ROS causes damage to cell membranes and other molecules such as DNA, carbohydrates, and proteins. Also referred to as free radicals.

Recommended Dietary Allowances (RDA) The set of nutrient intake goals for healthy individuals, derived from the Estimated Average Requirements.

Rectum The end portion of the large intestine.

Registered Dietitian/Nutritionist (RDN) A professional credentialed by the Academy of Nutrition and Dietetics who has undergone additional training after college or university graduation via an internship or combined master's degree program.

Retin-A A derivative of vitamin A used in the treatment of acne.

Retina The innermost area of the eye containing a pigmented layer and a thick layer of nerve tissue.

Rickets A condition found in children that may be caused by vitamin D and calcium deficiencies. Bones do not calcify as they should, resulting in growth retardation and skeletal abnormalities.

Saliva A mixture of secretions from the salivary and mucous glands of the mouth that lubricates chewed food, moistens the oral walls, and contains the enzyme amylase.

Salivary glands Glands that secrete saliva, including three pairs of large glands; the parotid, submaxillary, and sublingual.

Sarcopenia A degenerative loss of skeletal muscle mass and strength associated with aging.

Salt-sensitive Individuals who experience a rise in blood pressure because of excess salt consumption.

Satiety A feeling of fullness.

Saturated-Fatty acids A fatty acid that has hydrogen atoms attached to every available position on the carbon atom of the fatty acid chain.

Sebaceous gland The glands that produce the skin's natural oil.

SIDS Sudden infant death syndrome.

Simple diffusion A form of diffusion where molecules move freely through the cell membrane.

Simple sugar A group of sacharrides (sugars) consisting of the monosaccharides and disaccharides.

Small intestine The upper part of the intestine where digestion is completed and nutrients are absorbed by the blood. It consists of the duodenum, the jejunum, and the ileum.

SNAP The supplemental nutrition assistance program.

Sociological reasons for food choice External stimuli contributing to food selection, such as cultural and social attitudes.

Soluble fiber A polysaccharide that is soluble in water and may lower blood cholesterol levels.

Starch A polysaccharide used by plants for energy.

Steroid hormones Proteins that are synthesized from cholesterol and include testosterone and estrogen.

Sterols A lipid with multiple ring structures that functions in bile, vitamin D, and hormone production.

Stillborn Occurs when a fetus has died in the uterus.

Stomach The enlarged, saclike portion of the gastrointestinal tract that is located between the esophagus and the small intestine.

Subcutaneous fat The layer of fat under the surface of the skin.

Subjective-Evaluation of food The process involving the use of the senses in evaluating food.

Subthreshold The level at which an individual is unable to discern a taste although that taste may impact on another taste sensation.

Sucrose A disacarrhide found in table sugar and made up of glucose and fructose.

Sugar alcohol A nutritive sweetener containing one molecule of sugar and one of alcohol.

Supertaster An individual with a high number of taste buds.

Suppresion A reduction in the perceived intensity of a food by the presence of another substance.

Swallowing The voluntary process that moves food from the mouth to the stomach.

Synergism An increase in the perceived intensity of a food by the presence of another substance.

Target heart rate The speed at which one's heart should beat during exercise.

Thermic effect The energy needed to process consumed food.

Thrombin An enzyme found in plasma that catalyzes the conversion of fibrinogen to fibrin, and serves as the last step in the blood clotting process.

Tocopherol The chemical name for Vitamin E.

Tolerable Upper Intake Suggested upper limits of intakes for nutrients that may be toxic at excessive levels. When consumed at excessive levels, these nutrients are likely to cause illness.

Total energy needs The amount of calories an individual needs calculated by the BMR and a physical activity factor.

Toxicity The overabundance of a nutrient in the body that can potentially cause adverse health problems.

Trace minerals Essential nutrients found in the body in amounts less than 5 grams.

Trachea The tube to the lung, also known as the windpipe.

Transamination A reaction that uses nitrogen to make nonessential amino acids.

Trans-fatty acids Fatty acids produced through the hydrogenation process that have a negative health impact.

Triglycerides The fats that the body is able to utilize for energy and to store when not needed. These are made up of three fatty acids attached to a glycerol molecule.

Type I diabetes A form of diabetes caused by the insufficient production of insulin.

Type II diabetes A form of diabetes associated with the insulin resistance of a body's cells.

Umami Sometimes called the "fifth" taste, it is associated with the presence of free glutamate in food.

Undernutrition Malnutrtion resulting from suboptimal levels of one or more nutrients.

Unsaturated Fatty acids that lack one or more hydrogen atoms along the carbon chain of the fatty acid, and create a double bond between the two carbon atoms.

Vascular Tunic The middle layer of the eye consisting of the choroid, the ciliary body and the iris.

Villi Fingerlike projections of the small intestine that contain the microvilli. Villi are necessary to increase the surface area of absorption of the small intestine.

Visceral fat Fat located within the central abdominal area near the vital organs.

Vitamin Organic substances essential in small quantities to maintain normal body functioning.

Volatile A molecule that is airborne.

Water-soluble vitamins A category of vitamins consisting of vitamin B complex and vitamin C.

WIC A supplemental food program sponsored by the U.S. government for woman, infants, and children.

Xerophthalmia An abnormal dryness of the eye that can result in conjunctivitis.

Zygote The cell resulting from the union of an ovum and a sperm.

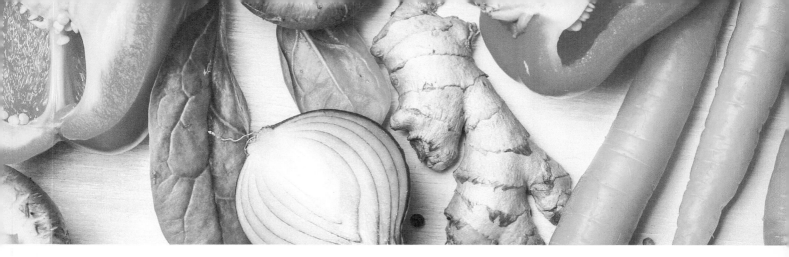

Index

Page numbers followed by f indicate figures; t, tables.